AF785711

Radiological Exploration of the Ventricles and Subarachnoid Space

By G. Ruggiero

J. Bories · A. Calabrò · G. Cristi · G. Scialfa
F. Smaltino · A. Thibaut

With the Cooperation of
G. Gianasi · G. Maranghi · Ch. Philippart
E. Signorini

With 90 Partly Coloured Figures
(279 Separate Illustrations)

Springer-Verlag
Berlin · Heidelberg · New York 1974

ISBN-13: 978-3-642-88033-9 e-ISBN-13: 978-3-642-88031-5
DOI: 10.1007/ 978-3-642-88031-5

This work is subject to copyright. All rights are reserved, whether the whole or part of the material is concerned, specifically those of translation, reprinting, re-use of illustrations, broadcasting, reproduction by photocopying machine or similar means, and storage in data banks.

Under § 54 of the German Copyright Law where copies are made for other than private use, a fee is payable to the publisher, the amount of the fee to be determined by agreement with the publisher.

© by Springer-Verlag Berlin Heidelberg 1974.
Softcover reprint of the hardcover 1st edition 1974

The use of general descriptive names, trade marks, etc. in this publication, even if the former are not especially identified, is not be taken as a sign that such names as understood by the Trade Marks and Merchandise Marks Act, may accordingly be used freely by anyone.

To the "Ecole de Saint' Anne"

Preface

A few evenings ago in the Hall of the Neurological Clinic of Bologna University Dr. HENRI HÉCAEN gave a lecture on the physiopathology of writing. As I was listening to his learned exposition, memories returned to me of times when my reaction to his work was not always the enjoyment of a quiet listener; namely, of the times when, ten years before, during the "séances du samedi" at the Neurosurgical Center of Saint' Anne Hospital in Paris, our meetings often consisted of disputes, in a sparkling tangle of alliances and hostilities, which would often result in clashes between TALAIRACH, AJURIAGUERRA, BRÉGEAT, M., and Mme DELL, KLOTZ (each one passionately pleading for his own speciality), with a brillant chorus of collaborators: CONSTANS, ABOULKER, DÉLIGNÉ, SADOUN, BANCAUD ... enlivening the scene. I remember the discussions on clinical cases, the "lettres au directeur et aux médicins soignants" in which GUILLY was a master of diplomacy, the biting hints at the administrators, the smiles between allies or lovers. And in that casbah-like uproar of students, doctors, patients, attendants, technicians, and spectators, the voice of the "Grand Chef," preceded by a slam on the table, ringing out loudly: "Nom de Dieu! Voulez-vous vous taire et nous foutre la paix?" Monsieur David was always able to humanize any abstract problem. Saint' Anne! An arena where we dealt with the latest findings of neurology, psychiatry, stereotaxis, neurosurgery, neurophthalmology, electroencephalography and neuroradiology.

I owe my career to having met Erik Lindgren and Marcel David. To the former I shall always be indebted for the rigor he employed in teaching me the basic elements of neuroradiology and the techniques of scientific research; the example of the latter still guides me in the difficult task of directing a large department of medicine with the goals of increasing humanity, indulgence, and humility.

It is unlikely that I will again find the ideal condition of cooperation with so many masters of the neurological sciences. If it were not for some of my works which are included in the vast bibliography of the "Ecole de Saint' Anne," I would perhaps wonder today if I merely imagined I was fortunate enough to have been one of its members. However, more than the works published and the honors achieved, it is my having in turn been able to establish a school of neuroradiology that perhaps makes me worthy of belonging to that circle of scientists.

This volume is dedicated to the "Ecole de Saint' Anne" and this preface is the only part signed by me alone. As a matter of fact, this work does not follow the traditional pattern requiring that each chapter be signed by its author; on the contrary, here the responsibility for every line belongs to all the authors. In this way, I wish to thank my pupils of that time, who are today my friends and colleagues, for accepting my advice and believing in my principles. My thanks also to those who, for reasons independent of our will, do not appear among the authors of this book.
Bologna, 1967

1971. The last four years have been hard for my country: continual strikes in hospitals, together with an organizational standstill, and often bitterness and discontent on the part of the Italian physicians. These are the essential reasons why this work has been delayed. I apologize to my foreign collaborators, hoping nonetheless that the revision of this book will appease their disappointment for the long wait.

End of 1972 GIOVANNI RUGGIERO

Acknowledgments

We wish to thank
Mrs. GIULIA RUGGIERO and Miss FULVIA BONOMO for the first draft of the English text.

Professor GIANCARLO PIAZZA for reviewing the English text.

Miss GABRIELLA GALLETTI for her secretarial work, with the cooperation of Mrs. ADRIANA LAFFI and Mrs. TAMARA FRASNEDI.

Mr. ANDREA COLINA R.T., Mr. CARLO DE GRASSI R.T., and Mr. QUINTO GASPERINI R.T. for their cooperation in preparing the radiographic and photographic material.

We are also indebted to the Administration of the Ospedale Maggiore of Bologna who helped to make this work possible by allowing us to call upon the assistance of some of the hospital personnel.

Introduction

RUGGIERO's monograph on fractional encephalography, published in 1957 (374), was based on the analysis of about 700 examinations collected over five years. One of the purposes of the present work is to record the progress achieved in this fundamental technique.

In the 1957 work the comparison between encephalography and ventriculography was the subject of an exhaustive discussion. Such a discussion is not included here, because this is a different kind of book, and especially because of the low incidence of ventriculography in our present material, where this examination is performed only in the rare cases of unsuccessful encephalography. However, as ventriculography still enjoys considerable prestige in other departments, its technique is still covered in this book.

A long chapter has been devoted to techniques with opaque contrast media, which have been used with considerable success in recent years, especially in neurological and neurosurgical centers not associated with departments of neuroradiology.

The neuroradiologist is a specialist in irradiation, not only by X-rays. Therefore, the exploration of fluid pathways by means of radioactive isotopes finds a suitable place in this book. The present monograph is limited to the technique, but, since the development of diagnostic methods is mirrored by technical progress, we do not hesitate to refer to clinical discussions, when we deem it useful to illustrate and justify an aspect of the technique itself.

Unless otherwise indicated, the material on which this work is founded—case reports and iconography—comes from the archives of the Divison of Neuroradiology of the Ospedale Maggiore of Bologna. This department performs neuroradiological procedures on the patients of two neurosurgical divisions, but it also has its own wards, reserved for patients applying directly to the department or coming from other areas for a diagnostic clarification. Thus, the neuroradiologist does not merely perform the examinations required by other specialists, he is also directly involved in the diagnostic problem (377, 382, 384), taking on himself the responsibility of the patient for the time he is under his care. In particular, this has contributed to an increased objectivity and validity of the chapters devoted to the clinical aspects of the examinations. In the preface we have stated that every part of the book reflects the opinion of all its authors. However, in cases where one of the authors has published some particular contribution his name is mentioned directly.

For the readability of the text, sometimes it was not possible to avoid such general expressions, such as "according to us", "we think", "it seems to us", etc. Obviously these terms refer to all authors; if one of them has a different opinion, his name is mentioned and the editorial "we" must be ascribed to GIOVANNI RUGGIERO. The term "our department" refers to the Division of Neuroradiology of the Ospedale Maggiore of Bologna, or, in the case of examinations performed by RUGGIERO with the Princeps 60, to the Clinic Villalba, also in Bologna.

Contents

List of Authors and Cooperators

Authors

Prof. Giovanni Ruggiero, Head of the Neuroradiological Department, Ospedale Maggiore Bellaria, Bologna, Italy.

Prof. Jacques Bories, Professor of Radiology, Head of the Neuroradiological Department, Hôpital de La Salpétrière, Paris, France.

Prof. Alberto Calabrò, Head of the Neuroradiological Department, Ospedale Cardarelli, Naples, Italy.

Dr. Gianfranco Cristi, Senior Assistant of the Neuroradiological Department, Ospedale Maggiore Bellaria, Bologna, Italy.

Dr. Giuseppe Scialfa, Assistant of the Neuroradiological Department, Ospedale Maggiore Bellaria, Bologna, Italy.

Prof. Francesco Smaltino, Professor of Neuroradiology, University of Naples, Italy.

Prof. André Thibaut, Professor of Neuroradiology, University of Liège, Belgium.

Cooperators

Prof. Giancarlo Gianasi, Senior Assistant of the Department of Anesthesia, Ospedale Maggiore Bellaria, Bologna, Italy.

Dr. Grazia Maranghi, Assistant of the Department of Anesthesia, Ospedale Maggiore Bellaria, Bologna, Italy.

Dr. Charles Philippart, Neuroanesthesist, Hôpital Universitaire of Bavière, Liège, Belgium.

Dr. Enrico Signorini, Head of the Neuroradiological Section of the Radiological Department, City Hospital, Perugia, Italy.

Chapter I. Fractional Encephalography

1. Introduction

The principle of fractional encephalography is the following: the endocranial cavities containing the cerebrospinal fluid (CSF) are studied radiologically by injection of moderate amounts of a gaseous contrast medium, usually air. The study is "fractional," i.e. the air, the volume of which is less than that of the ventricular system and the subarachnoid space, fills the different portions of these structures separately; the air is directed by suitable maneuvers on the principle that gas has an upward movement in fluids. These maneuvers consist of special variations in the body and head positions. The fundamental technique consists in letting the examination progress without necessarily following a set procedure in every case. In other words, as the first images (radiographic or televised) are examined, the operator decides how to continue, i.e. how to perform maneuvers and projections. The examination procedure depends on the condition of the patient, like any other clinical examination.

This subjectivity, which inspired the technique of encephalography in the "artisan" period, when the examination was performed with manually operated apparatus [374, 375], is still valuable nowadays in the "technological" era of sophisticated electronic and motorized apparatus [154, 383].

The title of this work already indicates the change: we call the technique *radiological* and no longer *radiographic*, as in RUGGIERO's 1957 monograph [374]. Radioscopic observation by means of an image amplifier in a closed television circuit [380, 381] constitutes a considerable technical advance [383] and, as we shall see later on, it has in turn led to other refinements, for example the use of urea [387, 388, 392]. But the main feature of the encephalographic technique remains the constant presence of the neuroradiologist beside the patient. His presence is even more necessary nowadays because the increased speed of the examination performed with modern apparatus makes it more difficult for the physician to correct any possible error in the technique. In modern encephalography the patient must be kept under continuous clinical supervision.

By October 1971, 4882 fractional encephalographies had been performed in our department on a total of 14836. patients.

We assembled 500 cases by extracting from our files the first 25 reports for each of the first 20 letters of the alphabet: there are 292 males and

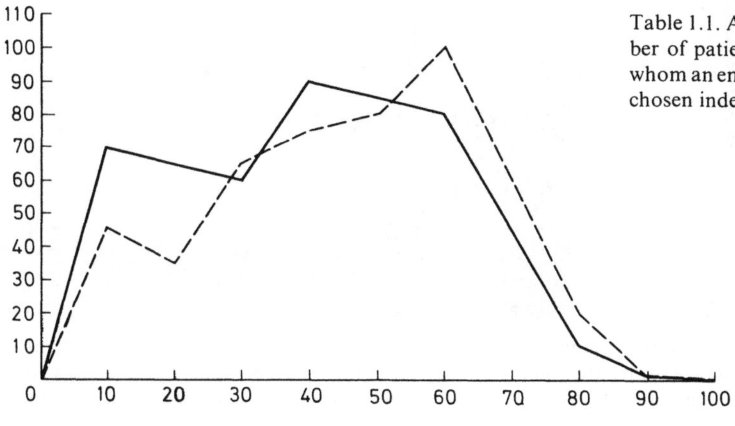

Table 1.1. Age in Encephalography. On the ordinate is the number of patients; on the abscissa, the age. Jull line: patients on whom an encephalography was performed; broken line: patients chosen independently of the encephalography

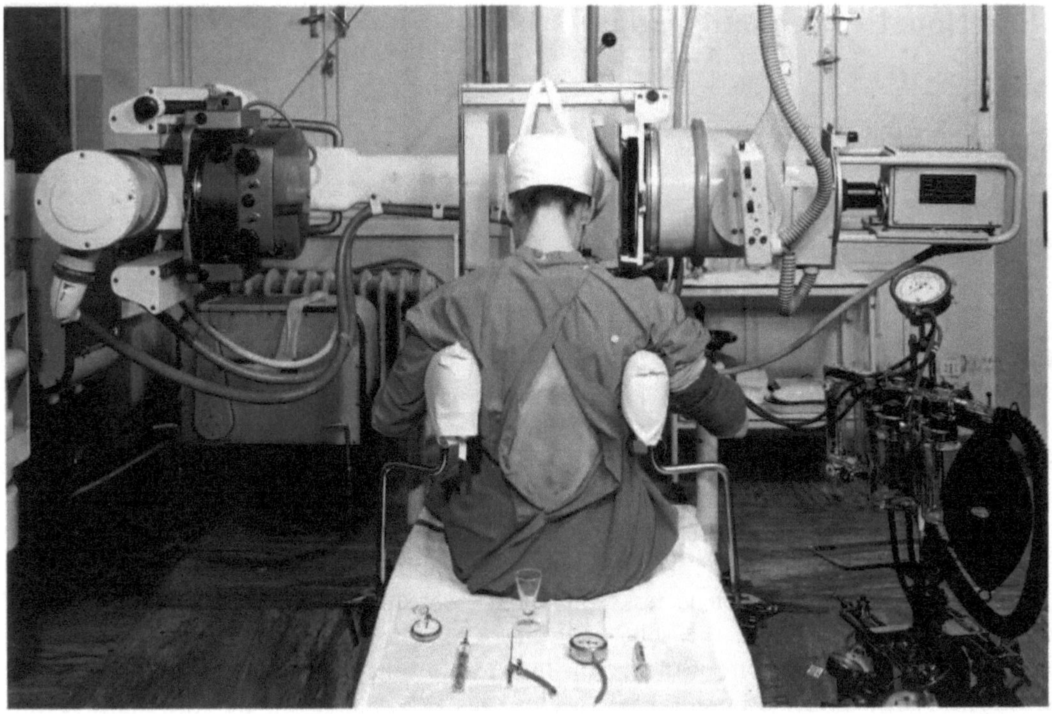

Fig. 1.1. *Examination with Mimer I.* The apparatus is ready for a lateral projection with the image amplifier and TV camera. On the table on which the patient is sitting, a chronometer, a lumbar puncture doubleway needle, and some syringes for the air and anesthetics injections are prepared on a sterile sheet. On the patient's arm is the sphygmomanometer armband

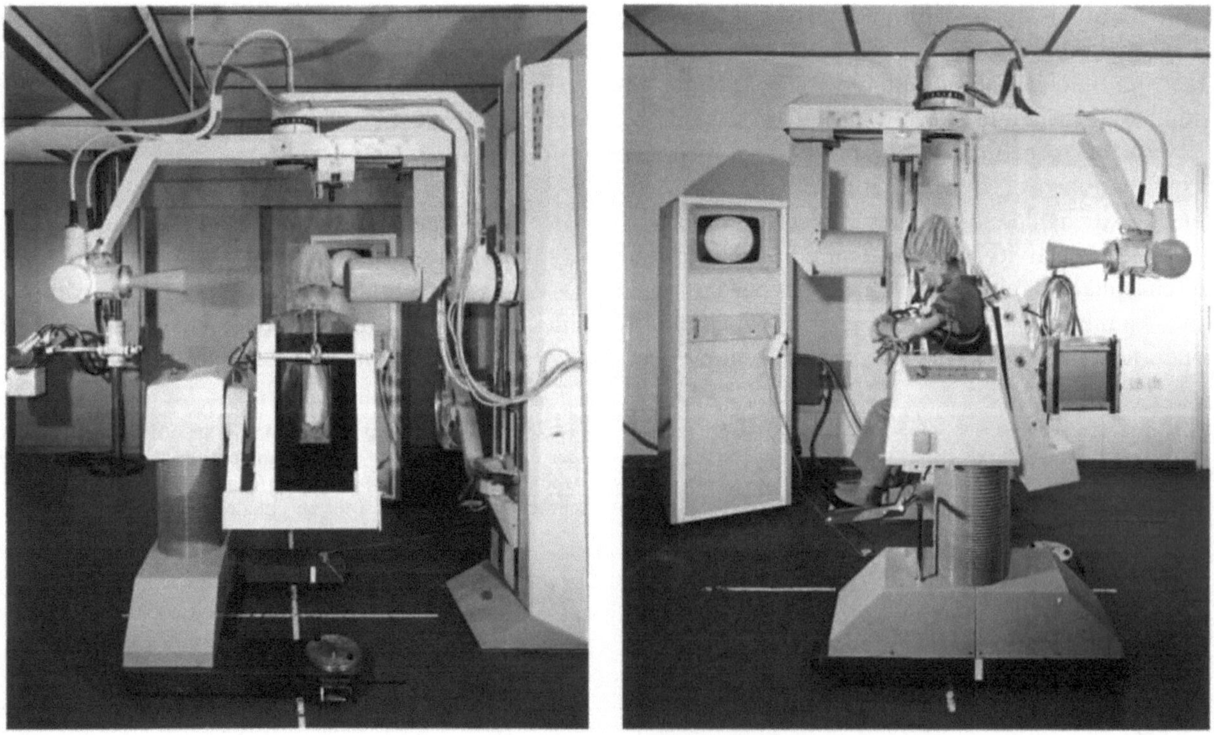

a b

Fig. 1.2a, b. *Examination with Princeps.* The patient is sitting on the rotating chair. The material necessary for the lumbar puncture, local anesthesia, and pharmacological assistance is prepared on the tray shown in Fig. 1.3. The fluoroscopic observation in the two orthogonal projections is possible without moving the patient, because either the tube or the chair can be moved

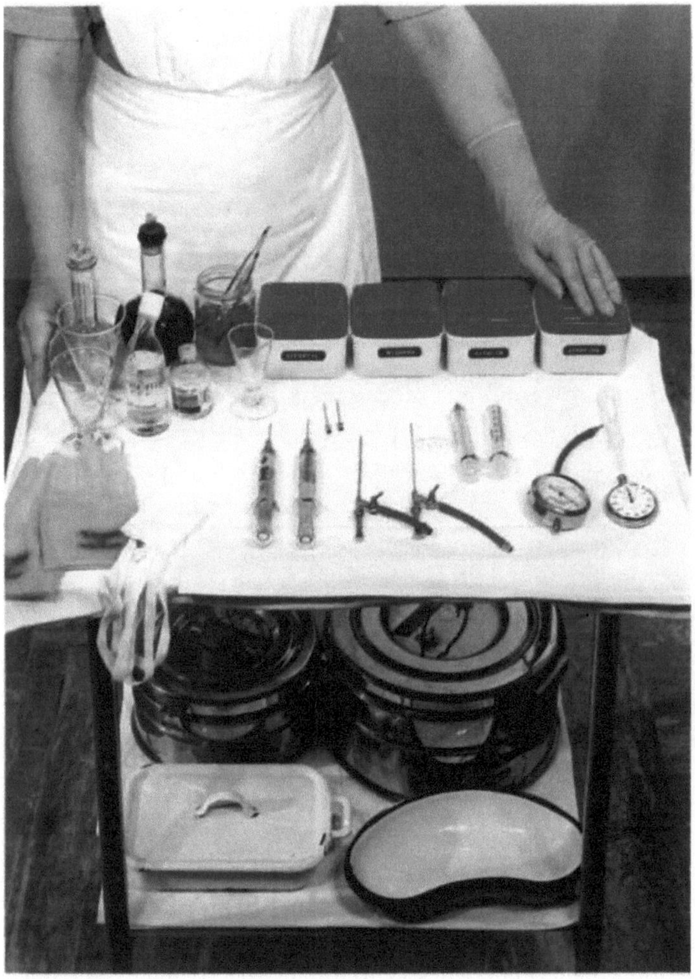

Fig. 1.3. *Material Necessary for the Encephalography*. On the tray are prepared sterile gloves, masks, two syringes for anesthesia and/or any other necessary intramuscular or intravenous injections of drugs, two 10-ml syringes, a Claude manometer, a sterile tube to collect the CSF for the laboratory, other beakers to collect CSF, iodine, alcohol, tweezers, ethyl chloride for local anesthesia, Novocaine for soft-tissue anesthesia, resuscitation material (Effortil, Micoren, etc.), sterile containers, and kidney basins

208 females of average age, respectively, 36 and 42 years. At the time of examination the oldest patient was 84 years old and the youngest 3 months. The excess of males reflects the predominance of the male sex in the population of our department. Every age is represented, but the first, fourth, fifth, and sixth decades predominate (Table 1.1). There is no constant relationship between these data and those observed on an equal number of patients selected on the basis of the same statistical criteria, apart from the fact of their undergoing an encephalography, or not.

2. Technical Equipment and Set-Up of Rooms

Figs. 1.1 through 1.3 illustrate the technical and medical equipment necessary for an encephalography. Two X-ray machines are shown, Mimer I and Princeps 60, of which the writes have personal experience. Fig. 1.4 is a comprehensive view of the room in which the examination is carried out. The picture shows a Mimer I, but the general set-up would obviously be the same with another apparatus.

The X-ray machine is set up for a lateral projection, with the patient in a sitting position. The central beam is selfcentering on the image amplifier. The chair is placed as shown in Fig. 1.1 to allow the patient to assume a sitting position. On the opposite side of the column of the Mimer or Princeps is the anesthesia apparatus, incorporating the manometer for checking blood pressure. On the same side is placed a lamp for illuminating the patient's back, thus facilitating the lumbar puncture and all the maneuvers relating to air introduction and CSF withdrawal. The sitting patient occupies

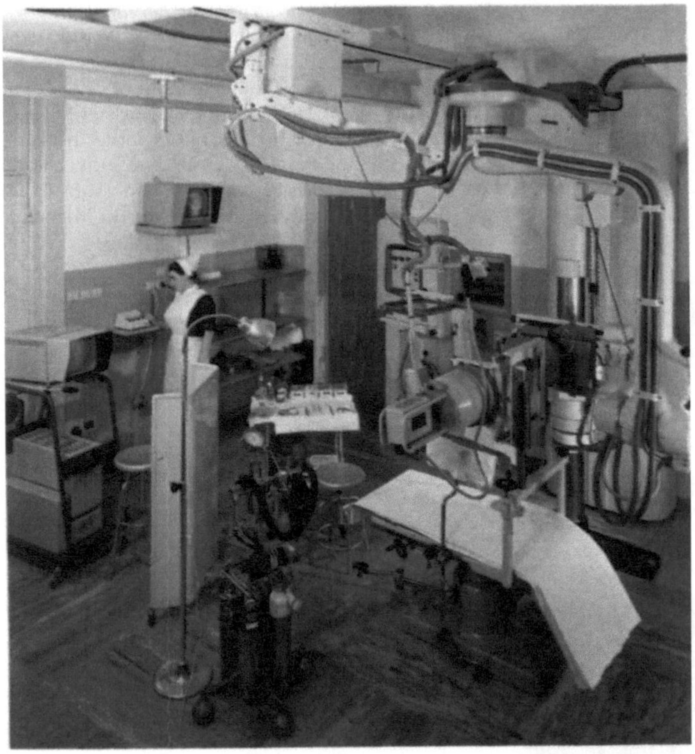

Fig. 1.4. *A General View of the X-ray Room in which Encephalography is Performed*

the front two thirds of the table; the rear third is covered by an aseptic sheet on which are placed the syringe containing the anesthetic liquid, the two-way needle for the lumbar puncture (as described in previous works [374, 375]), an aseptic test-tube for the collection of the CSF to be examined, and a graduated glass to measure the amount of CSF withdrawn, if any. Just behind the chair, on the side of the column of the Mimer, is a small table covered by an aseptic cloth holding all the equipment that might be needed: gloves, glasses, syringes, pressure gage, gauzes, drugs, etc. On the other side of the table is the TV monitor, connected by closed circuit with the image amplifier. In front of the monitor there is a rather high stool. Both monitor and stool are shielded by a movable lead protective device. When the doctor who is injecting the air wants to follow its progress on the TV screen, he can have the TV moved near his chair. However, he rarely does so because it is uncomfortable for the same person to handle the needle, check CSF pressure, and watch the screen at the same time. Generally in such cases, an assistant looks after the patient while the neuroradiologist responsible for the examination watches the TV screen. It is advisable for all the staff taking part in the examination to wear leaded overalls.

The monitor of the general TV network of the department is placed on a wall. However, this general network is no longer strictly necessary since the advent of the 90-second processing unit, which permits one to follow the examination directly on radiographs. These radiographs, fixed and dried, can be handled and transported very quickly.

Motorized Rotating Chairs

These chairs were introduced by GARCIA OLLER [161] and developed by TAVERAS [361, 453], POTTS [359–361], AMPLATZ [12], and others [175, 195, 259]. They make it possible without moving the patient to perform all the movements necessary to obtain the variations in air-fluid levels that are fundamental for the technique of encephalography. Usually, the patient is strapped to the chair and can be rotated in a complete somersault.

This type of chair was constructed for use with the various models of Princeps, Mimer, and Diagnost N. In the Neurocentrix the rotating chair is part of the apparatus itself. It is advisable to keep the duration of the somersault as brief as possible, especially the stage where the patient has his head down. This position is dangerous in the case of endocranial hypertension, as it produces an increase in the cerebral venous pressure. Moreover, it is impossible to monitor the patient's breathing when it is hampered by the pressure of the viscera and the diaphragm.

Recently ZIEDSES DES PLANTES [489] has emphasized the advantages of the somersault technique, which permits a complete examination (lateral ventricles, temporal horns, third and fourth ventricles, basal cisterns, subarachnoid space of the spine and brain) even without the use of a motorized rotating chair. The air is introduced by the suboccipital route. During the puncture, the patient lies on his back with the upper part of the body somewhat raised on a cylindrical cushion and the head in upright position. After partial filling and examination of the ventricular system, the temporal horns are filled by means of the forward somersault. A backward somersault is necessary to study the third and fourth ventricles from where, if there is no obstruction, the air passes into the spinal subarachnoid space, thus making it possible to perform a myelography. Finally the patient can be placed upright again for a further examination of the intracranial structures.

AZAMBUJA [18] and RUGGIERO [385] have expressed concern about the complete somersault technique because they have observed cases in which encephalography was poorly tolerated: these authors feel that the headaches and nausea persisting for many days were probably a result of the somersault.

The Neurocentrix

At least some of the drawbacks just described could disappear with the Neurocentrix, a new apparatus (Fig. 1.5), designed by BORIES and ZECQUES [48, 52]. The rotating chair is incorporated in this machine, which moves on a giant wheel and can be fixed at any desired inclination between 0 and 180°. The apparatus is also adjustable and can turn on itself, or be moved in a longitudinal, lateral, or vertical direction.

The center of the patient's head is the center of the wheel. All movements are radio-controlled, and radiographic exposure is automatic. The Neurocentrix is provided with an image amplifier and a seriograph which, according to RUGGIERO, could be useful for subtraction in encephalography (see Chap. I, p. 50).

Camera 70-mm

SIMON *et. al.* [429] reported two years' experience with a 70-mm camera attached to a craniograph of Diagnost N or Mimer III Type. The photographs reproduce exactly the picture shown by the image amplifier. The main advantages are that the examination is shortened by the elimination of the use of cassette, and photographs may be taken in rapid succession. The disadvantages are that the more peripheral portion of the injected structures is deformed by the curve of the amplifier and that it is difficult to study small or poorly contrasted structures.

3. Staff

The staff comprises doctors, nurses, technicians, and attendants.

When suitable equipment is available, one neuroradiologist is generally sufficient. An assistant may be necessary in special cases: with anxious patients for whom anesthesia is not practicable; when it is necessary to proceed very quickly; and above all, when following on the TV screen the air movement that we have already mentioned. In a very busy department, once the stage of encephalography in the sitting position (which is the most awkward) is finished, the neuroradiologist frequently entrusts the rest of the examination to an assistant, freeing himself for other tasks.

Theoretically, one nurse is sufficient to look after the patient during the examination and to hand the neuroradiologist the things he needs. However, for some years now we have found it better to have two nurses who can perform their duties without haste and therefore with less possibility of error. The operations connected with modern encephalography are numerous: checking blood pressure and CSF pressure, recording on special forms the amount of air injected and of CSF withdrawn, the speed of air injection, drugs administered, etc., not

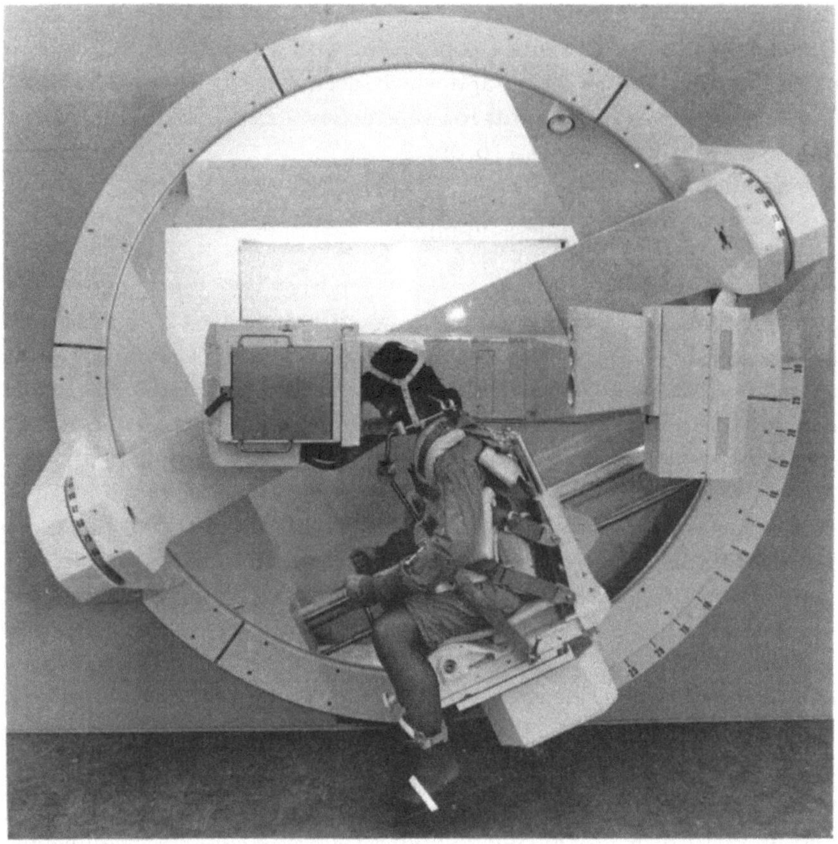

a

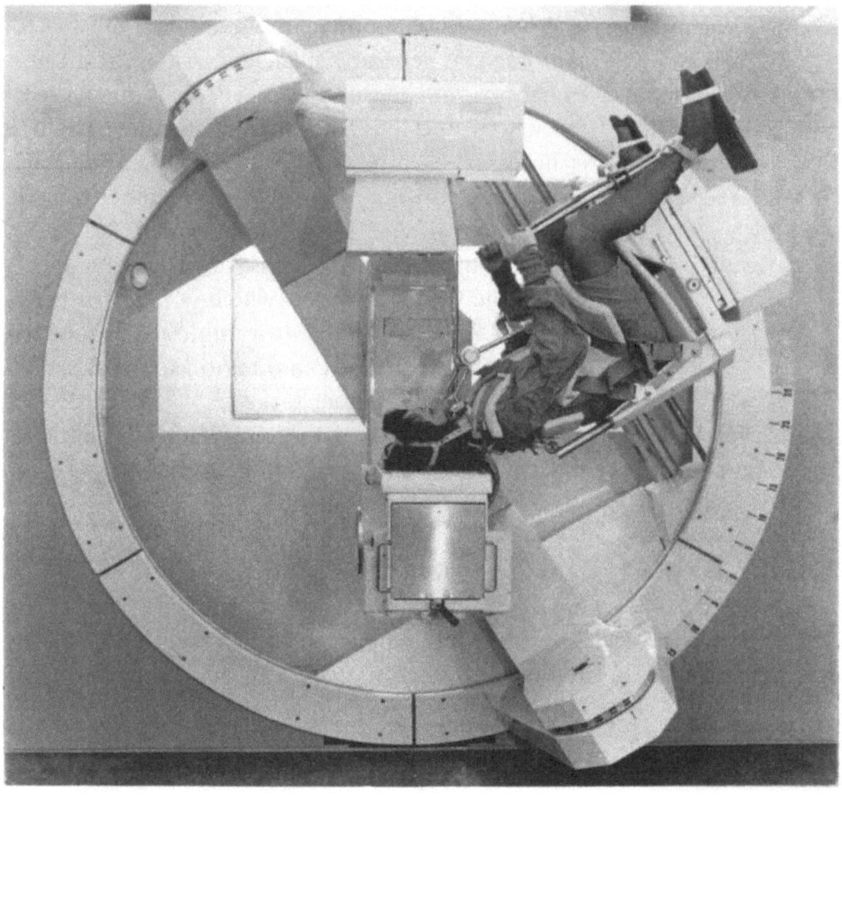

b

Fig. 1.5a, b. *Neurocentrix*. a) Positioned for the examination of the posterior fossa; b) positioned for the examination of the frontal horns to mention assisting the anesthetist when the examination is performed under general anesthesia or on patients in poor general condition.

The number of radiographers needed depends on the quality of the equipment available. With apparatus such as the Mimer III or Princeps 60, with motorized rotating chairs, one radiographer is sufficient. Otherwise (with Mimer I, for example, or with a normal craniograph) a second radiographer is often necessary to help in moving the patient and generally speeding up the maneuvers. For instance, one technician might manage the chair, the other move the amplifier.

The radiographer's only duty is to handle the X-ray apparatus. The attendants see to it that the cassettes are taken mechanically or manually to the darkroom, where they are entrusted to specialist technicians.

4. Preparation of the Patient

The problems relating to premedication and anesthesia are discussed in Chap. I, p. 87.

The patient wears a very large special jacket, with an opening at the back corresponding to the region, where the lumbar puncture will be made (Fig. 1.1). Until a few years ago, in our department aseptic measures were limited to painting the patient's back with iodine and disinfecting the doctor's hands with iodinated alcohol, but for three years now both doctors and nurses have worn gloves and masks. This measure was introduced following an incident which might have had tragic consequences. One of our colleagues, a neurosurgeon who had taken part in a stereotaxic operation on a Parkinsonian patient, was infected with encephalitis. These precautions are not only for the doctor's protection, they also contribute to the patient's safety. In addition, the patient receives 100 mg of Theramycine at 8 p.m. on the evening before the examination; a further 100 mg is given 1 hour before encephalography, and then twice a day for 1 or 2 days after the examination. In the three years we have used this treatment we have found that the fever which usually follows encephalography has diminished and in many cases even disappeared.

To ensure a correct position at the beginning of the examination, certain rules must be observed:

1. The dorso-lumbar spine must be bent in the classic position for lumbar puncture.
2. The head must be slightly flexed and positioned in such a way as to be perfectly centered in the field of the image-amplifier set up for a lateral projection. With the Princeps we make use of the special head support; with the Mimer I the head leans on the Potter, with a small cushion chosen from a series of various thicknesses placed between the Potter and the patient's forehead.
3. The patient must be comfortable in the chair. This is ensured by supports placed under his armpits. When a motorized rotating chair is used, the patient is strapped in by means of parachute belts. The cuff of the manometer for measuring blood pressure which is incorporated in the anesthesia apparatus, is attached to the patient's arm. The bloood pressure is generally checked three times: before the examination, at the end of the stage in the sitting position, and at the end of the examination. Other checks may be carried out as necessary, according to the patient's condition and in case of abrupt variations in CSF pressure.

5. Encephalography Today. Schematic Outline of an Examination

The advent of rotating motorized chairs has simplified many aspects of the encephalographic technique. Such chairs, however, are not universally available because of their high cost. It is for this reason that we describe here an examination performed without a rotating chair, by illustrating movements which the patient performs to order and/or maneuvers carried out by the doctor. With a rotating chair, the same projections are obtained by varying the position of the chair without moving the patient.

We have summarized schematically the different stages of the examination, describing a "negative" examination, without particular difficulties or complications, in a patient with a normal ventricular system and a normal subarachnoid space. Figs. 1.6 through 1.10 illustrate the radiographic images and explain how the air penetrates into the ventricular system and the subarachnoid space, according to

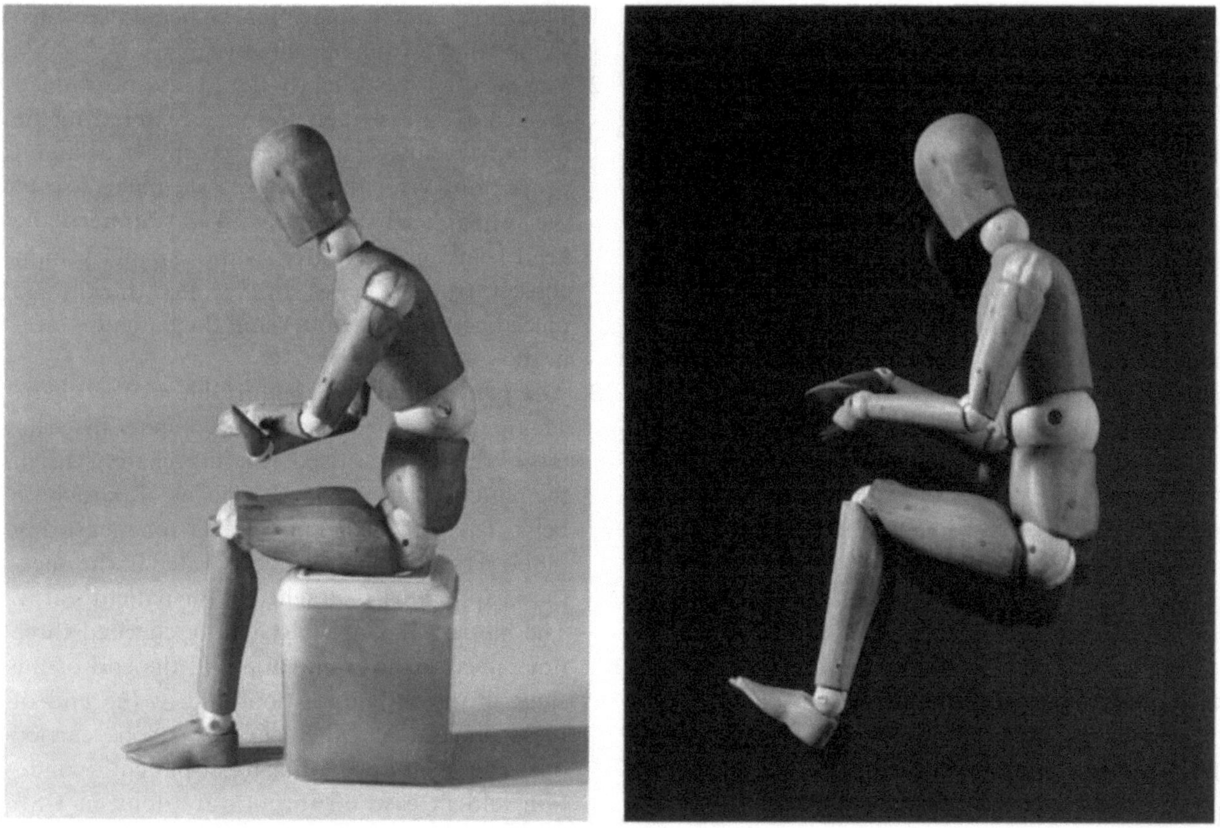

a b

Fig. 1.6a, b. The examination begins. The patient is positioned in order to fill the ventricular system. a) Without the rotating chair; b) with the rotating chair

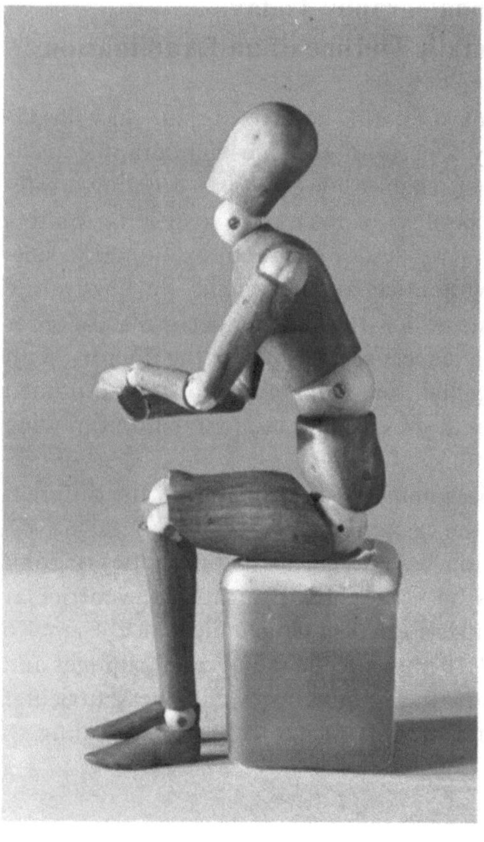

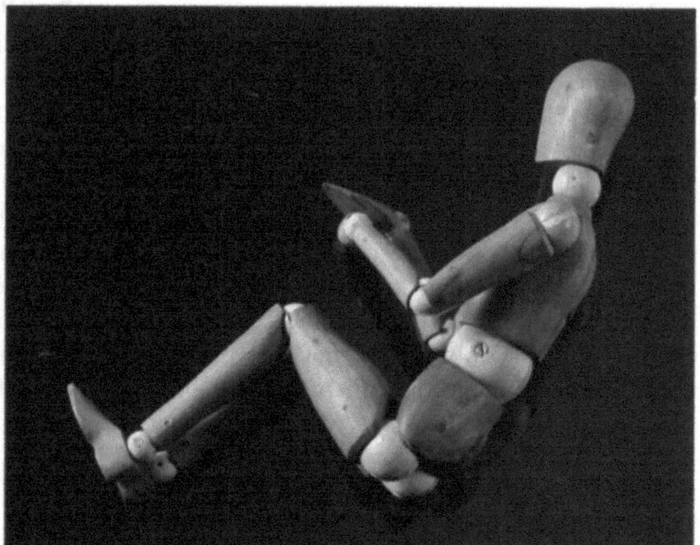

b

a

Fig. 1.7a, b. *Filling of the Subarachnoid Space*. The air present in the fourth ventricle, the aqueduct, and the posterior part of the third ventricle passes, to a great extent, into the lateral ventricles. a) Without the rotating chair; b) with the rotating chair the different positions of body and head. To make everything as clear as possible, we have replaced the patient by a jointed manikin.

Subtentorial Structures

Immediately following the lumbar puncture, 10 ml of air is injected in 30 seconds before any fluid is withdrawn; at the end of the injection the position of the contrast is checked on the TV screen. The air should normally occupy the cisterna magna, the fourth ventricle, the aqueduct, and the posterior portion of the third ventricle. Then the head is extended, another 10 ml of air is introduced in 15 seconds, and the head is flexed again at the end of the injection. Another TV check is made: this time the contrast fills all the cisterns of the posterior fossa and brain stem, also the lateral ventricles into which it passed on extension of the head from the subtentorial portion of the ventricular system. Generally sufficient air remains in the aqueduct and in the fourth ventricle, but the filling of these structures is completed by injection of a further 5 ml with the head flexed. After a further TV check, radiographs are taken in lateral and postero-anterior half-axial projections. These will show the sub-

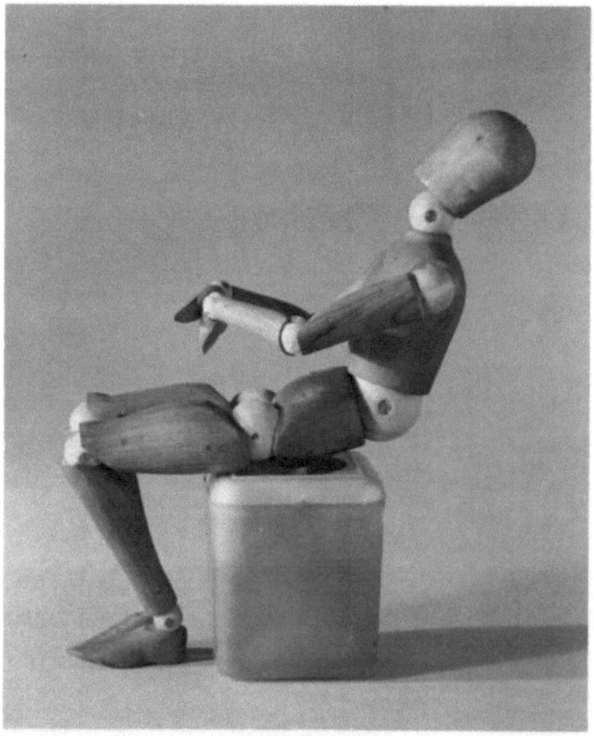

Fig. 1.8. *Examination without the Rotating Chair*. Before the needle is withdrawn, the body and head are extended. In this position the air present in the subtentorial structures passes into the supratentorial structures; the degree of filling is checked on a TV screen. With a rotating chair this maneuver is unnecessary, since the needle can be left *in situ* until the end of the examination

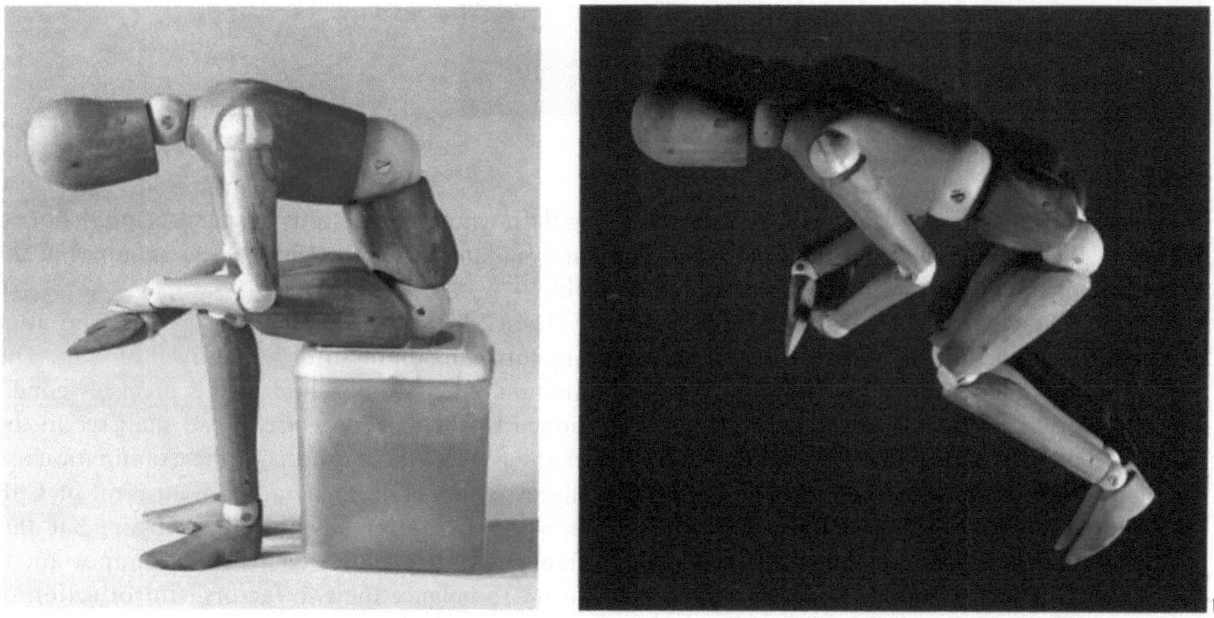

a b

Fig. 1.9a, b. Position of the patient for the examination of the occipital horns. a) Without the rotating chair; b) with the rotating chair

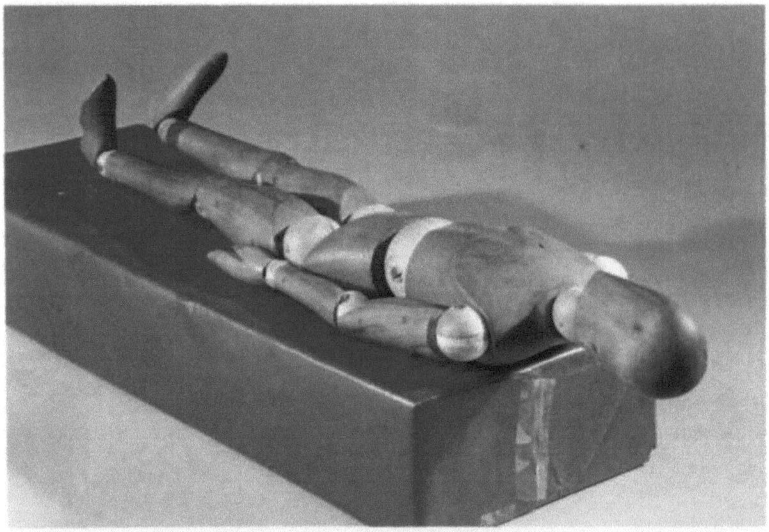

a

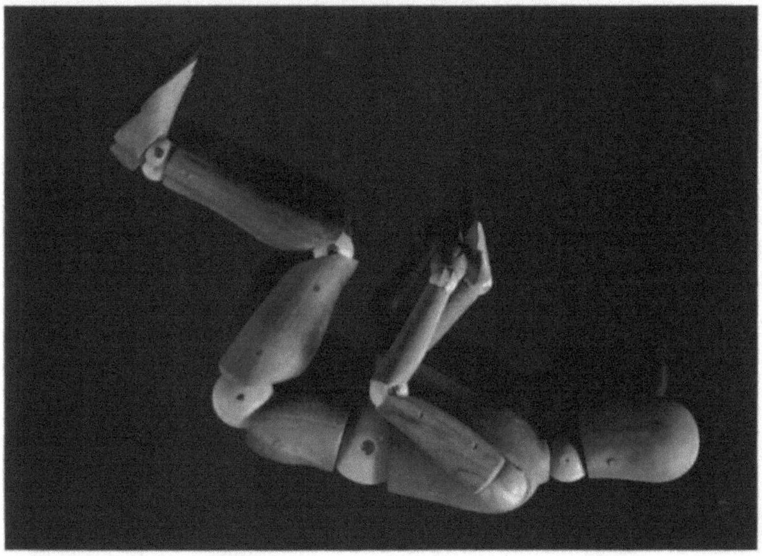

b

Fig. 1.10a, b. Position of the patient for the examination of the anterior supratentorial portion of the ventricular system and subarachnoid space. a) Without the rotating chair; b) with the rotating chair

tentorial portion of the ventricular system, the bodies of the lateral ventricles, the cisterns of the posterior fossa, and the brain stem injected at the same time. Then the head is again extended so that all the air contained in the ventricular system can pass through the foramina of Monroe into the lateral ventricles, allowing an evaluation of their volume, the extent of their filling, and the symmetrical distribution of the air in each of them. Likewise, the contrast leaves the cisterns of the posterior fossa to fill the suprasellar cisterns, those of the Sylvian fissure, and the subarachnoid sulci of the convexity. Generally the needle is removed at this point. However, in dubious cases it can be left in situ and withdrawn after the study of the occipital horns, or even later if a motorized rotating chair is available.

The CSF pressure is measured before and after any introduction of air or withdrawal of CSF. The amount of CSF to be withdrawn is precisely conditioned by the CSF pressure, as we shall see in the chapter where these aspects of the examination are discussed in detail. Generally, about 3 ml of CSF is withdrawn after any injection of air, but this figure is purely indicative. What is important is to try to balance the two factors—introduction of air, and withdrawal of CSF—and before removing the needle to leave the CSF pressure at the desired level, which is generally slightly higher than the initial one.

Occipital Horns

The patient remains in the sitting position; his trunk is inclined far forward, and his head is also bent forward. After a TV check, radiographs are taken in lateral, straight, and half-axial postero-anterior projections.

Frontal Horns

After a blood-pressure check, the patient is placed in supine position for the study of the frontal horns, which are examined in three traditional projections: lateral, antero-posterior, and half-axial antero-posterior. This concludes the examination. Throughout its course the examination has been, so to speak, "charted" on a form that summarizes its essentials (Fig. 1.11). In the following chapters we discuss the main points of this technique and any variations and/or innovations with respect to our earlier work [374, 375], also special procedures for the study of certain anatomic regions or special pathologic situations.

6. Lumbar Puncture

The lumbar puncture is performed under local anesthesia. This is carried out in two stages: first, the skin is cooled with ethyl chloride, second, the soft tissue situated in the path of the needle toward the meninx is anesthetized by both subcutaneous and intramuscular administration of Novocaine.

This technique makes the whole procedure of the lumbar puncture painless, enabling the patient to tolerate the examination. However, with good premedication of the patient (see Chap. I, p. 87) and if the lumbar puncture is made by an expert, the Novocaine injection is unnecessary. Sometimes we tell the patient he is "going to feel the prick for the anesthesia," whereas instead we perform the lumbar puncture.

The lumbar puncture is a fundamental part of encephalography. It is desirable to puncture the arachnoid only once and to go right across the subarachnoid space as near as possible to the midline to avoid painful contact of the needle with nerve roots.

Generally, the first introduction of air is made without withdrawal of CSF. However, this is only theoretical. When the manometer measuring the CSF pressure is inserted in the needle, some CSF, though a very small quantity, must necessarily escape from the subarachnoid space in order to reach the manometer. However, it is possible to introduce air into the subarachnoid space without letting even a drop of fluid come out if the syringe plunger is depressed just before the needle tip enters the subarachnoid space. Experts in encephalography are able to distinguish between the "feeling" of puncturing the dura mater or the arachnoid. Anyway, it is possible to tell whether the needle is in the subarachnoid or in the subdural space by performing the lumbar puncture with the manometer connected to the needle once the tip is located in the subdural space. At this point it is enough to push the needle gently; after a few millimeters the positive pressure will indicate that the tip of the needle has reached the subarachnoid space (Fig. 1.12).

There is another way of knowing when the subdural space has been reached: after penetration of the skin and muscles, the mandril is withdrawn and a drop of saline is put on the graft cone. The needle is then pushed gently forward. When the needle tip penetrates the subdural space, the drop of saline is sucked into the needle.

The time during which the needle indicates negative pressure is very short, generally not more than a few seconds, after which the manometer again moves toward zero. This may be because the subdural space inspires the air contained in the needle, thus reestablishing the pressure balance. Sometimes, after a quick movement toward negative pressure, the pointer returns to zero and then suddenly moves without interruption toward positive values, *even if the position of the needle has not been modified.* This probably happens when the subdural space is very narrow: in such cases the needle tip pierces the dura mater and the arachnoid at almost the same time, thus establishing a communication between the subarachnoid and the subdural space.

Ospedale Maggiore, Bologna
Neuroradiological Department

Fractioned Encephalography (Form)

Date: January 23th 1967

Patient	*Doctors*	*Technicians*
Name: C. Umberto	*Operator:* Prof. G. Ruggiero	Agostina
Chart N°: 6764	*Assistant:*	Bertozzi
Serial: 2633	*Anesthesist:*	

Time	Procedure	CSF Removed	AIR Injected	CSF Pressure	B. P.	P.
12.20	P. L.		VS* 10 in 30″	46 95	145/90	92
12.25			VS 10 in 30″ ∅	40 74		
12.34		4		42 38	110/70	
12.40			SS** 5 in 10″ °°	44 57		
12.42	Needle out			42		
13	End of exam				130/80	92

* Ventricular system.
** Subarachnoid space.

NOTES

∅ Mild headache, rapidly subsiding.

°° Severe headache, due to rapid injection of air, subsiding in 1 – 2 minutes.

Conclusions:

Patients' condition
at the end of procedure:

Very good
× Good
Fair
Poor

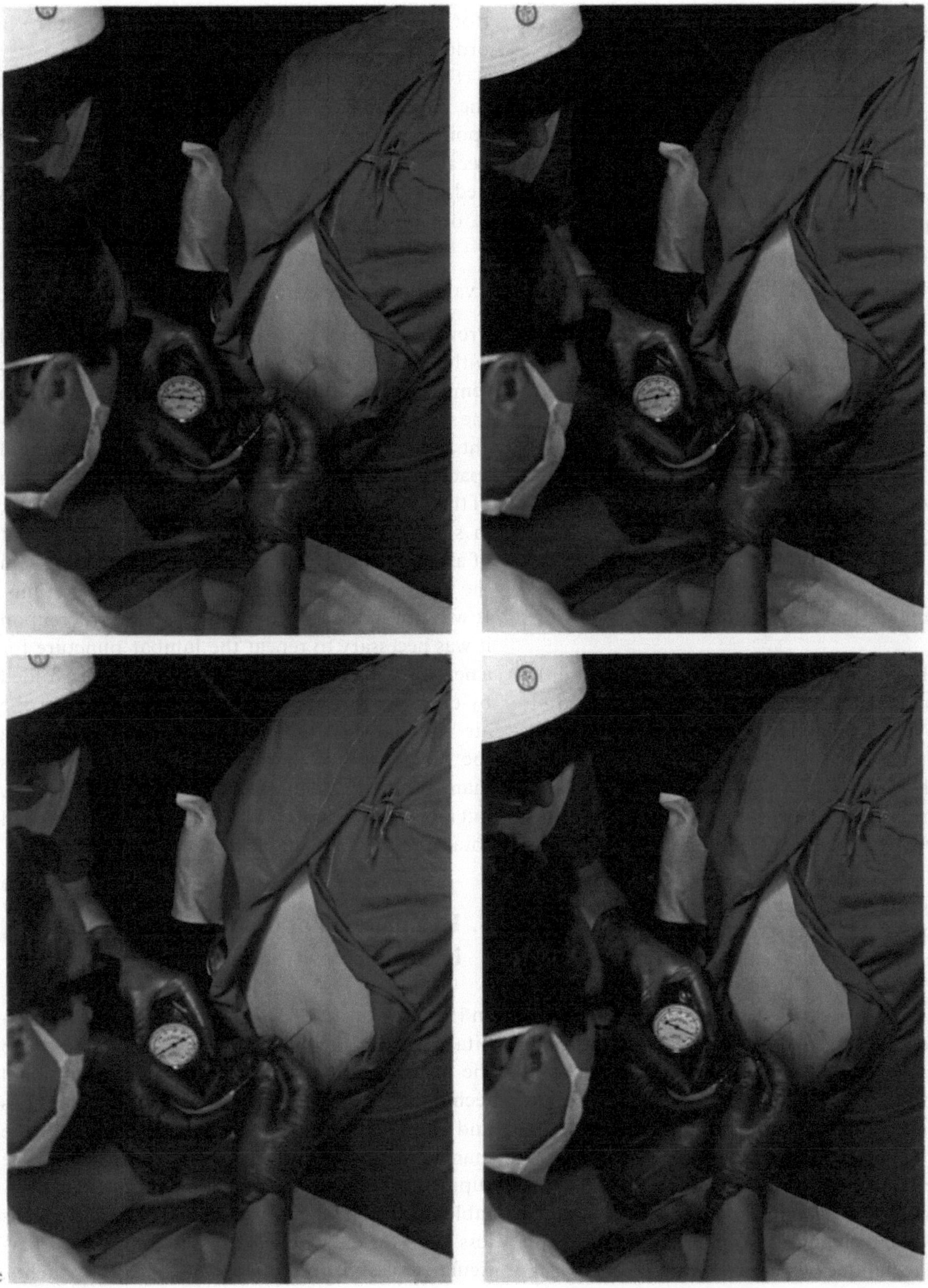

Fig. 1.12a–d. *Manometric Control during Lumbar Puncture.* a) Needle has just entered the dura mater. Negative pressure: −4. b) Needle in the subdural space. Pressure: −10. c) Needle advances into the subdural space. Pressure: −18. d) Arachnoid perforated: the needle is in the subarachnoid space. Positive Pressure: +62

◅ Fig. 1.11. Form summarizing the main aspects of the examination

7. Image Amplifier with Television Control

Radioscopic exploration in neuroradiology coincides with the advent of the image amplifier. In 1964 Ruggiero [380] emphasized its importance by presenting to the French Society of Radiology a film illustrating many aspects of the technique described in the present paper. Later on, the utility of the amplifier-TV system was confirmed by the same author [383] on the basis of much statistical material. His material currently includes more than 3000 examinations. With the exception of a few special cases (but never when a tumor is suspected), all our encephalographies are now monitored by TV. This technique constitutes a technical advance for two reasons: it shortens the examination, and it virtually eliminates errors in judging the amount of contrast to be injected.

Shortening of the Examination

In the absence of TV monitoring, the four fundamental stages of the encephalography are the study of 1. the subtentorial portion of the ventricular system, 2. the cisterns of the posterior fossa, 3. the occipital horns, and 4. the frontal horns. These stages are separated from each other by the time necessary to process the radiographs. With the amplifier-TV, this dead time is considerably reduced. The extent of filling of the different structures is observed on the screen and, if it is considered satisfactory, one can take the pictures and pass on to the next steps of the examination while they are being processed. We have calculated from the records on our special forms the average time taken for the stage of the examination carried out in the sitting position in 20 negative encephalographies performed by the same neuroradiologist, with and without TV monitoring. The result was 10 minutes with the amplifier and 20 minutes without it; the difference is even greater in pathological cases or when special techniques are employed, for example the urea technique, which requires repeated checks before the needle is removed. It is particularly useful to check on TV at the beginning of the examination whether or not the air is entering the ventricular system, or to observe the result of special maneuvers (for example, the filling of one temporal horn) in order to avoid making useless radiographs.

The only drawback of using TV may be when the processing unit breaks down. A mislaid or spoiled radiograph could not then be repeated because subsequent maneuvers would have modified the position of the air in the skull. But this is, obviously, an exceptional event.

Evaluation of the Amount of Contrast

Previously, when the examination was performed without television, it was necessary to decide before removing the needle (at the end of the stage in the sitting position) whether the quantity of air present in the ventricular system and the subarachnoid space was sufficient for the correct visualization of the supratentorial structures to be examined later in supine and prone positions. Before the advent of automatic processing machines in the darkroom the decision was sometimes made from the films. It was not unusual to make a mistake, whereupon it was necessary to repeat the lumbar puncture for a new injection of air. Such a mishap can be avoided by checking on the TV screen the position of the air after an extension of the head, and allowing the air to collect in the lateral ventricles. This maneuver is ticklish when the needle is inserted, but it becomes simple, as we shall see, if a motorized rotating chair is available.

8. Examination of the Occipital Horns in Sitting Position

In 1964 Ruggiero [383] suggested studying the occipital horns in the sitting position, as opposed to the prone position employed in the conventional technique. The use of the sitting position simplifies and shortens the examination as it eliminates the maneuvers involved in moving the patient from the supine to the prone position. This is more comfortable for the patient, who is not jolted, and means less work for the whole staff. The technique is particularly useful for obese and heavy patients, patients in poor general condition, and those liable to complications like nausea, vomiting, headache, etc. Moreover, it is easier for the anesthetist to assist a patient in the sitting position than in the

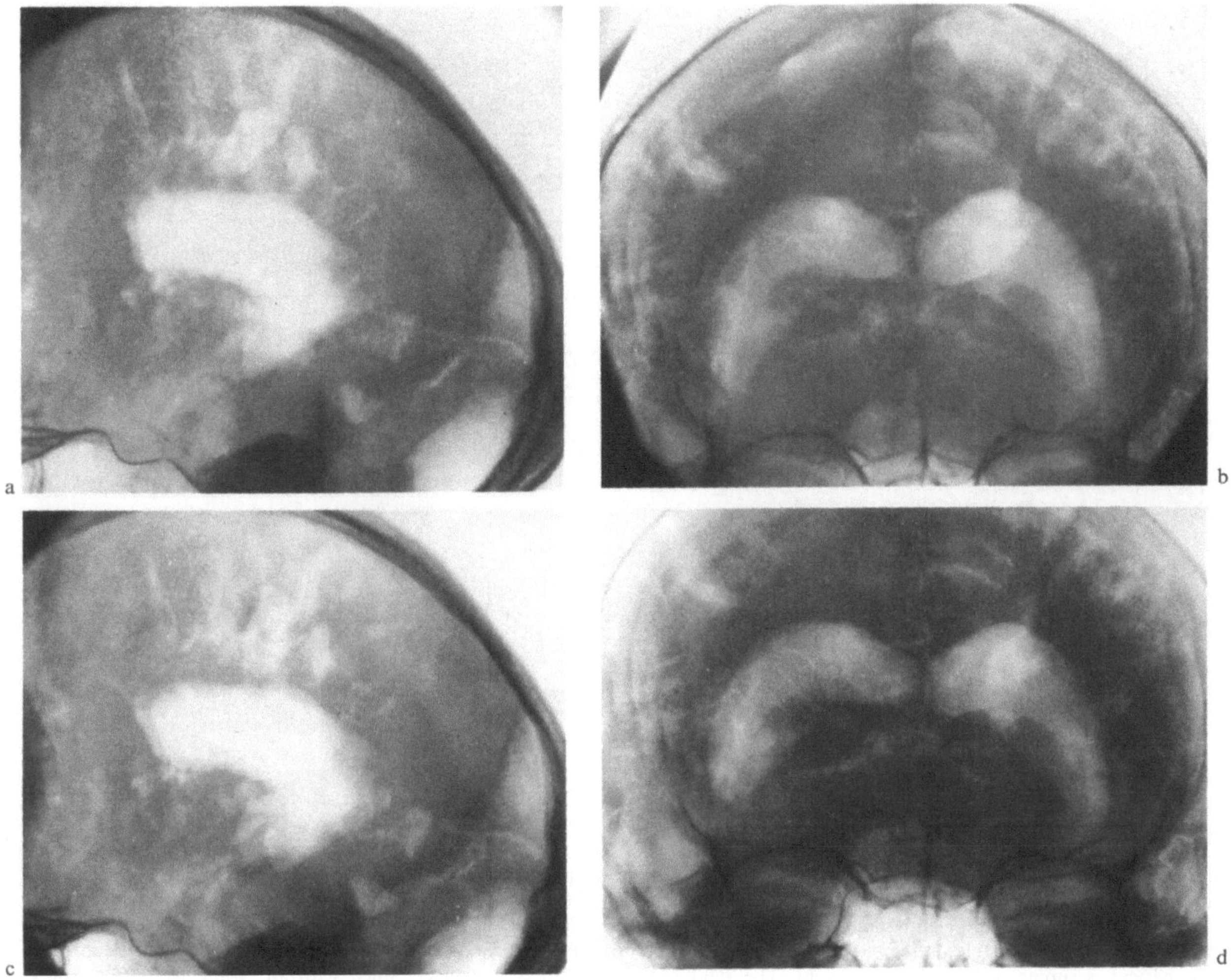

Fig. 1.13a–d. *Aspect of the Occipital Horns Examined in the Sitting Position.* a, b) Orbito-meatal line perpendicular to the cassette; c, d) orbito-meatal line tilted 25° caudally. In (c) the air-fluid level appears oblique

prone one. Sometimes, with obese or patients with short necks, it may be difficult or even impossible to flex the head sufficiently to orient the long axis of the ventricles perpendicular to the horizontal plane. It is usually possible, however, to obtain satisfactory views of the occipital horns, even when head flexion is incomplete; the only difference from a true postero-anterior projection will be that, on the lateral view, the air-fluid level will appear more or less oblique (Fig. 1.13), but this does not affect the diagnostic value of the radiographs.

9. Examination of the Temporal Horns

Two conditions must be fulfilled for correct examination of the temporal horns:

1. The patient must be supine in order to obtain complete filling of the anterior portion of the temporal horn which, in laterial projection, will then be radiographed with the central beam set horizontally.
2. In lateral projection each of the two temporal horns can be studied separately. It is very important to look carefully at the upper and lower walls of the ventricle to observe any possible infiltration of a slowly growing, expansive process. Such lesions are usually astrocytomas or cicatricial tissue. The separate visualization of the two temporal horns in lateral projection will show even the slightest changes, which are not visible when the two ventricles are superimposed. The separate visualization of the temporal horns may be effected in two ways: they can be filled

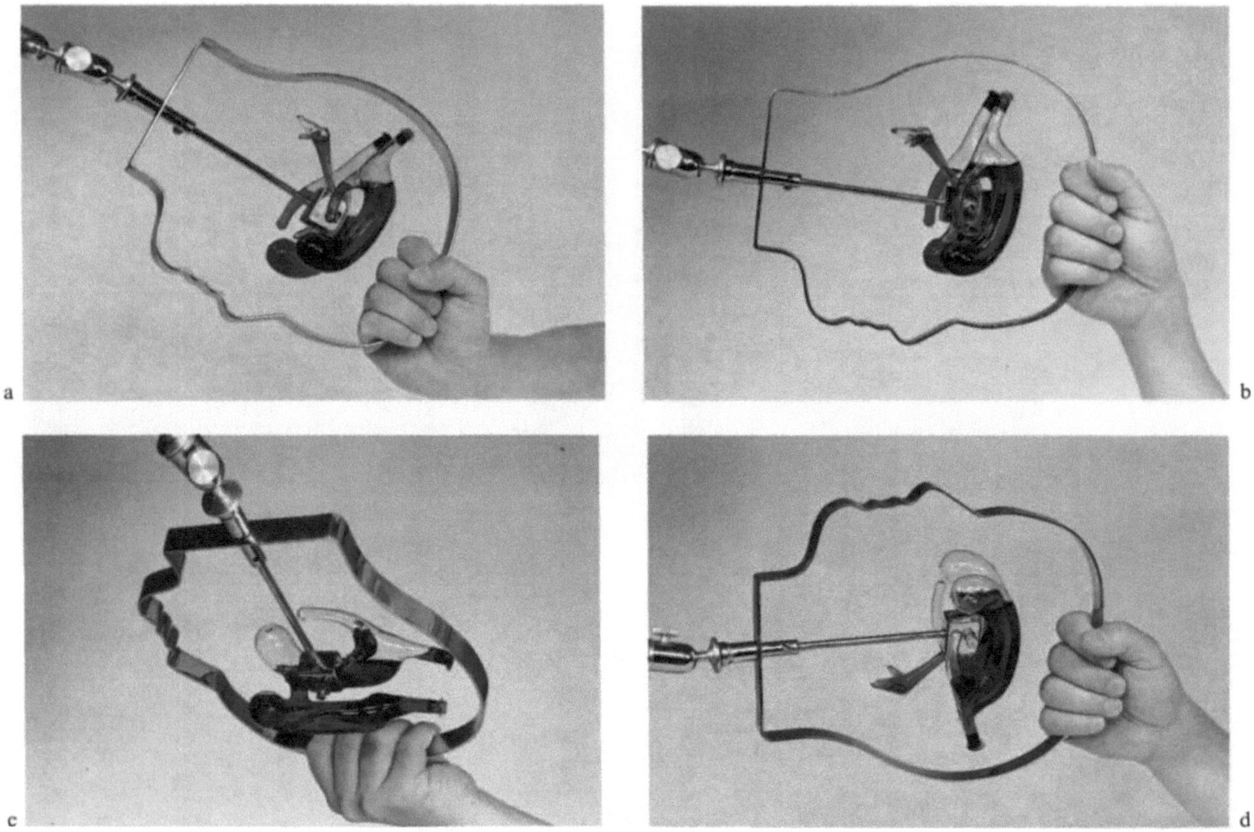

Fig. 1.14a–d. LINDGREN'S *Maneuver for the Examination of the Right Temporal Horn.* a) After the examination of the occipital horns, the patient is prone. The amount of air present in the two ventricles is almost the same on each side, while both temporal horns are filled with CSF. b) The head is moved downward and slightly to the right. c) Rotation increases. CSF moves toward the left ventricle, while the right frontal and temporal horns are filled with air. There is some air also in the left temporal horn, which is hardly visible on the picture owing to the superimposition of the ventricular body. d) Rotation is accomplished. The patient is supine, with his head straight. The right temporal horn is completely filled with air, while the left temporal horn is poorly filled. Also the right frontal horn contains more air than the left one

one at a time, taking care to empty the temporal horn which has already been examined, or they can be filled simultaneously and tomograms made. The first way requires special maneuvers with the direct intervention of the neuroradiologist; for the second, the motorized rotating chair is generally used.

Maneuvers for the Filling of a Single Temporal Horn

In LINDGREN'S [254] classical maneuver (Fig. 1.14), the temporal horns are studied after the occipital horns. The patient is moved from the prone back into the supine position. During this rotation of the body, the head is positioned such that the temporal horn to be examined is always at a higher level than the corresponding frontal horn. When both temporal horns are to be examined, this maneuver is repeated, of course, on the other side. The patient therefore undergoes the following changes of position:

1. from prone to supine,
2. from supine to prone,
3. from prone back to supine.

It is not necessary to emphasize the inconvenience to the patient of all these movements, which also increase the duration of the encephalography. We [383] have suggested a maneuver allowing one to examine the temporal horn directly in the supine position. This maneuver is the natural consequence of our technique of examining the occipital horns in the sitting position, which would obviously lose some of its advantages if the patient had to be moved to the prone position for any reason. Our

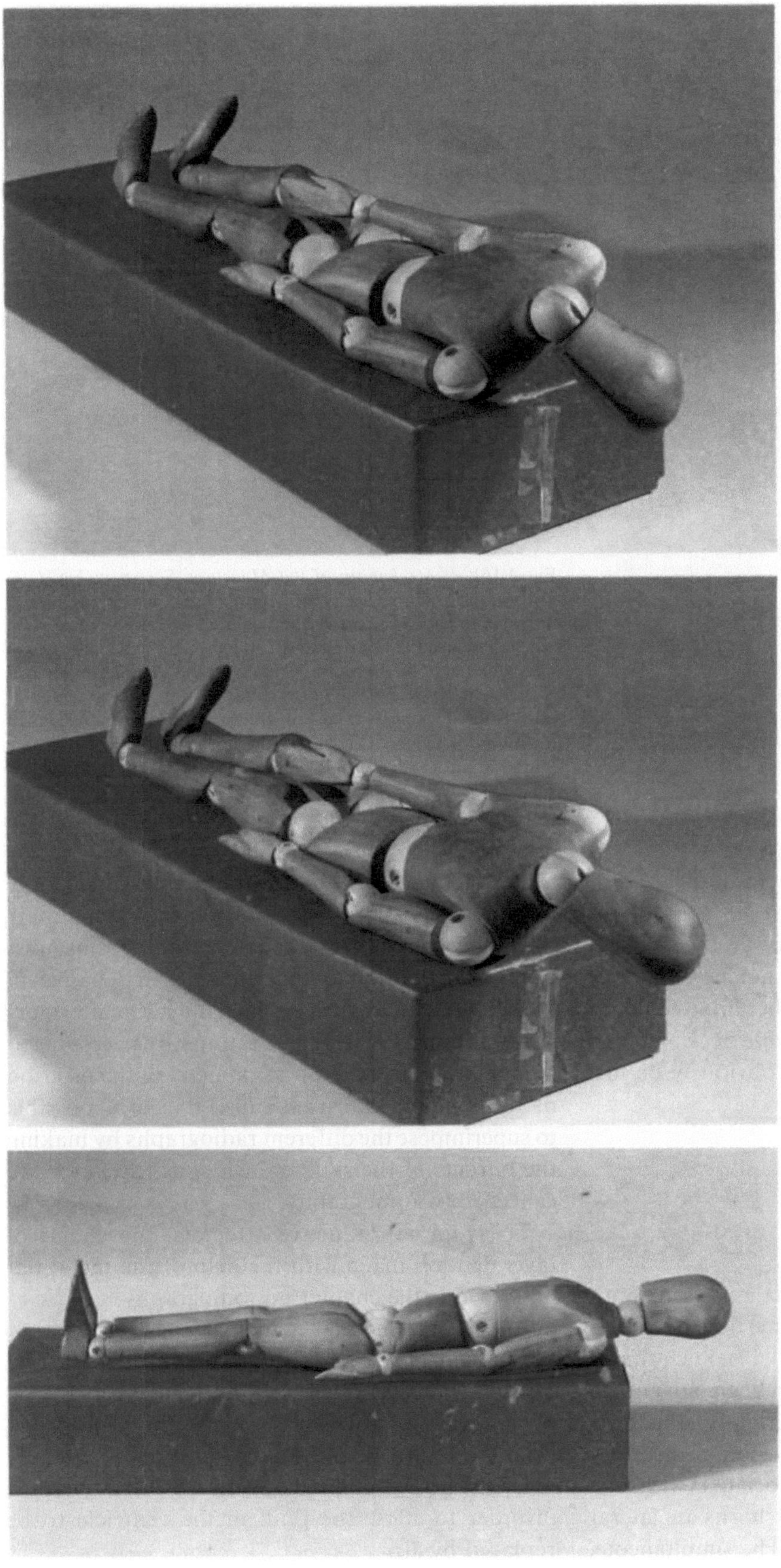

a

b

c

Fig. 1.15a–c. RUGGIERO'S *Maneuver for the Examination of the Right Temporal Horn.* a) The patient is supine, the right shoulder elevated. The head is markedly lowered and rotated to the left. b) The right shoulder is lowered. The head is elevated but still rotated to the left. c) The patient is again in the supine position; the head has been rapidly straightened

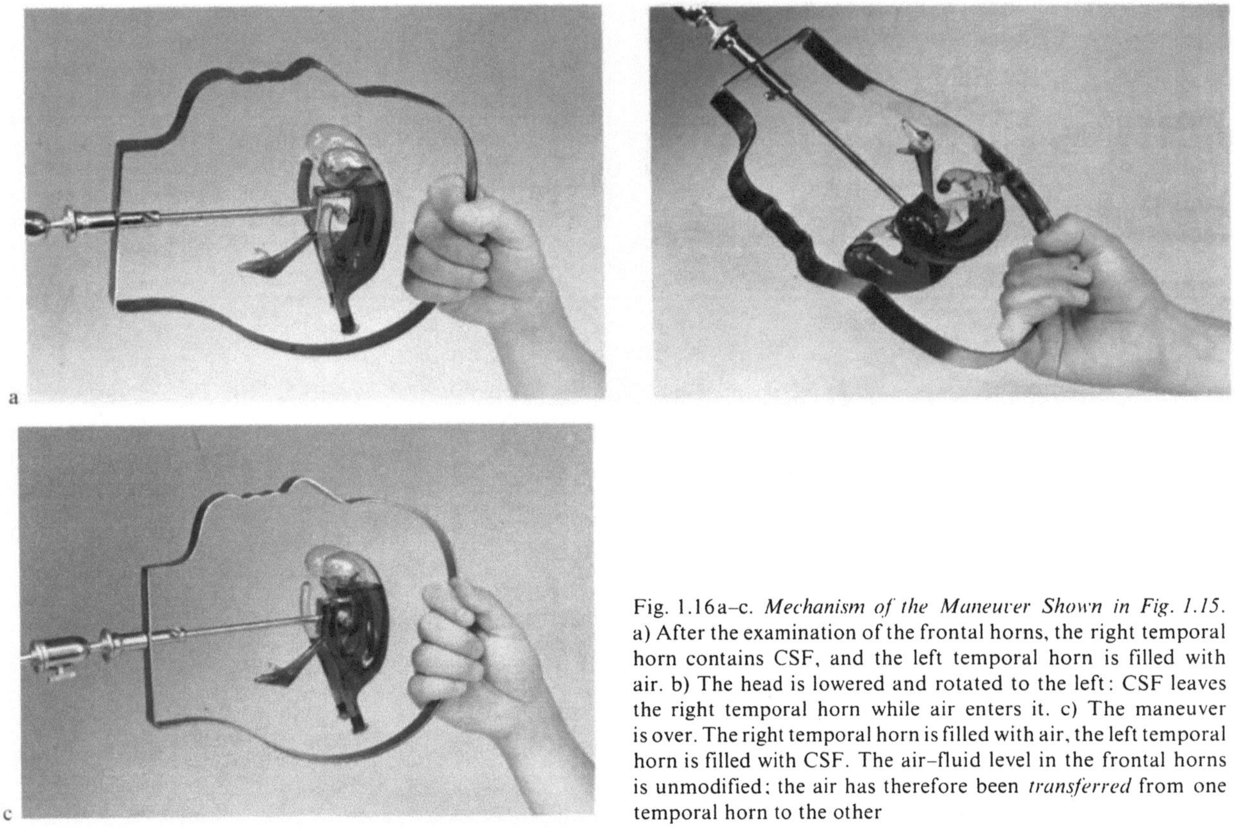

Fig. 1.16a–c. *Mechanism of the Maneuver Shown in Fig. 1.15.* a) After the examination of the frontal horns, the right temporal horn contains CSF, and the left temporal horn is filled with air. b) The head is lowered and rotated to the left: CSF leaves the right temporal horn while air enters it. c) The maneuver is over. The right temporal horn is filled with air, the left temporal horn is filled with CSF. The air–fluid level in the frontal horns is unmodified; the air has therefore been *transferred* from one temporal horn to the other

maneuver is illustrated in Figs. 1.15 and 1.16 and described in the legends. It must be carried out slowly and most precisely, otherwise the replacement of the fluid by the air will not be complete. The maneuver may prove to be impossible in patients with a short or unextensible neck; in such cases LINDGREN's maneuver will obviously be utilized.

Simultaneous Filling of the Two Temporal Horns

When the motorized rotating chair is used, both temporal horns are filled at the same time by means of the somersault technique (Fig. 1.17). Such simultaneous visualization is considered an advantage by many authors [175, 195]. Certainly, the time saved is considerable, but in our opinion this does not offset the disadvantage associated with the superimposition of the temporal horns in lateral projection, as mentioned above. The simultaneous filling of the two temporal horns is justified only if there is a possibility of studying them separately by tomography. A series of lateral tomograms must be made carefully so that there is no change in the centering of the head, which must remain rigorously stationary. These precautions are necessary to demonstrate any possible asymmetry in the position of the temporal horns because it is not possible to superimpose the different radiographs by making the borders of the skull coincide, as the latter are cancelled by tomography.

To avoid unproductive attempts, the choice of layer depth is made with the help of the metal bar described in the chapter on tomography.

As with the manual maneuvers, the rotation of the patient in a motorized chair must be carried out with due care. While the speed may be increased during passage from the supine to the prone position, the return to the supine position—especially when the head is pointed downward—must be slow in order to allow the fluid in the ventricle to be replaced by air.

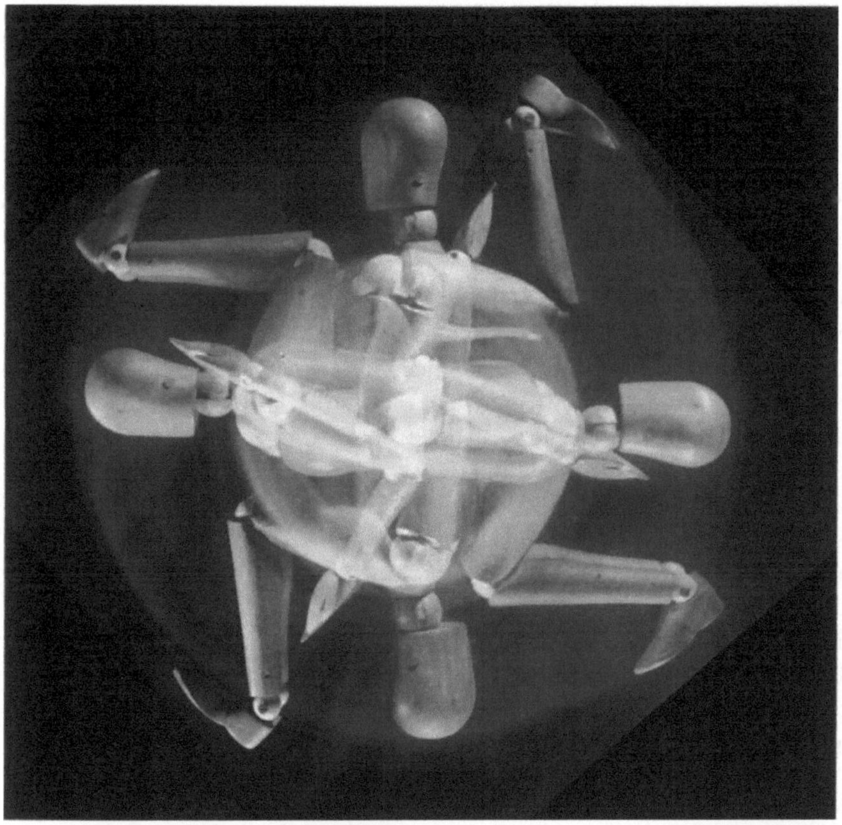

Fig. 1.17. *Somersault to Fill Both Temporal Horns Simultaneously*. Arrows point to the rotation direction. The circle indicates the beginning and finishing positions

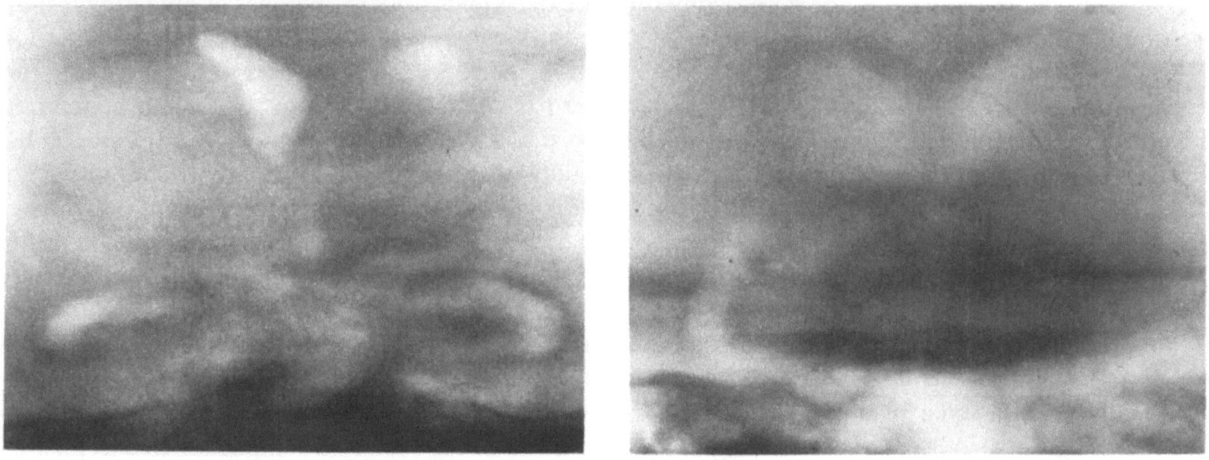

a b

Fig. 1.18a, b. *Unsuccessful Somersault Maneuver with a Motorized Rotating Chair*. Only the right temporal horn is visualized (a). A manual maneuver has been necessary to fill the left temporal horn, which appears visualized together with the right one (b)

Finally, it must be emphasized that in exceptional cases one of the temporal horns may not fill (Fig. 1.18). This generally occurs in pathological conditions. We had one case of an intraventricular tumor in which the somersault maneuver was unsuccessful three times. The lesion was finally demonstrated with our maneuver.

10. Tomography

Literature

The history of tomography of the ventricular system starts with JANKER's work [233] in 1936; he (first on a cadaver and later on a living subject) obtained a tomogram of the third and lateral ventricles in the antero-posterior projection.

In 1937 CARILLO, ORIBE, and MALENCHINI [74] published a lateral tomogram of the midline that clearly visualized the fourth ventricle, the aqueduct, and third ventricle. Not until 1940 did the technique come into neuroradiological practice with LUTZ and TURNER's paper [267] on tomography applied to pneumoencephalography and ventriculography. Six years later EPSTEIN and DAVIDOFF [141], on the basis of experience acquired in 45 cases, recommended sagittal stratigraphy as the routine procedure in cases where it was necessary to visualize the structures of the midline. These authors stressed the use of stratigraphy in tumors of the posterior fossa, as it gives better visualization of the third and fourth ventricles, the aqueduct, the pontine cistern, and the cerebellar sulci. Unfortunately, they did not use a fractional technique for the encephalographies but made stratigrams of patients in the supine position with only lateral projection.

In 1935 POPPEL *et al.* [353], after a study of 62 cases, confirmed that tomography was superior to the conventional techniques and/or stereoscopy for the examination of midline structures.

In Europe, tomography as an adjunct to pneumoencephalography was introduced in 1952, at the Symposium Neuroradiologicum in Stockholm, by a group of Italian and French neuroradiologists, including VALLEBONA, MASCHERPA, and FISCHGOLD [53, 285].

On the same occasion, GROS [183] proposed tomography for the study of cisterns, using an old technique that nevertheless anticipated present trends, as the injection of 20 ml of air was not accompanied by the removal of cerebrospinal fluid. One year later, a so-called "tomocisternography" was proposed by PALEIRAC *et al.* [326]: again 20 ml of air was injected with the patient's head extended, but an equal quantity of CSF was removed. Further contributions on tomography in pneumoencephalography [41, 42, 244] were given by the Strasbourg school, and a technique for the simultaneous study of cisterns and ventricles was proposed by BÉTOULIÈRES *et al.* [40]: 20 ml of air is injected with the patient's head extended, the head is straightened and the contrast moves from the cisterna magna into the ventricles, which are then examined, together with the cisterns, by means of tomograms in quick succession.

All these authors obtained stratigrams with apparatus designed for routine use in general radiology [285], therefore without the advantage of the craniograph. As far as we know, the first attempt to use conventional tomography together with correct encephalographic technique was made by VALENTINO [464] in 1956. In 1957 MANFREDI and KRUSE [276] maintained that tomography was particularly useful when encephalography was performed with small quantities of air, allowing better visualization of the desired structure. Their work, like that of SHIPSS and RAAT [421] published one year later, is of no value at present since their technique cannot be applied with the patient in the sitting position, and this is fundamental in the encephalographic technique. In Italy tomography was also adopted by LENZI who, with CANOSSA and BASSANI, [251] published an atlas in 1959.

In 1960 autotomography was proposed again: this technique had been suggested by VALLEBONA [465] 30 years before and was applied for the first time to pneumoencephalography by ZIEDSES DES PLANTES [485] in 1937, in hopes of obviating technical difficulties in the encephalographic examination of the posterior fossa. ZIEDSES DES PLANTES did not write a special paper on this work, but he referred to it in articles dealing with the ventriculographic study of the third and fourth ventricles [485–487]. It is not clear who reintroduced autotomography. The paper by SCHVARCZ [411] appeared in 1959; but, according to the 1962 editorial [17] in the *British Journal of Radiology* devoted to this method, it was SCHECHTER [400–402] who demonstrated the technique to SCHVARCZ [411] at the Serafimerlazarettet. Before SCHECHTER, this method had been used by SIMON [428], who applied it to encephalography after seeing slides shown by CREZÉE [93] at the Scientific Exhibition of the IV Symposium Neuroradiologicum, in 1955. It seems that it was SIMON who coined the term "autotomography." At about the same time SWANN [445] introduced autotomography at the National Hospital for Nervous Diseases, London, where SCHECHTER learned the technique and developed it in England, and later in the United States. SCHECHTER described it in detail in papers written jointly with JING [401], STRENGER [402], and GUTIÉRREZ-MAHONEY [400].

TOLPEZHNIKOV [458] and CAMPBELL [71] made contributions to autotomography. Some authors [104, 220, 226, 318, 449] proposed that the movement of the head, either made spontaneously by the patient or imposed by the doctor through bridles, be replaced by the movement of the whole body on a rotating chair.

In the United States the importance of tomography was emphasized by DI CHIRO in two atlases [116, 123] on normal and pathologic pneumoencephalography. He also suggested [118, 119] reintroducing VALLEBONA's technique [465] of transverse axial tomography, as applied to the skull by VALLEBONA's pupils and later to pneumoencephalography by TAKAHASU *et al.* [448].

This concludes the first period of the history of tomography in pneumoencephalography: clinical contributions without any special technical improvements were made by FAURÉ with several coworkers [144, 248], JEFFERSON and LEWTAS [238] on "subdural tomography" in fractures, LEFÈVRE *et al.* [248] on gliomas of the brain stem, BONKALO [47] on pituitary adenomas, and finally WACKENHEIM who, with several co-workers [80, 455–457], emphasized the use of tomography for the study of the brain stem and the atrophic lesions of the cerebellum. Included in this group are the publications of KADRNKA [221], SUBIRANA and VROUSOS [442], ALBERTI *et al.* [6], BERNEY and WERNER [38], BETZ [43, 44], BRADAC and WACKENHEIM [55], HANAFEE and LECKY [198], KANEKO [223], MARIN, ANDRIOLI E ZACCHI [280], POTTHOFF and SCHMIDT [357, 358], ROBERTS [370], WEYER *et al.* [410, 479], and NEUMANN [310].

The second period of tomography starts with the introduction of the new power-driven craniographs: the Swedish Mimer [182, 260] and the French Princeps [133] in their successive models, and more recently, the Franco-Dutch Diagnost N. With these machines, especially the Mimer III and the Princeps 60, the switch from TV to the standard radiograph and tomography is very rapid. This considerably reduces, though it does not eliminate (as we shall see later) the negative aspect of tomography, i.e. prolonged examination. The best work with the Mimer III was done by GREITZ, reaching its peak in the excellent reports made in collaboration with CORRALES [86–88, 181] on the anatomy of the fourth ventricle, the results of which were confirmed by CRISTI [94]. The best results with the Princeps 60 seem to have been obtained by BORIES and his colleagues [50, 51], who for some years have been making improvements to this apparatus. METZGER and FISCHGOLD with various collaborators [146, 147, 302, 303] have described tomography with hypocycloidal movement, which in their opinion is far better than linear movement. This opinion is supported by MCLACHLAN [294], AMUNDSEN *et al.* [14], and STEARS and SANDERS [434]. The last two authors have made a special study of the opto-chiasmatic region. Similar studies were done by FISCHGOLD *et al.* [147]; FREDY also published a thesis [151] on the subject.

Linear tomography has recently been suggested by HAMMER and SCHERRER [197] for the study of the anatomy of the cerebellar vallecula, and by FREDY and BORIES [152] for the careful examination of the temporal horns. The latter authors feel that only by tomography is it sometimes possible to demonstrate very small tumors in the temporal region. RUGGIERO's experience dates back 10 years. After he had used autotomography in his department for a short time, he performed the examination with one Mimer I equipped with the additional tomographic device, and a second in conjunction with TV. The author recently had a Princeps 60 at his disposal, which prompted him to employ tomography more often, and for some structures in every case. The Princeps 60 and the Mimer III are easy to use; but the images obtained with the tomographic device of the Mimer I are also of good quality, as proved, we think, by the illustrations in the present work.

In spite of his considerable interest in encephalography, RUGGIERO acknowledged the contribution of tomography rather late. For this reason he has sometimes been criticized as an opponent of tomography, but this is not true. In 1959 in his book *Neuroradiologic Technique* [375], he included a short chapter on tomography in encephalography. He stated that there were two reasons for questioning its use: the difficulty of obtaining images with sufficient contrast in tomograms of thin layers, which were the only ones possible at that time, and the impossibility of performing tomography without abandoning the correct technique of fractional encephalography. With today's apparatus and with the introduction of zonography [477], these difficulties have been overcome, and excellent results have been obtained, as RUGGIERO had always hoped. However, the author is still convinced of the uselessness of employing new terms. There is only one technique of fractional encephalography but it has many aspects, of which tomography is one.

Technique

Autotomography

The foregoing analysis of the literature should make any further discussion on autotomography redundant. If we continue —and in a rather exhaustive manner—it is for a practical reason: machines like the Mimer III or the Princeps are certainly not within the range of all neuroradiological budgets. On the other hand, autotomography ordinarily gives excellent results, provided that the patient's head is moved with sufficient precision (Figs. 1.19 and 1.20). Therefore, in departments having limited specialization or activity, use of normal, nonmotorized craniographs can be justified, for instance, the still valuable craniograph of LYSHOLM, and the technique of autotomography may be resorted to when tomography is indispensable for the study of the midline structures.

The technique consists in taking radiographs of the head while the head is rotated about the axis that passes through the median longitudinal plane of the brain. In other words, the tomography is achieved by keeping both the roentgen source and the radiographic cassette stationary while the object moves. The rotating movement of the head can either be made by the patient himself, who is given appropriate instructions, or it can be imposed by the hand of an operator protected by a leaded glove, or even by means of reins (SCHVARCZ [411], SCHECHTER and STRENGER [402]), or special mobile devices attached to the craniograph (DAVIDSON and CLARK [104], BURROWS [67]) that can be maneuvered without exposing the hand of the operator in the field.

One possibility suggested by some authors (POTZ [359], AMPLATZ [12], TANAKA [449], NOVAK [318]) is to turn the patient on a rotating chair, whether motorized or not, so that the patient is not obliged to move his head, thus easing the problem of centering the head. Another advantage of a rotating chair is that it is easier to give an exact definition of how to rotate the head, which seems to be an essential point in autotomography. IWABUCHI and SUZUKI [220] wrote papers on this subject, but we were unable to have direct access to their works.

According to SCHECHTER *et al.* [400–402], the clearest tomograms are obtained by rotating the head through 10°, but it is possible to obtain equally satisfactory results by rotating the head through 5° to one side, and then moving it back to the midline. In some cases, however, it may be necessary to increase the rotation. It seems that the speed of head rotation does not play an important role; what is essential is that the rotation be gentle and uniform.

NEW and WEBSTER [313] contributed an excellent paper on the theory of autotomography, analyzing the geometric and anatomic aspects connected with this technique. Their conclusions can be summarized as follows:

1. The rotation axis must pass as close as possible to the anatomic region being studied. In autotomography this rotation axis is represented by the odontoid process. The position of the head, therefore, influences the quality of the autotomographic image. Let us consider examination of the third ventricle, the aqueduct, and the fourth ventricle. Of these median structures, the fourth ventricle is the most posterior; therefore for its best visualization the head should be inclined slightly forward. For the aqueduct, and even more for the third ventricle, the head should be slightly extended so that the rotation axis can move forward.
2. The focus-film distance must be as long as possible.
3. Bilateral rotation gives better results than unilateral.
4. The rotation angle should not be wider than $\pm 5°$.

Conventional Tomography

There are four factors to be considered:

1. choice of apparatus
2. type of cancellation
3. thickness of layer
4. choice of layers to be tomographed according to their depth and the position of the head

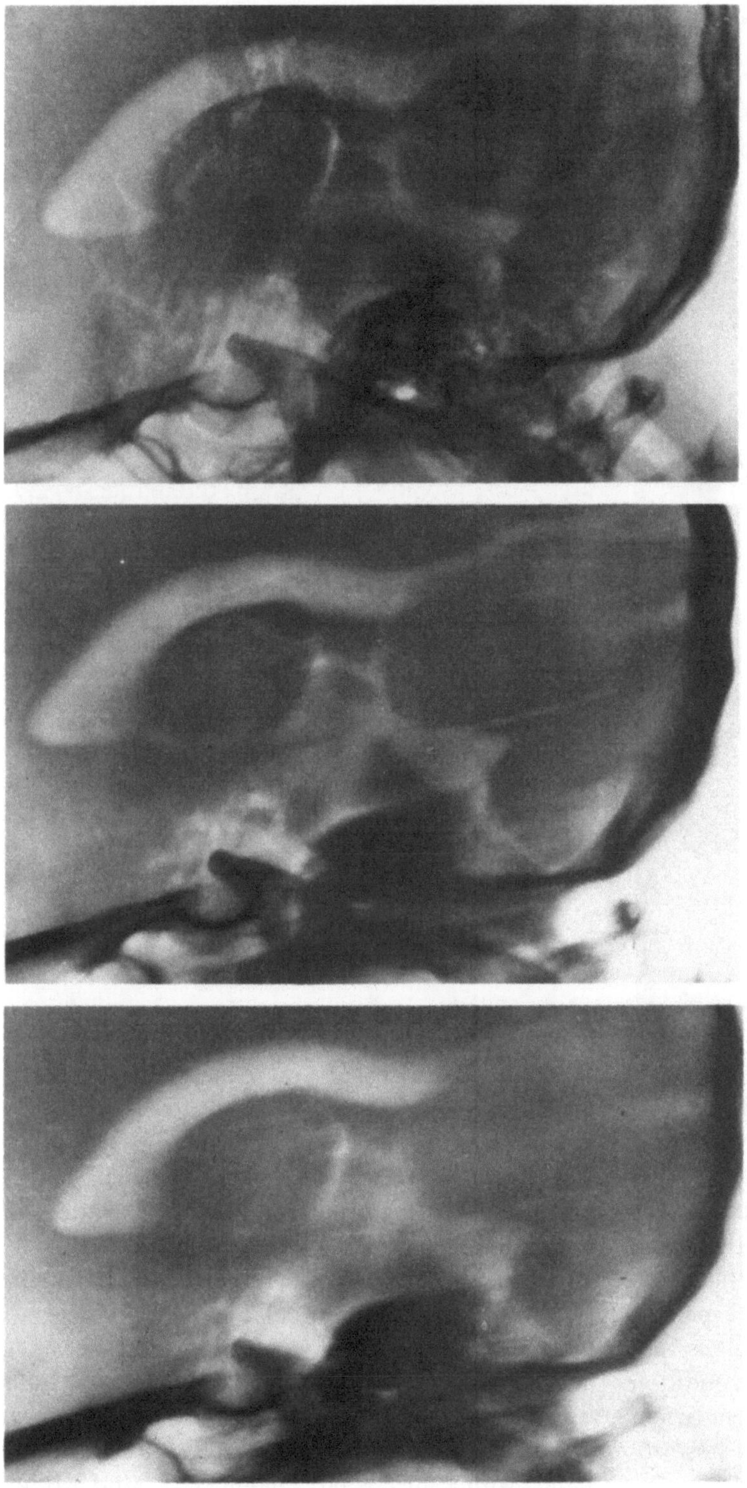

a b c

Fig. 1.19a–c. *Negative Encephalography*. a) Standard radiograph. b, c) Autotomography, in which the midline structures are better visualized, especially in (b), where the focal plane passes almost exactly through the midline. In (c) the rotation of the head has been imperfect and the focal plane is somewhat lateral; consequently certain structures, such as the foramen of Magendie and the posterior portion of the third ventricle are less clearly visualized than in (b)

Equipment

The fundamental requirement of a tomograph for encephalography is the ability to make tomograms in lateral and postero-anterior projection with the patient in the sitting position. With conventional tomographs this is possible only by means of some technical arrangements that are inconvenient for the patient, because he must be moved on passing

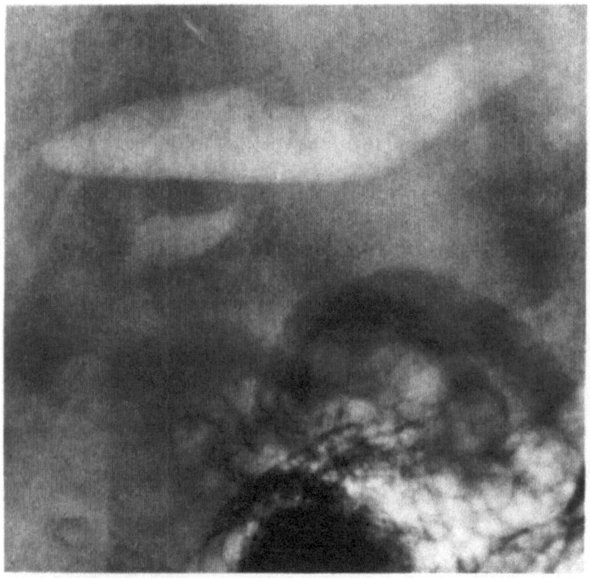

a

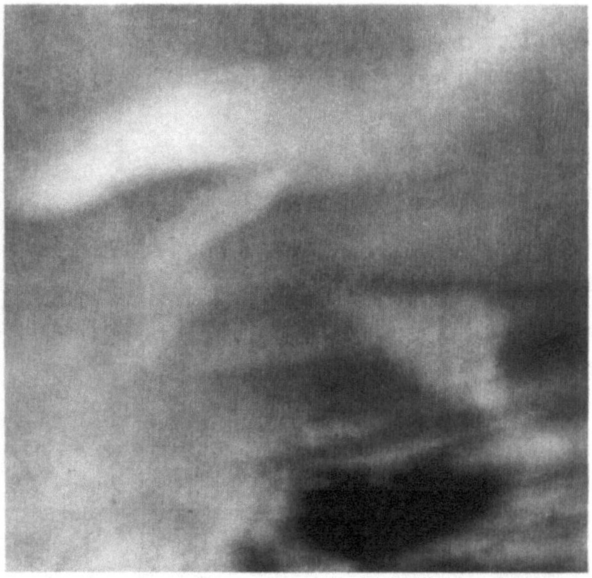

b

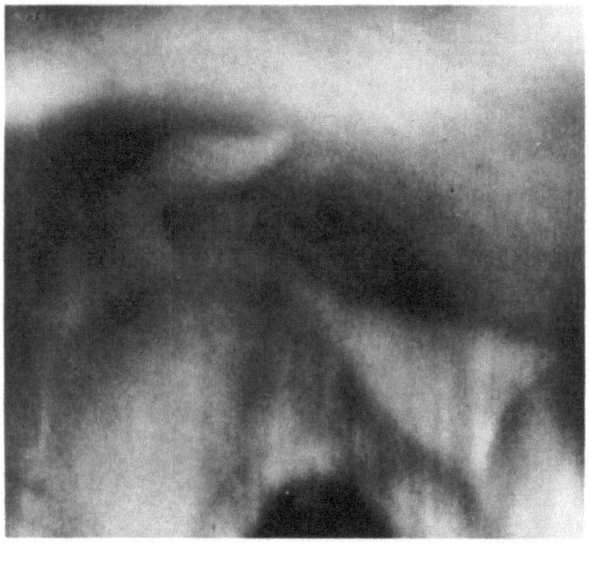

c

Fig. 1.20a–c. *Negative Encephalography*. a) Standard. b) Autotomography. c) Tomography with Mimer. The third ventricle and the aqueduct are easily visible also in (a), though perhaps less clearly. The fourth ventricle is more easily visible in tomography. In practice, there is no difference between the autotomography (b) and the midline tomography with the Mimer (c)

from one projection to the other. Di Chiro's atlas [116] shows some excellent tomograms that were obtained with the Siemens planigraph; however, Fig. 5 of that book, illustrating how the patient is positioned, clearly indicates the difficulties that would be encountered if patients in poor condition were examined with this apparatus. It is sufficient to mention the difficulties of centering in posteroanterior projection, especially with the patient under general anesthesia.

Additional tomographic devices have been suggested for the Lysholm craniograph, both the original model of Elema Schönander and others derived from it. However, they are not always simple to use and the results are usually not of high quality. It is pointless to describe these at the present time, when first-class craniotomographs exist, such as those often mentioned in this chapter.

A tomographic device can be attached to the Mimer I, allowing tomograms with the patient in the sitting, supine, and prone positions. With the patient supine or prone, tomography can be obtained by a linear or circular movement, whereas when he is sitting only linear movement is possible. The images are good; however, there is one serious drawback: it is impossible to pass quickly from TV monitoring to the tomography. On the other hand, with Princeps 60, Diagnost N, and Mimer III this problem is solved, though these apparatuses allow only a movement of linear cancellation. In the Mimer III, under special technical conditions, it should even be possible to see the tomographic image during fluoroscopy.

Type of Cancellation

Which is the best tomographic technique in encephalography? This question may be answered by comparing a series of different elements: theoretical factors, difficulty of technical realization, and bulk. The most modern craniographs adopt the system of linear cancellation, but this may well change in the future. In fact, from the technical viewpoint, linear cancellation is perhaps the least suitable. In 1957 STIEVE [438] by his experiments on dummies proved that, at the same angle of pendulation, linear movement gives tomograms of poorer quality than those obtained by multidirectional movements. In 1935 GROSSMANN [189] stated that linear movement was superior, provided that the angle of pendulation was double than that of other movements. However, in encephalography the necessity of radiographing rather thick layers forces one to adopt a narrow angle of pendulation, which creates disturbing shadows due to the shading of images above and below the ventricular or cisternal structure that is the object of the study. The most complex multidirectional movement, but also the one allowing the most precise tomograms almost without disturbing shadows, is the hypocycloidal movement, that is, the one obtained with the Polytome, designed by SANS and PORCHER [396] in 1949. However, the size and bulk of this device is such that the present model, at any rate, cannot be included in craniographs. If the Polytome is used, it is necessary to bring the patient to it after the examination has been begun on another apparatus. This procedure was followed by METZGER *et al.* [302], to study the chiasmatic cistern, for which they consider the Polytome almost indispensable. These authors, however, are aware of the drawbacks of this procedure, chiefly its longer duration. We cannot evaluate to what degree, in certain cases, the use of hypocycloidal cancellation is indispensable, for we have no direct experience with it; incontestably, the images obtained with the Polytome represent the highest level of tomographic quality so far attained. This seems to be the opinion of AMUNDSEN [13] and AMUNDSEN *et al.* [14], who have suggested a special armchair to facilitate the use of the Polytome in encephalography.

In theory, better images than those obtained with linear movement could also be obtained with circular tomography; in fact, though disturbing shadows are considerably reduced, the ventricular images are deformed (Fig. 1.21).

In 1970 EDHOLM and QUIDING [136] examined the different methods used to eliminate shadows in linear tomography; they described a system of TV circuits and filters admitting high-frequency beams while retaining soft ones. This theoretical work is not applicable to encephalography, but it could be a cue for the future. For the moment, linear tomography is the technique most easily applicable to craniographs and by far the most often used. A problem with linear tomography is the choice of direction—horizontal or vertical—of the cancellation movement. BORIES *et al.* [50] prefer horizontal movement for tomography in lateral projection and vertical movement for tomography in frontal projection. According to RUGGIERO, vertical movement is also to be preferred for tomography in lateral projection, as this seems to reduce the disturbing shadows of the petrous bones, especially as they encroach upon the posterior part of the fourth ventricle. In any case, the differences are not great, as Fig. 1.22 shows.

Layer Thickness

The choice of layer thickness presupposes some knowledge of the theoretical aspects of tomography. The present work does not call for a detailed discussion, but we deem it useful to mention and summarize them as simply and clearly as possible. For this purpose we have recorded a conversation between authors A and B.

A. We have been hearing for some time about zonography in encephalography. Is it to be preferred to tomography? And if so, in which cases? BORIES *et al.* [50, 51], for example, seem to be quite certain: tomography in frontal projection, zonography in lateral projection. WESTRA [477], who has written an excellent monograph on zonography, thinks that zonography is always better when an air-containing structure is to be examined, thanks to the larger "free zone" that WESTRA defines as "an area devoid of image-producing particles, situated between the object to be seen and the nearest parts which produce disturbing shadows."

B. The free zone leads on to the problem of the shading of the tomographic image, and hence to the problem of the type of movement of the tube.

A. This is correct. On the other hand, it is precisely because of the infrequent use of multidirectional movements in cranial tomography that zonography has not been used very much up to now, for zonography is obviously made easier by the multidirectional, or rather hypocycloidal, movement of the tube. But perhaps it is better to start from the beginning. As is often the case in the field of radiographic technique, and of tomography in particular, it is again the name of ZIEDSES DES PLANTES that we find among the early researchers. His first work dates back to 1931 [483] and deals with planigraphy with "light shading." Other authors are mentioned in WESTRA's monograph [477], and we report their works in our bibliography [90, 262, 349, 444, 476, 478]. Let us be clear that zonography, planigraphy with light shading, and tomography with a narrow angle of exposure are synonyms. From the theoretical and geometric viewpoints, there is no qualitative difference. In tomography the larger angle of exposure (30° and more) enhances the shading of the layers above and below the focal plane to the extent that they appear almost completely cancelled; in zonography the narrower angle of exposure reduces the shading of the layers above and below the focal plane along fairly large thicknesses; this means we have the tomography of a zone rather than of a plane. According to SUTHERLAND [443], with an angle of exposure between 5° and 10° this thickness ranges between 2 and 6 cm, whereas in tomography, using angles of exposure of 30°, we obtain sections of 1.3–1.5 mm thickness. But, I repeat, the differences are quantitative and not qualitative.

B. However, WESTRA [477] maintains that the image is formed in a different way...

A. For me there is no doubt: zonography is to be preferred in pneumoencephalography as it allows the central beam to hit tangentially a gaseous layer having sufficient thickness to give a well-contrasted image (Figs. 1.35 through 1.38). But, above all, the examination is quicker, as it involves fewer exposures for a complete exploration. In this connection let us recall that, to speed up the examination, it may also be useful to make tomographs with multifilm cassettes. Anyway, we are far from reaching conclusions about tomographic technique. There is no paper that compares zonographs and tomographs obtained with the same parameters—type of tube motion, projection, etc. Our experience, too, is very limited.

B. It would be useful to explain why multidirectional movement is to be preferred in zonography even more than in tomography.

A. I will try to express myself in simple words. The narrower the angle of exposure, the more necessary it is to cancel the "out-of-zone" parts that are capable of casting disturbing shadows; obviously, this is more effectively obtained by multidirectional movement. For the same reason, in all types of tomography, with both large and narrow angles of exposure, hard rays are to be preferred because they reduce the radiographic contrast of the structures that produce disturbing shadows. Moreover, it is obvious that, when short-wavelength beams prevail, the risk of an uneven absorption along the different planes of the "zone" is reduced. As regards projection, I would like to stress one point; from the theoretical viewpoint, tomography should be done by orienting the central ray in the direction of the main axis of the desired structure (this does not mean axial projection). However, for many parts of the ventricular system and subarachnoid space, this approach entails the great problem of the superimposition of bony structures. Let us consider, for example, the fourth ventricle: to study its floor, tomography with the incidence of the central beam perpendicular to it while passing through the shadow of the fastigium, would be ideal. However, the petrous bones would then be superimposed, giving rise to an enormous quantity of disturbing images. A compromise is perhaps represented by the method suggested by SUTHERLAND [443] for zonography, which is to place the film obliquely in the cassette holder. It seems that this is also the opinion of FREDZELL *et al.* [153] as regards the zonographic study of the optic chiasm.

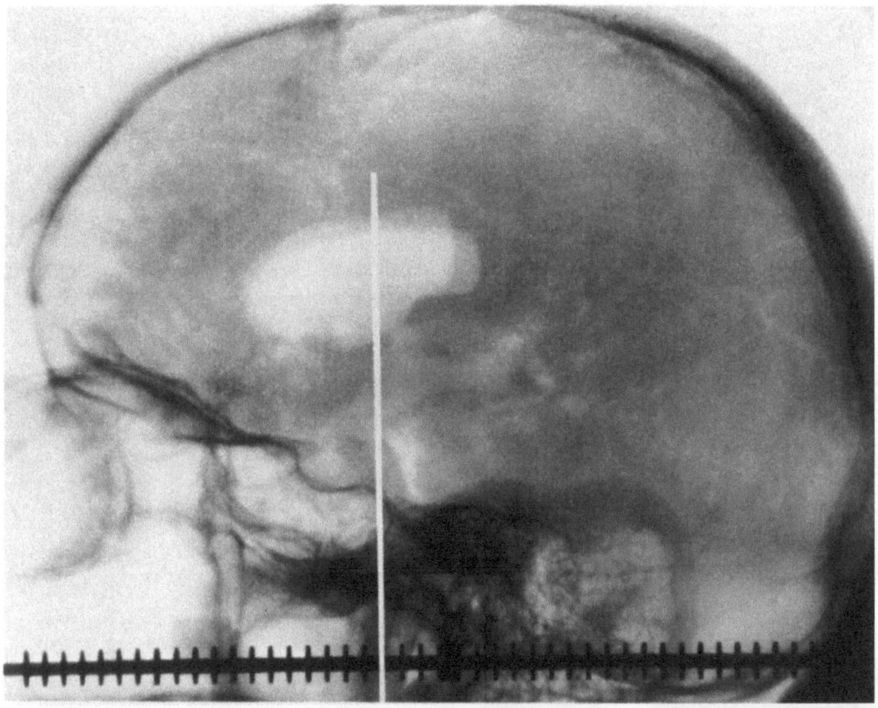
a

Fig. 1.21a–c. *Linear (b) and Circular (c) Tomograms.* The focal plane passes through a plane cutting the third small bar before the large central bar visible on the lateral radiograph A (↑). The third ventricle and septum pellucidum are better visualized on circular tomograms (c); however, the lateral ventricles appear slightly distorted

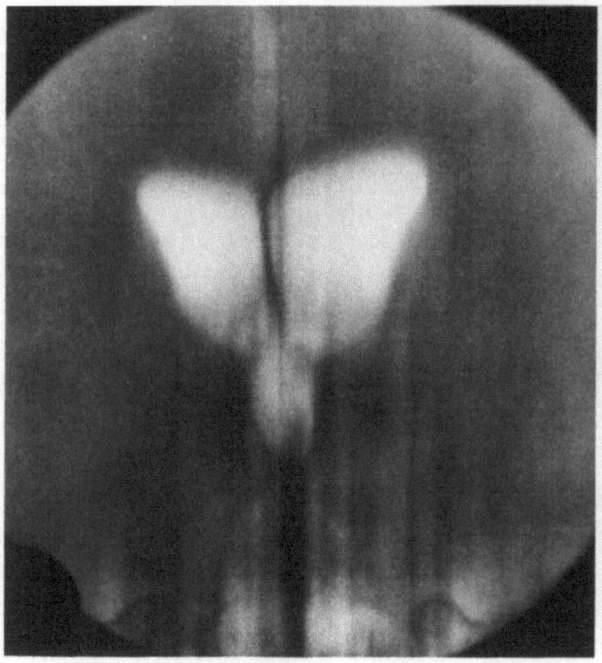
b

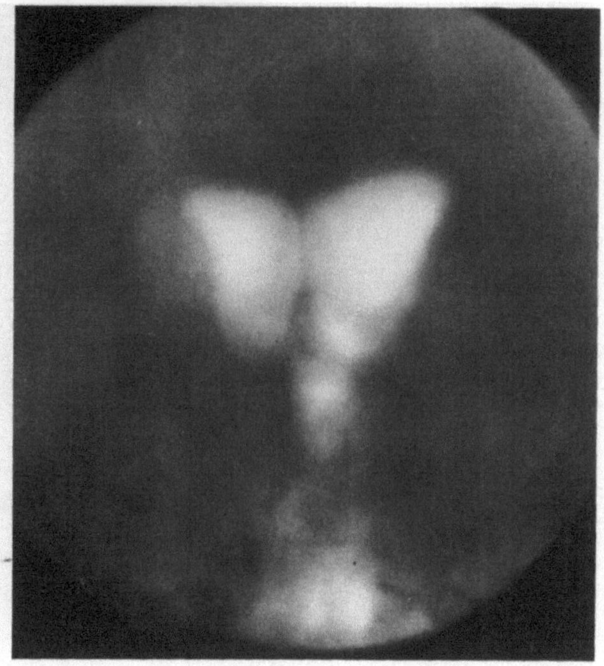
c

B. However, hypocycloidal movement would tone these shadows down considerably.

A. Certainly. I am very much of the opinion of Metzger [302], and Amundsen *et al.* [14]: the future seems likely to bring new developments in several directions.

Choice of the Cutting Plane

An important problem is the relationship between the desired structures and orthogonal planes, i.e. the position of the head with respect to the central beam. This is most important for the study of the posterior fossa where, to avoid the disturbing shad-

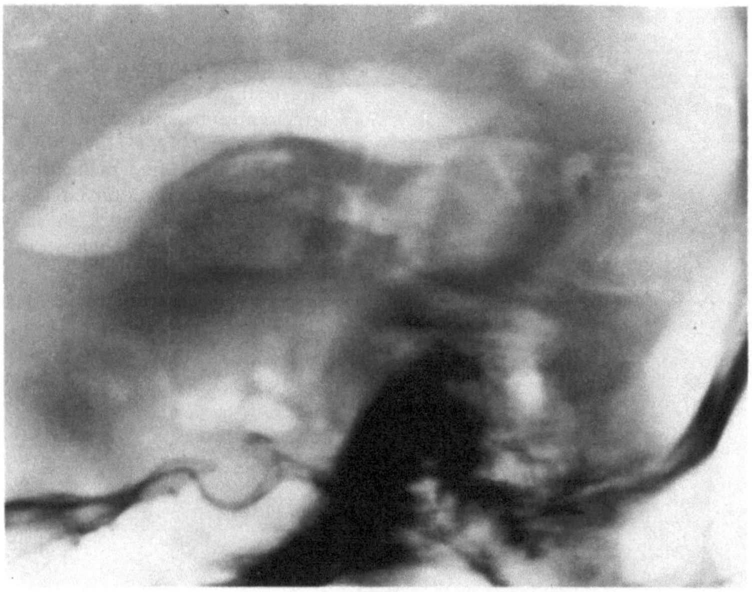

a

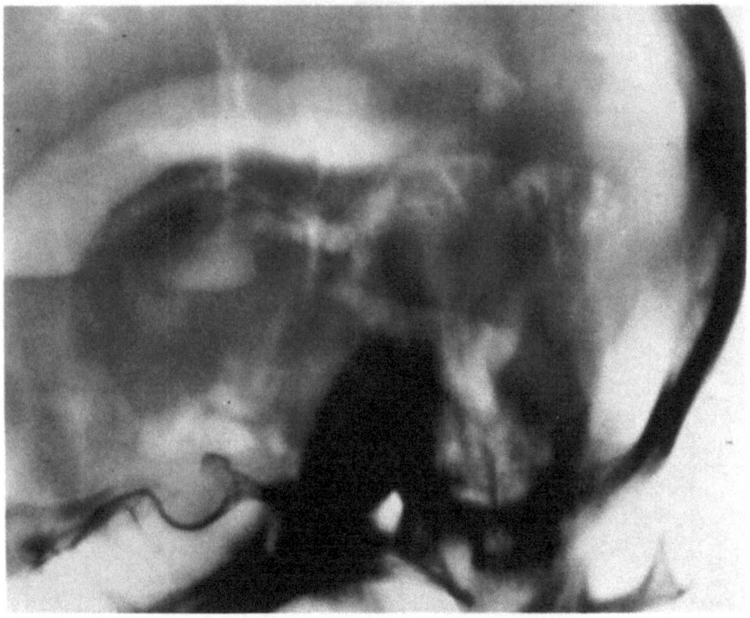

b

Fig. 1.22a, b. *Midline Zonography Obtained by Horizontal (a) and Vertical (b) Cancellation.* Layer thickness 2, 5–3 mm. The image in (b) is sharper, especially at the level of the floor of the fourth ventricle because of the absence of the disturbing horizontal shadows, which instead appear in (a). Moreover, in (b) the fastigium can be dissociated from the superimposed postero-superior recesses more easily than in (a), where the posterior part of the cistern of the corpus callosum is less clear

ows due to the facial bones, it is necessary to resort to half-axial projections.

For the study of the brain stem, for example, Bories *et al.* [50, 51] advise flexing the head in such a way that the orbito-meatal line forms an angle of 30–35° (33° on average) with the horizontal plane; this angle must be increased to 55° for the study of the cerebellum. To calculate the flexion, the authors use a special goniometer (Fig. 1.23).

According to Greitz [181], for the accurate study of the anatomy of the fourth ventricle two conditions must be fulfilled:

1. The ventricle should be completely filled with air: this can usually be attained when the head is markedly flexed and the top of the fourth ventricle lies at the level of the aqueduct.
2. The central beam must be aimed exactly at the desired structure.

Most authors (and we used to be among them) calculate the cutting plane starting from the external auditory meatus. This method is open to various objections. First of all, it is not precise: the external auditory meatus is not a good point of reference as its aspect depends on the ear shape, which is

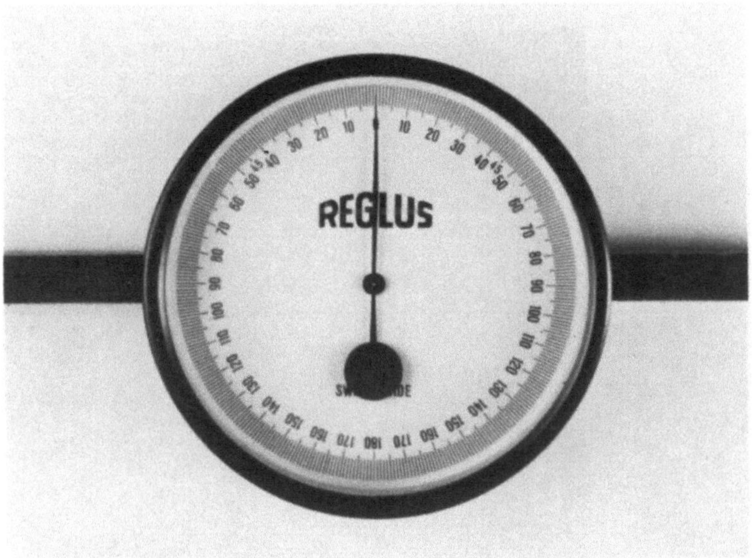

Fig. 1.23. *Goniometer Used by* BORIES *and Collaborators for Chosing the Right Angle of Inclination of the Head for Tomography in Encephalography*

variable; on the other hand, it is easy to recognize this aspect on radiographs. Furthermore, it does not take into account the normal variations of cerebral and cranial structures, and of their relationships, which cannot be known beforehand. Therefore, it is always necessary in practice to perform numerous tomograms with consequent protraction of the examination. These difficulties increase considerably in pathological cases, where one structure—for instance the fourth ventricle—may well be displaced by several centimeters in respect to its normal location. RUGGIERO started some time ago to test a very simple method based on the principle of choosing the cutting plane according to a foreign structure that can be visualized clearly. He uses a metal rod similar to the one described in a previous paper to demonstrate the usefulness in cerebral angiography of antero-posterior projections with different degrees of inclination of the central beam. This bar is a straight line crossed by a number of short bars, spaced at 3-mm intervals, with a larger bar marking the midpoint. For frontal tomography, the desired cutting plane is chosen so as to pass through one of the bars visible on the radiograph in lateral projection, and vice versa. According to the apparatus in use, the metal rod will be placed on the radiographic cassette, on the grid, or on the head-rest. To choose the cutting plane in frontal tomography, it is then sufficient to calculate on radiographs in lateral projection which bar is crossed by the plane perpendicular to the metal rod that coincides with the desired structure (Fig. 1.24).

For lateral tomograms an analogous procedure will obviously be followed, calculating the cutting plane on frontal images (Fig. 1.25).

Finally, let us say that absolute precision in the choice of the cutting plane is generally not essential (Fig. 1.26).

Uses of Tomography

Knowledge of the anatomy of the ventricular system and subarachnoid space has become more "refined" with the advent of tomography. It is mainly a recent advance: before the advent of modern apparatus, the use of tomography was generally limited to midline structures—the third ventricle, the aqueduct, and the fourth ventricle—but recently it has been extended to the study of lateral ventricles (chiefly the temporal horns) and the subarachnoid space. Tomographic examination is currently made not only in the lateral, but also in the frontal projection. A detailed description of the normal and pathologic tomographic pictures of the cerebrospinal fluid pathways goes beyond the limits of this work, which deals only with technique. It is sufficient to recall that tomography is particularly useful to emphasize structures which are poorly visualized on standard radiographs, owing to their unusually small volume (Fig. 1.27), or whose image is disturbed in some way by the superimposition of bone

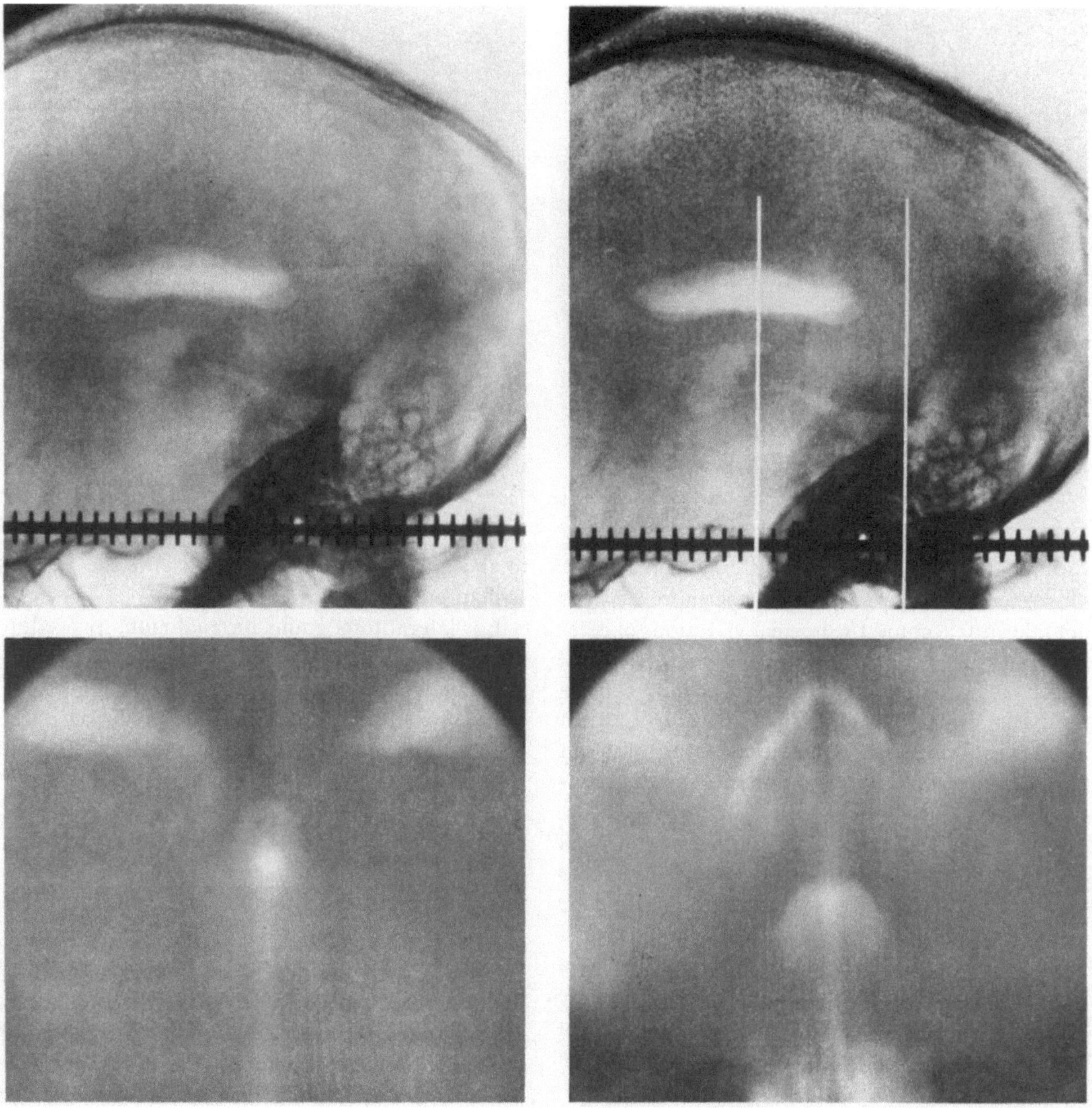

a b c d

Fig. 1.24a–d. *Choice of Focal Plane.* a) Represents a lateral view in sitting position visualizing the posterior part of the third ventricle, the aqueduct, and the fourth ventricle. The metallic rod is easily visible in (a). In (b) are traced the perpendiculars passing, respectively, two bars before and six bars behind the large central bar. Therefore tomograms pass exactly through the upper portion of the aqueduct (c) and the fourth ventricle at the level of the upper medullary velum (d)

or of air contained in other parts of the ventricular system or subarachnoid space. This is the case, for example, with mastoid cells for the fourth ventricle (Fig. 1.28); petrous bones for the cerebello-pontine angle cisterns (Fig. 1.29); the lower border of lateral ventricles for the cisterns venae magnae Galeni and of the superior vermis; the anterior border of the foramen magnum and the odontoid process for the vallecula and the bulbar cistern (Fig. 1.30); the Sylvian fissure for the anterior part of the third ventricle (Fig. 1.31); and the interpeduncular cistern for the anterior part of the temporal horns (Fig. 1.32). But, apart from these superimpositions, tomography may be useful because it reveals or better emphasizes anatomic details (Figs. 1.33 and 1.34). This is best exemplified by the recesses of the fourth

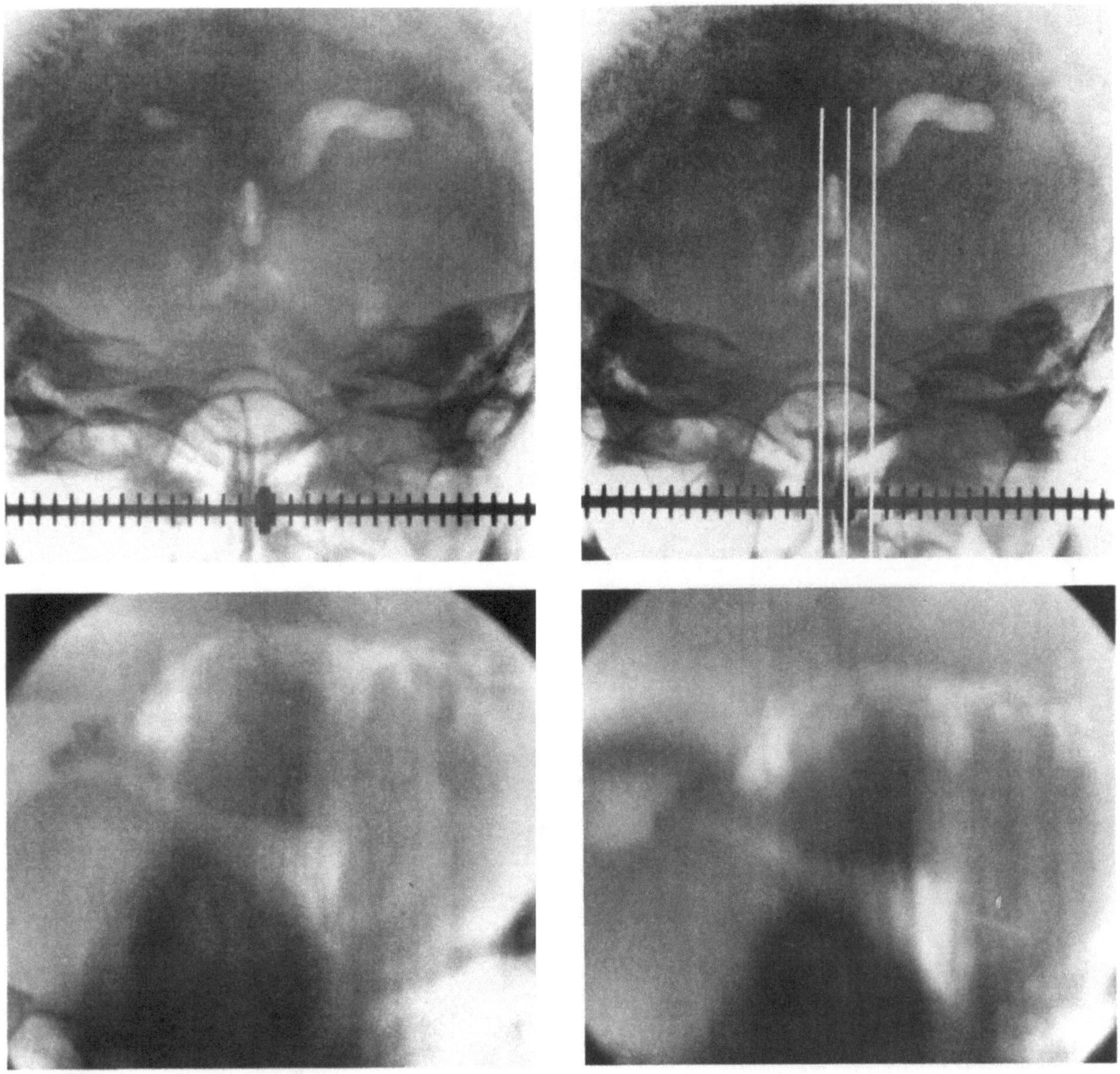

a b c d

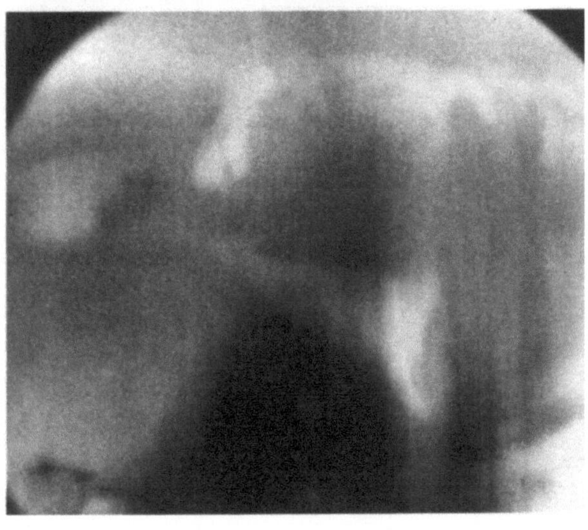

e

Fig. 1.25a–e. *Choice of Focal Plane.* a) Represents the postero-anterior view of the structures described in Fig. 1.24. The metallic rod is easily visible and in (b) are traced the perpendiculars passing, respectively, by the central bar and the bars lying at the close left and right of it; they indicate the focal planes of tomograms illustrated in (c, d) and (e) respectively

Fig. 1.26a–c. *Lateral Tomography with Horizontal Cancellation.* Layer thickness is 1.4 mm. In (a) the focal plane is on the midline, in (b) and (c) it is 0.5 cm to the left and the right of the midline, respectively. There is no considerable difference in the aspect of the fourth ventricle, the aqueduct, and the third ventricle in these three pictures. The subarachnoid space of the prevermis is slightly more clearly visible in (a)

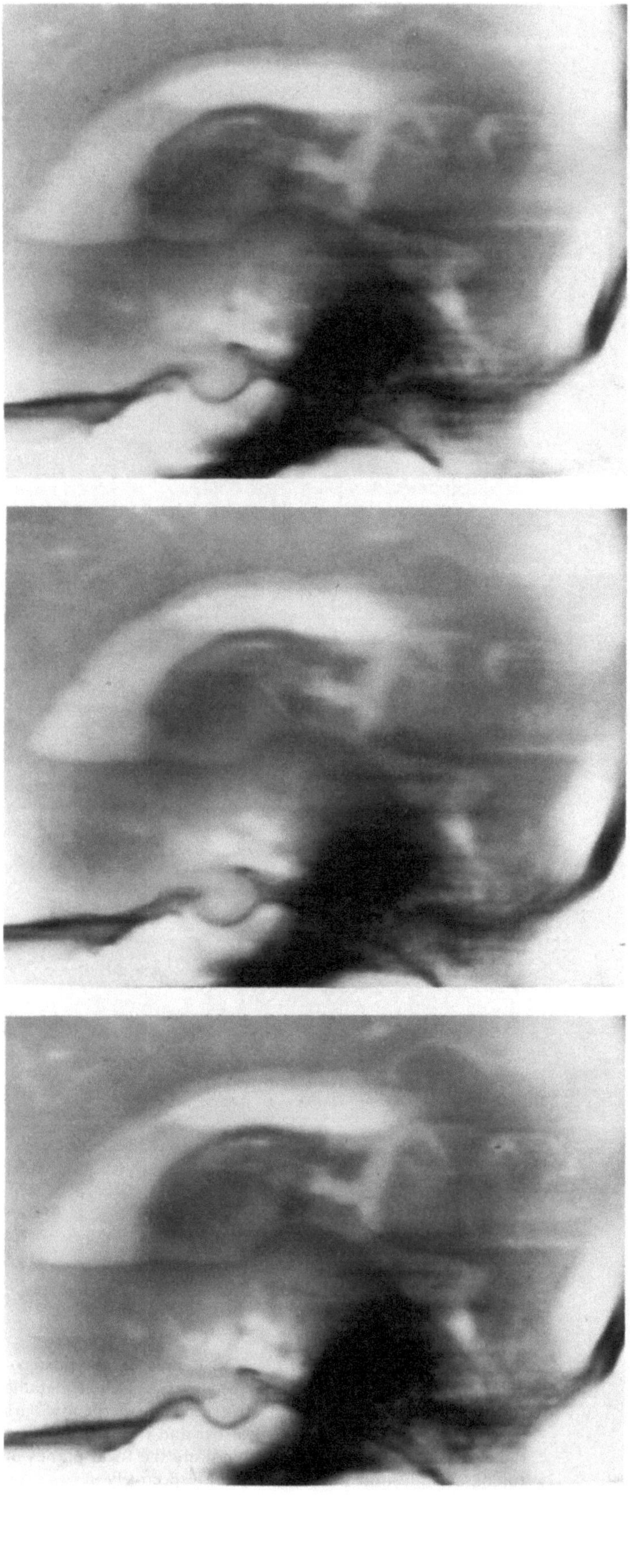

a

b

c

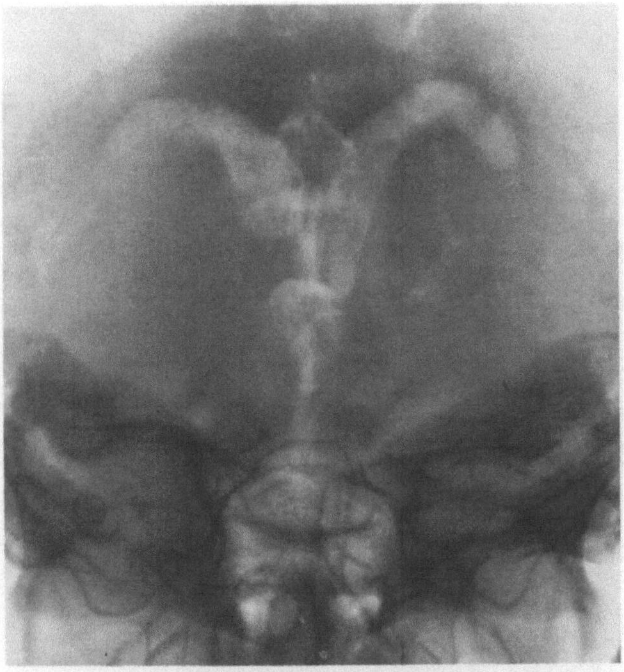

a

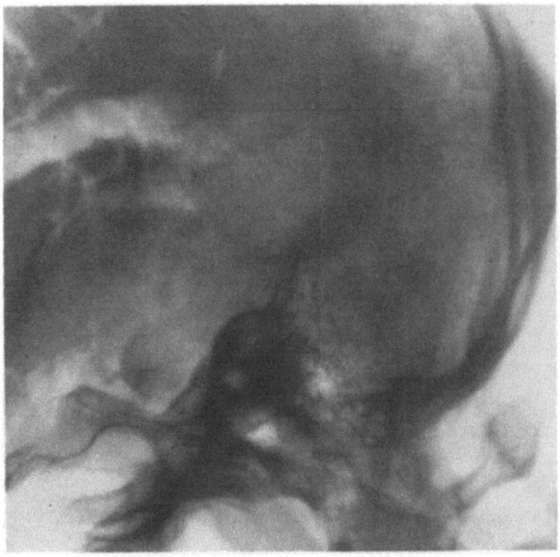

b

Fig. 1.27a–c. *Negative Encephalography. Tomography of the Midline Structures of the Posterior Fossa in Lateral Projection.*
On the standard lateral radiograph (b) the aqueduct and the fourth ventricle are poorly visible, probably because they are unusually small, as shown by (a). The following portions are rather clearly visible:
1. the inferior portion of the aqueduct;
2. the superior portion of the fourth ventricle;
3. the subarachnoid cervical space bordering the medulla;
4. the intracranial part of the cisterna magna;
5. the cisterna interpeduncularis;
6. the very thin cisterna pontis;
7. the cisterna venae magnae Galeni.

On the tomography of the midline (c) all these structures are likewise well visualized. The following portions are better demonstrated:
1. the posterior portion of the third ventricle;
2. the superior portion of the aqueduct;
3. the inferior portion of the fourth ventricle with the foramen of Magendie;
4. the extracranial portion of the cisterna magna;
5. the vallecula;
6. the posterior portion of the cisterna corporis callosi;
7. the sulci of the upper portion of the vermis cerebelli

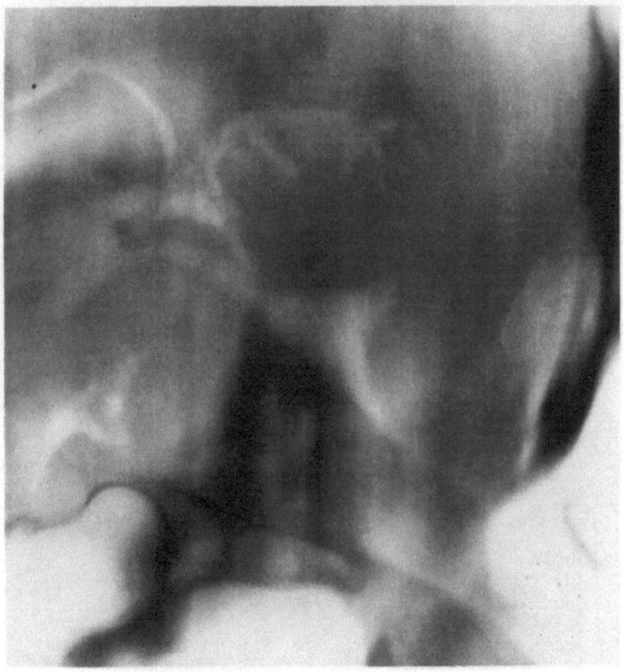

c

ventricle (Figs. 1.35 through 1.38), which we learned to recognize on the standard radiograph [94] precisely with tomography. Finally, there are cases, though rare, where the standard radiograph shows structures which are not seen in tomography, for example, the cisterna corporis callosi (Fig. 1.31), and cases where the standard image is "richer," as when it shows a filling defect in cisterns, and vessels that do not appear in tomography because of the small quantity of air crossed by the central ray.

But we think that, for the moment, this drawback has no practical implications as it may be eliminated by zonography or multiple tomograms taken at different levels.

Tomography undoubtedly improves the quantity and quality of anatomic information, but it rarely proves to be fundamental for diagnosis. In our experience this has occurred in very few cases, certainly

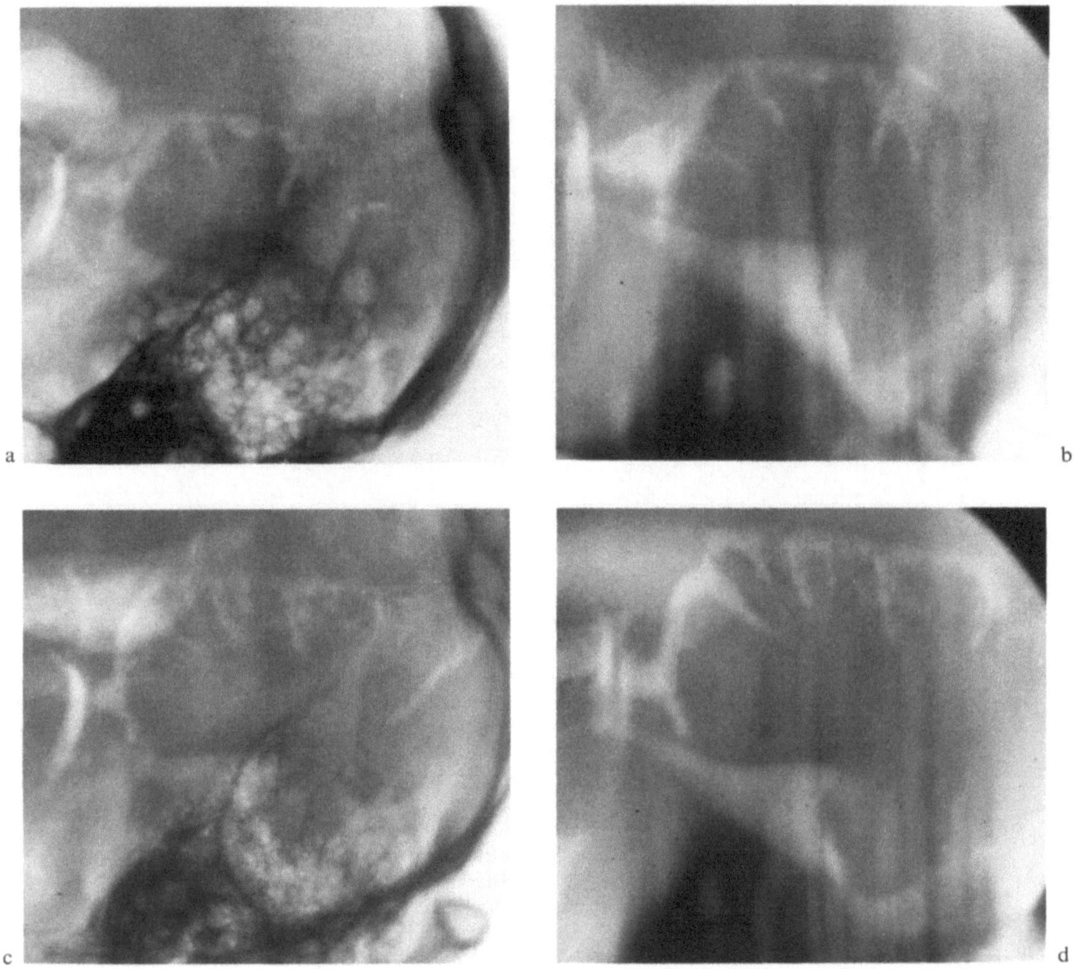

Fig. 1.28a–d. *Two Cases of Negative Encephalography*. On the standard radiographs (a, c) the fourth ventricle is partially concealed because of the superimposition of the mastoid cells. This structure is much better visualized on tomograms (b, d), as well as on the subarachnoid sulci dividing the superior vermian lobules

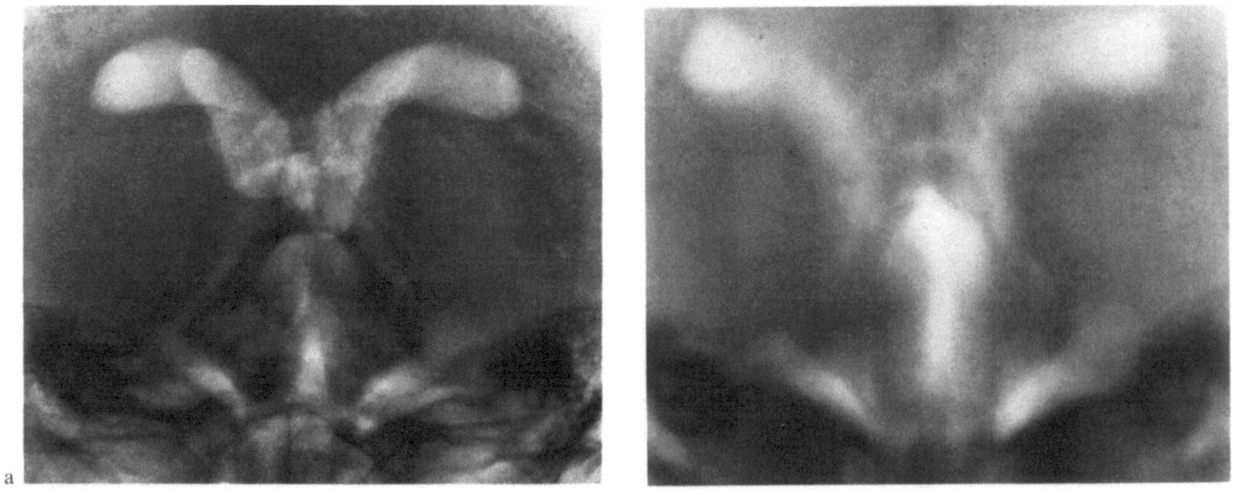

Fig. 1.29a, b. *Negative Encephalography*. Standard radiograph (a) and tomogram (b) are equivalent, but the contours of the cerebello pontine angle cisterns, especially the right one, are more easily recognized on the tomogram

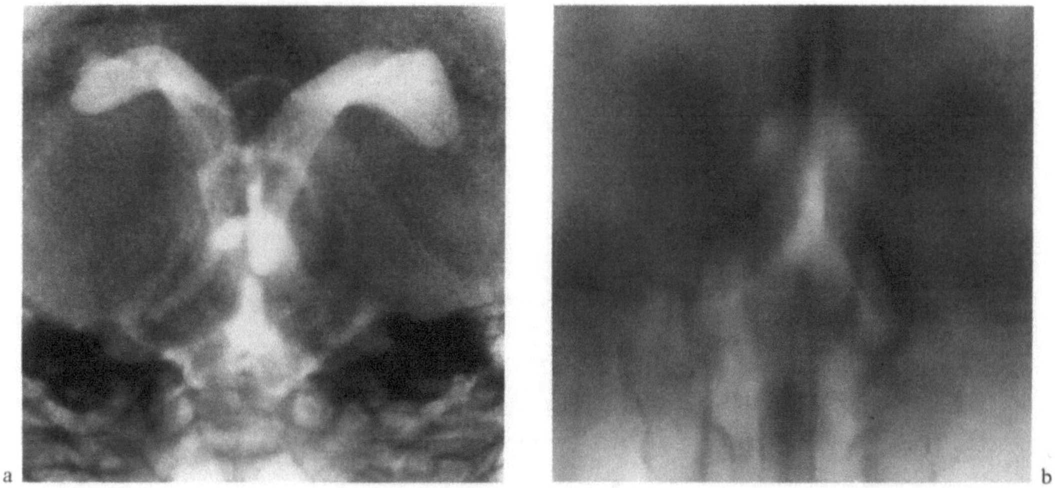

Fig. 1.30a, b. *Negative Encephalography*. The standard radiograph (a) is excellent, but the superimposition of the foramen magnum and the odontoid process disturbs the visualization of the vallecula and the medullary cistern. These structures are perfectly demonstrated with tomography (b), where the negative image of the bulb and the superior portion of the cervical cord is evident

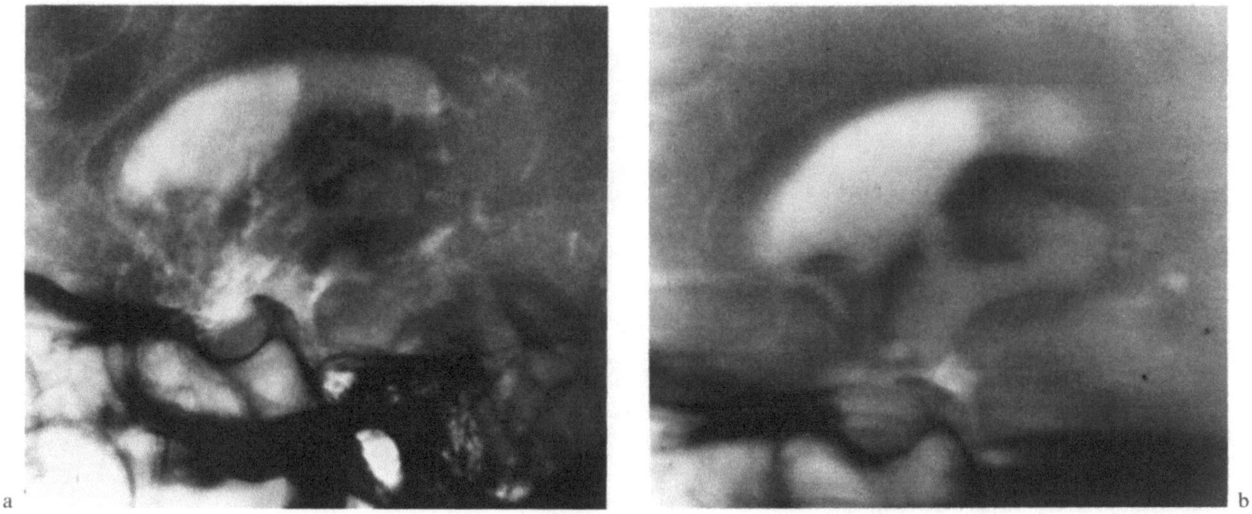

Fig. 1.31a, b. *Negative Encephalography*. The anterior portion of the third ventricle is better visualized on the tomogram (b) than on the standard radiograph (a), where it is concealed by the superimposition of the horizontal portion of the Sylvian fissure. The cistern of the corpus callosum, on the contrary, is better visualized on the standard radiograph

not more than five (Fig. 1.39 and 1.40). This may seem a low incidence in more than 5000 examinations, but beside these exceptional cases where tomography is indispensable to reach a diagnosis, there are many more cases where tomography offers greater security and more details on which to base a diagnosis (Figs. 1.41 through 1.50).

Conclusions

The distinctive features of an "ideal" tomography in pneumoencephalography are the following:

1. zonography, within certain limits
2. hard rays (high kilovoltage or enhanced filtration)
3. movement of multidirectional cancellation
4. central ray in the direction of the main axis of the structure to be examined, possibly without producing on radiographs disturbing shadows that lower the quality of diagnosis
5. choice of cutting plane by reference to a metal bar
6. a rational procedure, avoiding useless prolongation of the examination.

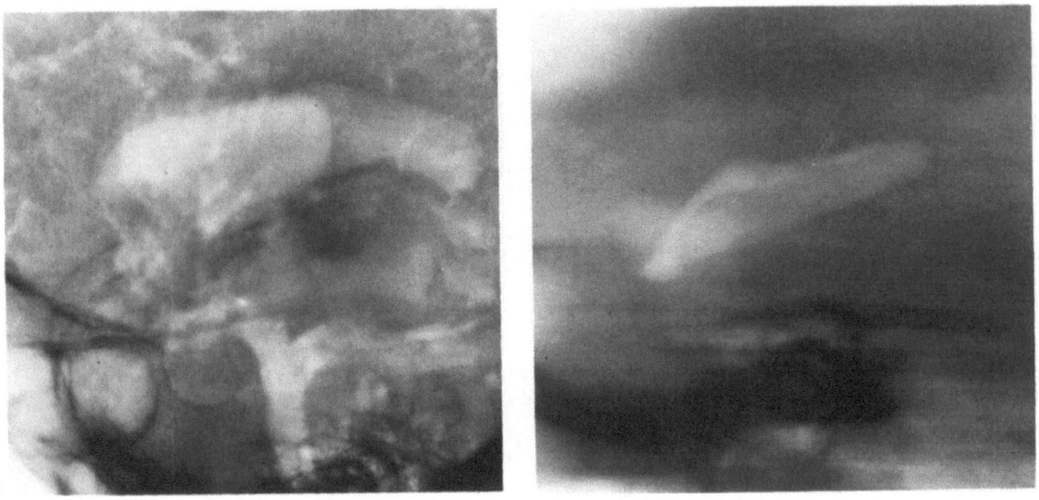

a b

Fig. 1.32a, b. *Negative Encephalography. Examination of the Temporal Horn.* On the standard radiograph (a) the anterior portion of the temporal horn is superimposed on the superior portion of the cisterna pontis and on the cisterna interpeduncularis, and its morphology is not clear; on the other hand, this is perfectly demonstrated on the tomogram (b), 3 cm from the midline

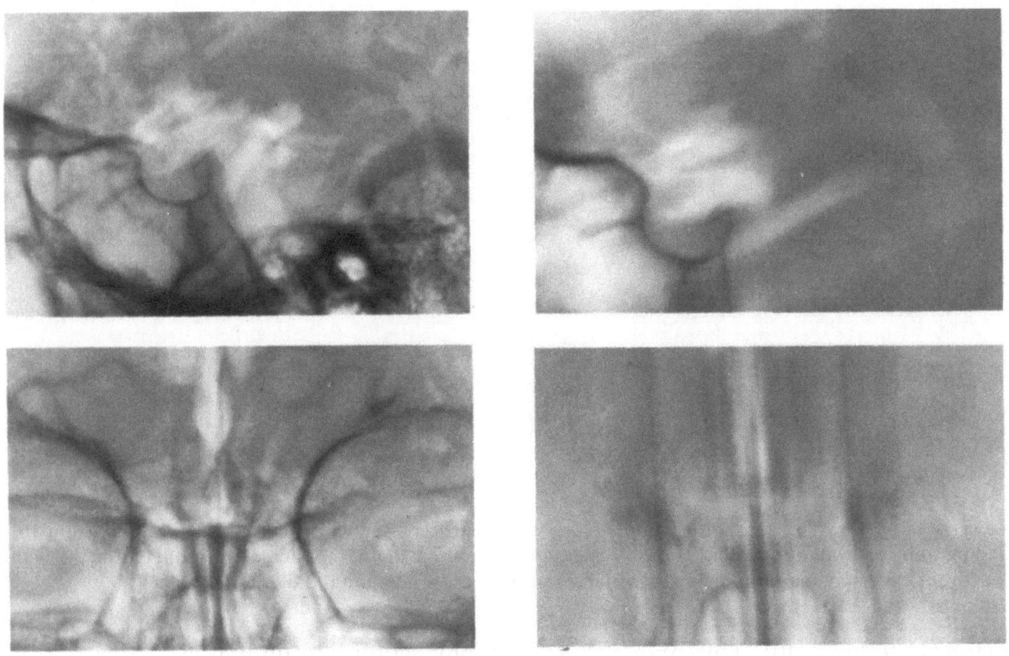

a b c d

Fig. 1.34a–d. *Negative Encephalography. Examination of the Chiasmatic Cistern.* In the lateral view, on the standard radiograph (a), the negative image of optic formations is hidden by the superimposition of the contrast in the cisterns of the Sylvian fissure; on the contrary, it is easily recognized on tomogram (b). In the antero-posterior view the chiasma is visible only on tomogram (d)

▷

Fig. 1.33a-f. *Negative Encephalography. Examination of the Cisterns of the Posterior Fossa and of the Brain Stem.* The great cistern, the cisterns of the cerebello-pontine angles, the pontine cistern, and the interpeduncular cistern are very well visualized on standard radiographs (a, c). In the postero-anterior view the negative image of the basilar artery and its terminal branches is better visualized on the tomogram (f). In the lateral view the basilar artery is better visualized on tomogram (b), whereas the origin of the posterior cerebral arteries is visible only on the standard radiograph (a). The cistern of Galen is better visualized with tomography, especially in the postero-anterior view, on which there are also visible the retro-pulvinaric cisterns. The superior vermian cistern is better visualized with the tomogram, both in lateral (b) and in postero-anterior (d) views. The anterior bulbar cistern is better demonstrated in the lateral view by tomogram (b), whereas in the postero-anterior view it is demonstrated only by tomogram (d)

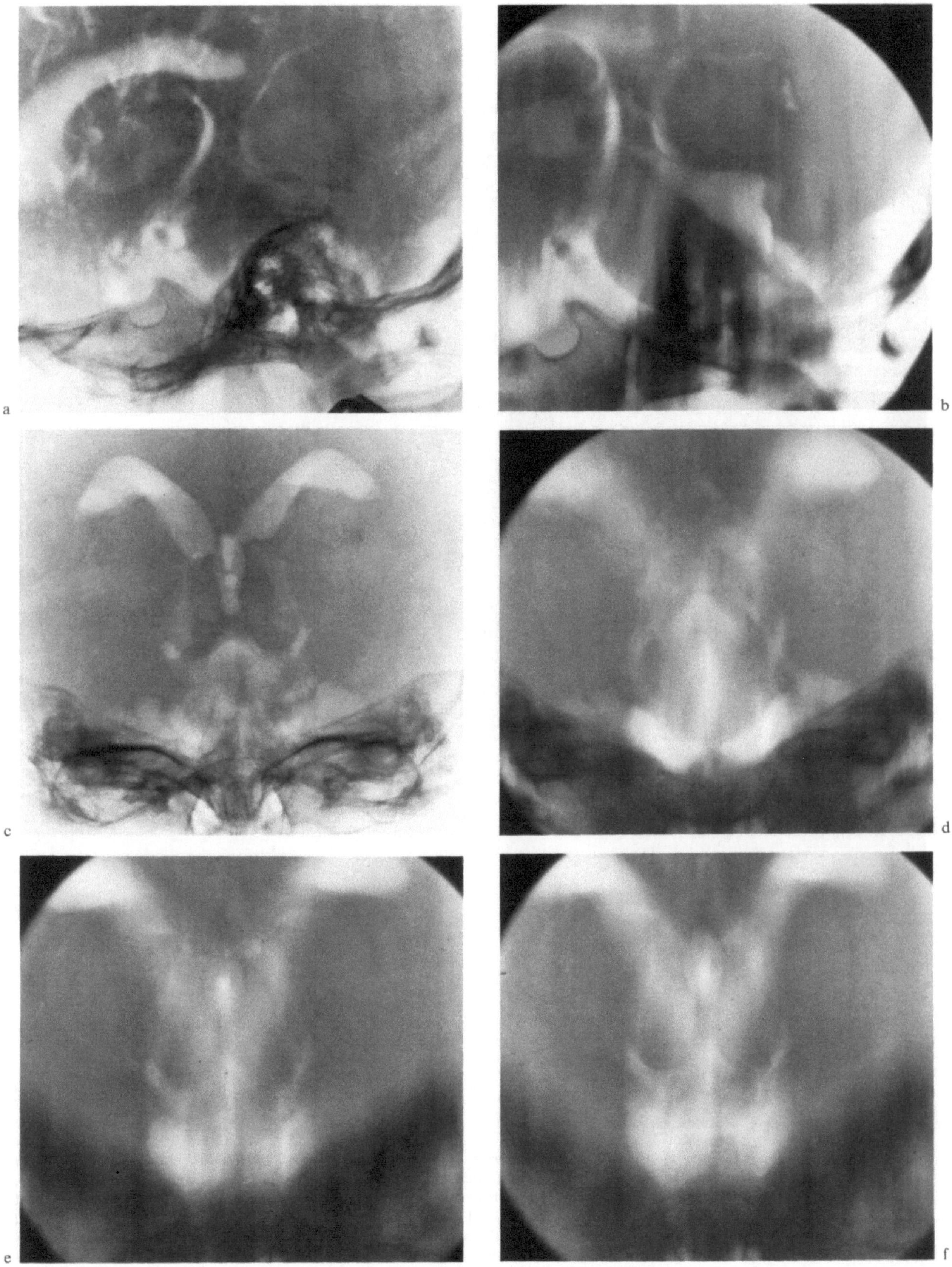
a
b
c
d
e
f

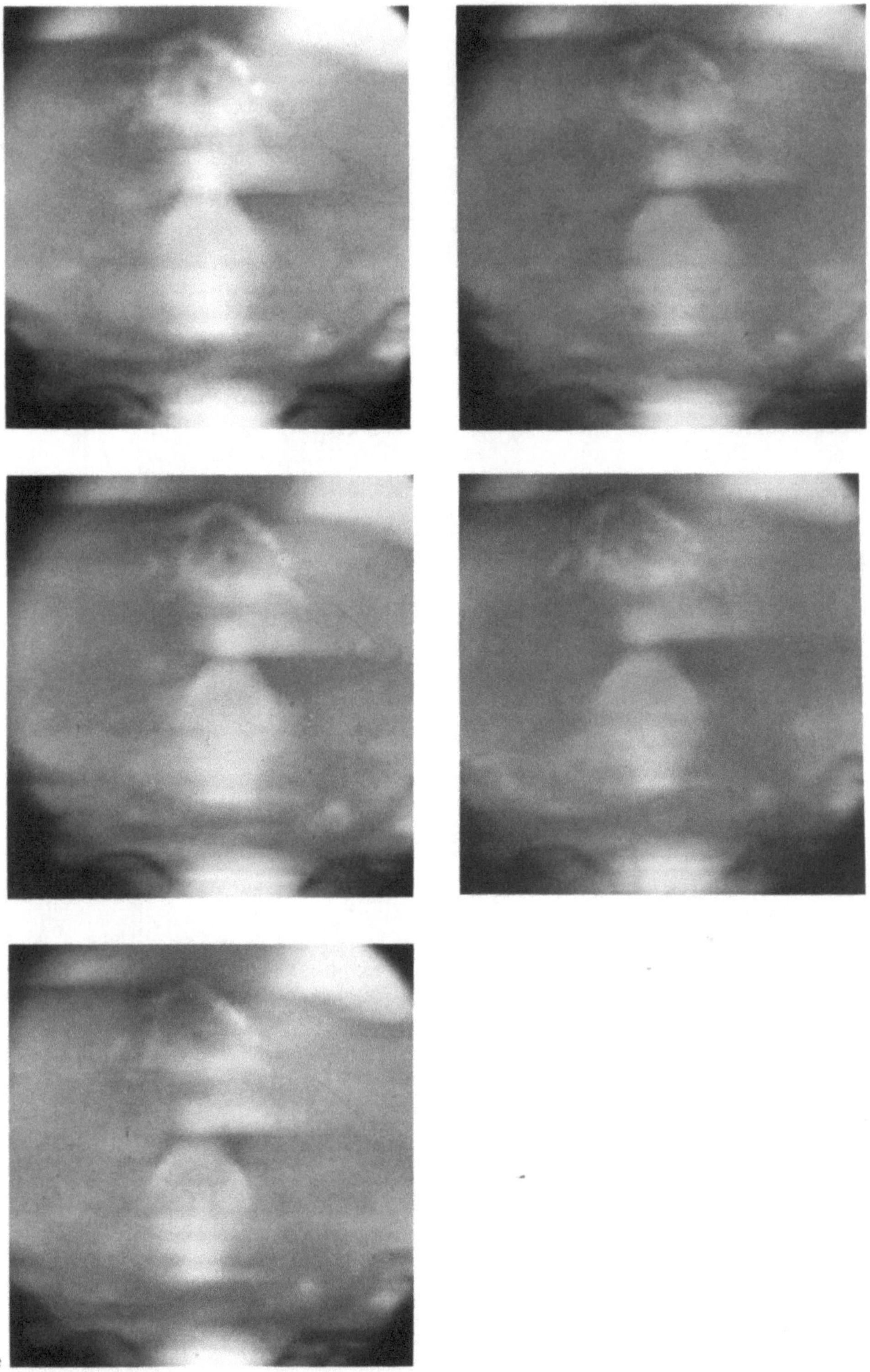

a b c d e

Figs. 1.35a–e and 1.36a–e. *Tomography in the Postero-Anterior Projection of the Fourth Ventricle with Horizontal (Fig. 1.35) and Vertical (Fig. 1.36) Movement of Cancellation.* In (a) the focal plane passes through the external auditory meatus. In (b), (c), (d), and (e) the focal plane passes 2, 4, 6, and 8 mm, respectively, behind the external auditory meatus. The images of Fig. 1.36 seem to be slightly sharper than those of Fig. 1.35. However, some structures, for example, the upper portion of the roof of the fourth ventricle with the indirect image of the superior medullary velum, appear more evident in the images of Fig. 1.35, whereas the postero-superior recesses of the fourth ventricle seem to be better demonstrated in Fig. 1.36

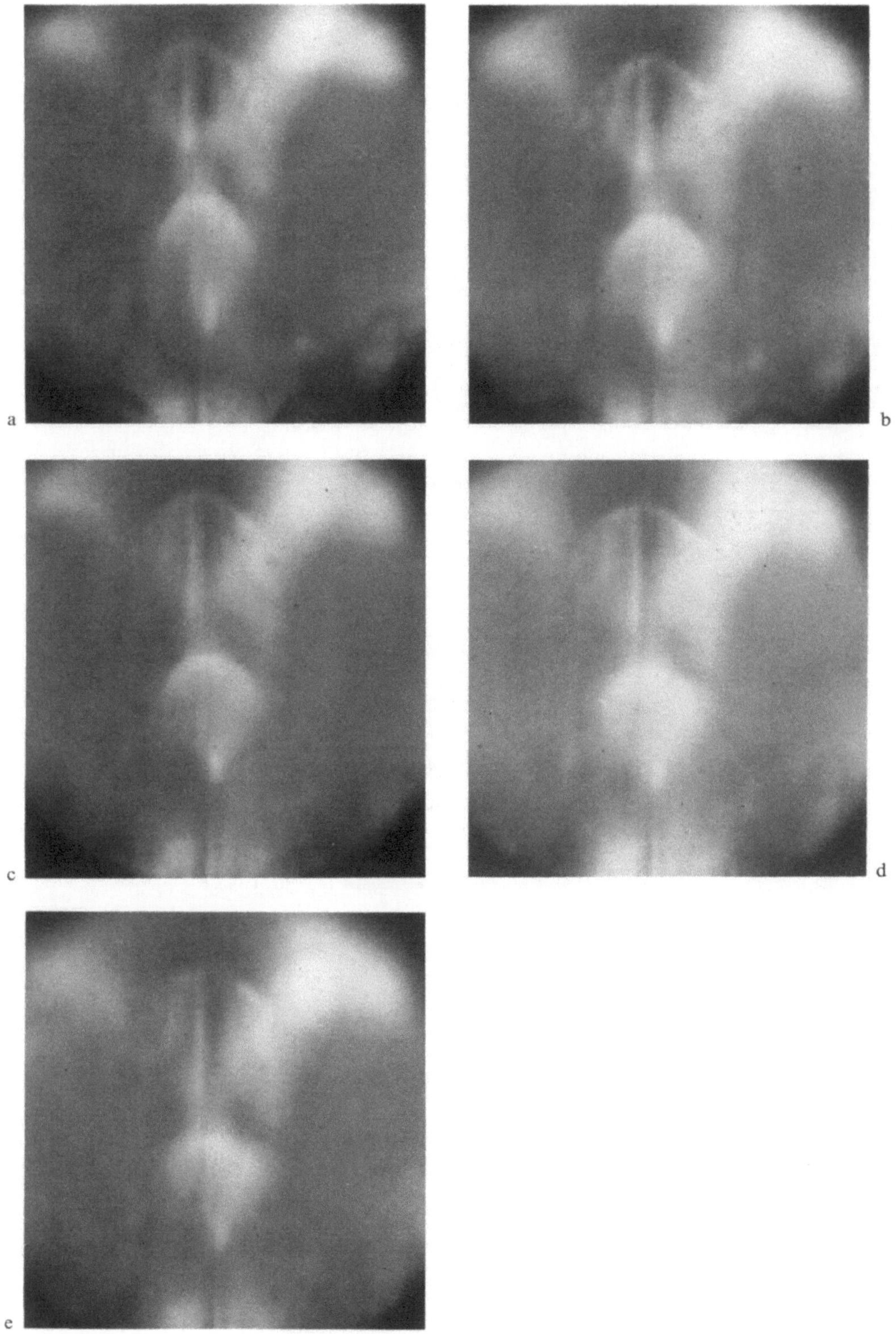

Fig. 1.36

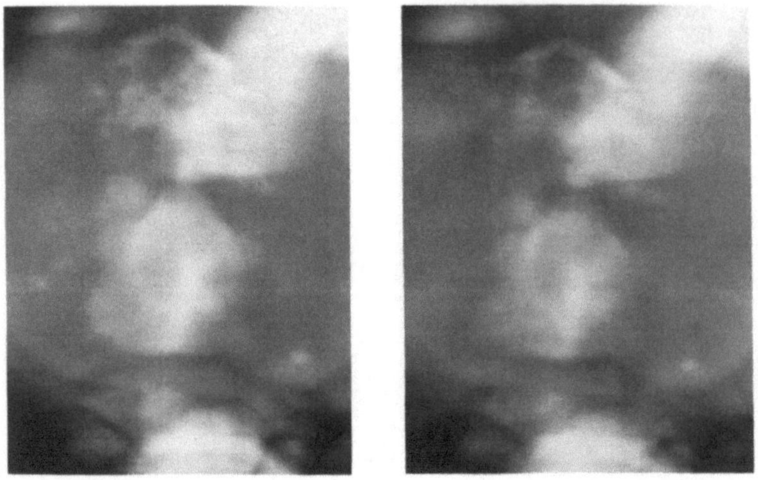

a b Fig. 1.37a, b

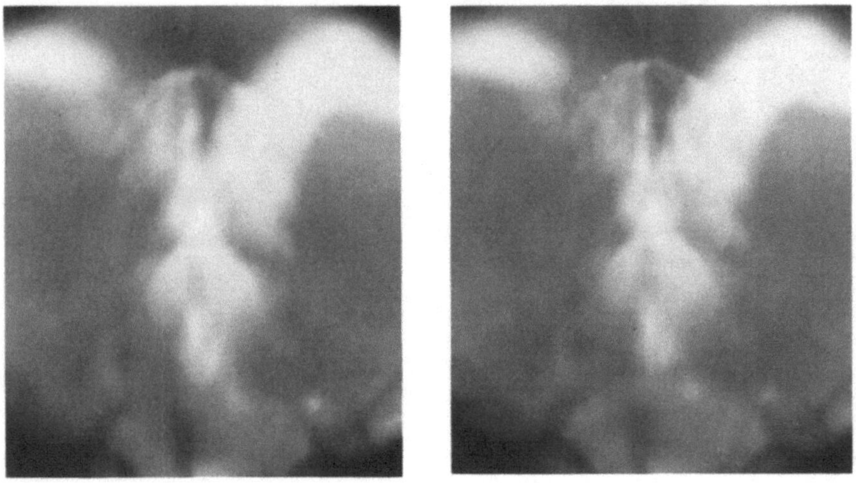

a b Fig. 1.38a, b

Figs. 1.37a, b and 1.38a, b. *Zonography of the Fourth Ventricle with Horizontal (Fig. 1.37) and Vertical (Fig. 1.38) Movement of Cancellation.* In (a) and (b) the central ray is directed, respectively, 4 and 8 mm behind the external auditory meatus. As in tomography (Fig. 1.35 and 1.36), and also in zonography the image of the postero-superior recesses is sharper when adopting a vertical movement (Fig. 1.38). The indentation produced by the nucleus dentatus, for instance, is very well visible in Fig. 1.38, but not as well, and only on the right side, in Fig. 1.37

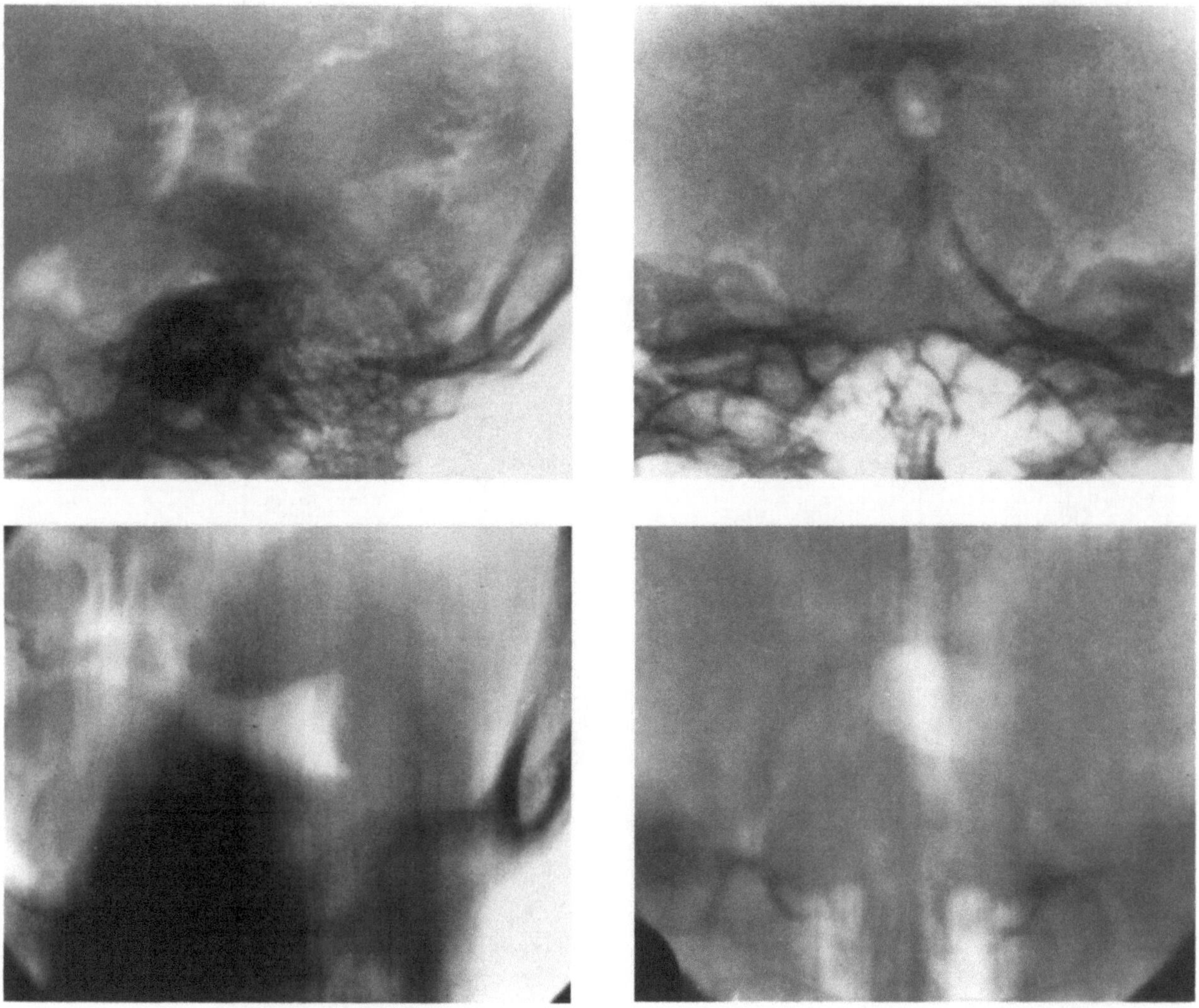

Fig. 1.39 a–d. *Verified Tumor in the Right Lower Portion of the Floor of the Fourth Ventricle.* a, b) Standard radiographs. c, d) Tomograms. The fourth ventricle is much better visualized with tomography, chiefly in the postero-anterior view, where its right lower limit appears stretched and raised, and the upper portion of the lateral recess is pushed upwards and sideways (especially in d). In this case tomography has been determinant for the diagnosis

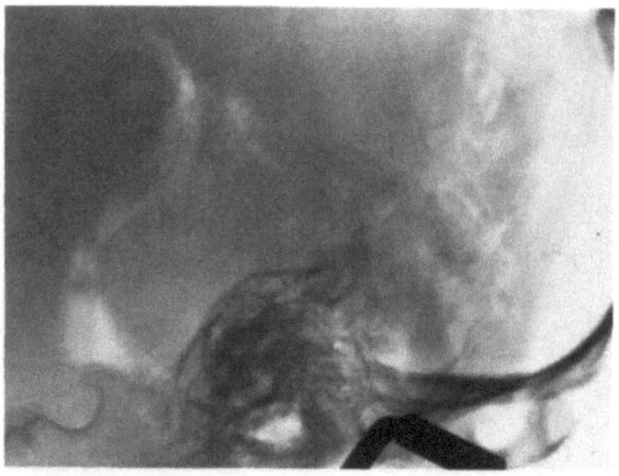
a

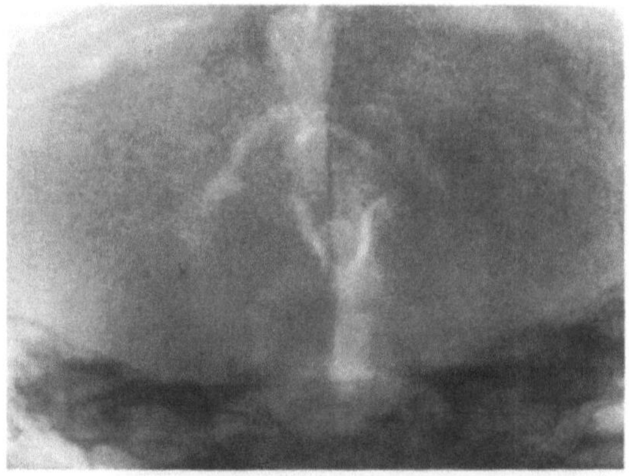
b

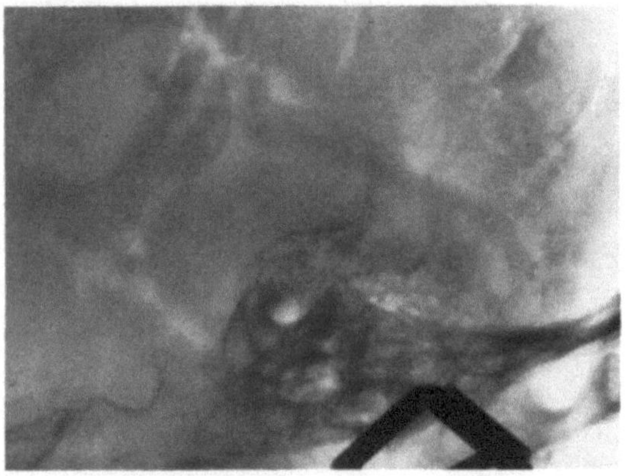
c

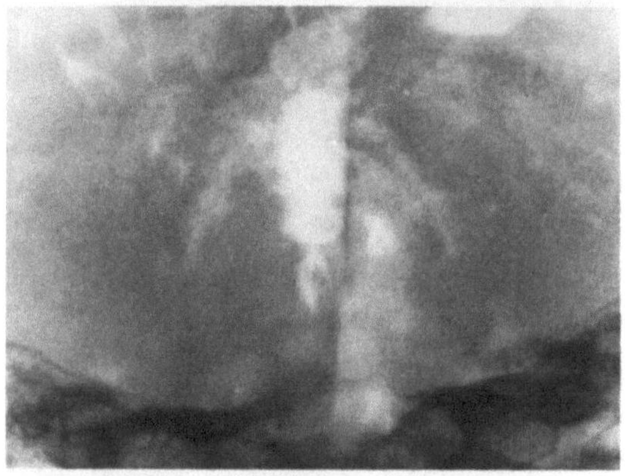
d

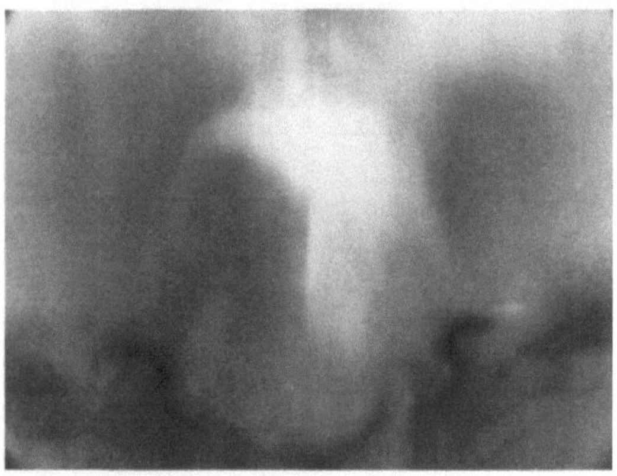
e

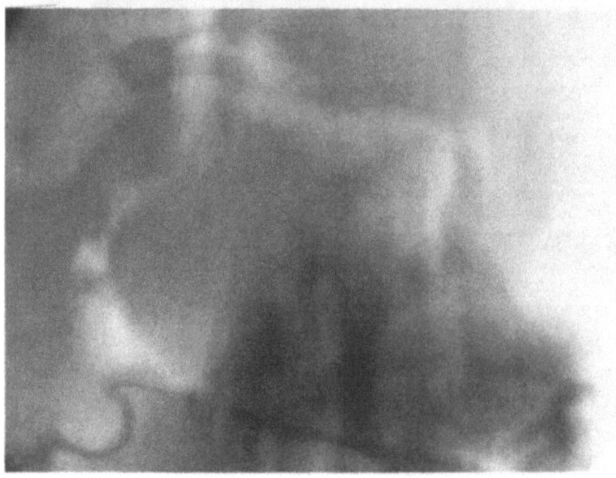
f

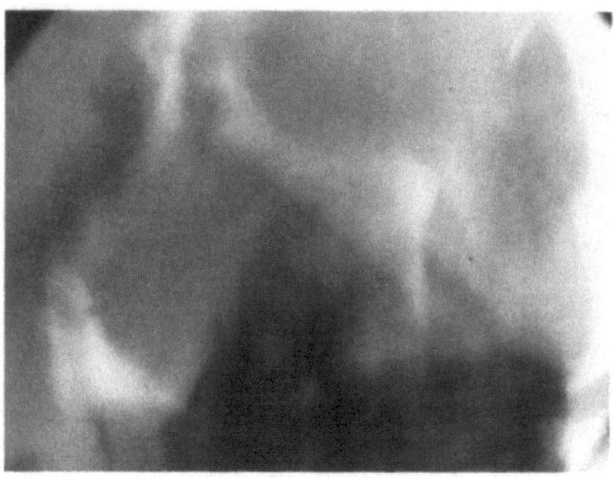
g

Fig. 1.40a–g. *Bulbar-Pontine Spongioblastoma.* The lesion infiltrates the right middle and inferior cerebellar peduncles, as well as the right inferior portion of the fourth ventricle. Encephalography (a, b) points to a tumor in the posterior part of the posterior fossa, probably more extended on the right side. With urea (c, d), the contrast enters the ventricular system, but the filling of the fourth ventricle is insufficient for its exact valuation. On the contrary, this is possible with the help of tomography (e, g): in the postero-anterior projection it is quite evident that the fourth ventricle is affected on the right side, where the right lateral recess is displaced upward and to the right. Note, in the lateral projection, the normal aspect of the floor of the fourth ventricle on the tomogram passing 0.5 cm to the left of the midline (g), whereas this floor appears most deformed on the tomogram passing 0.5 cm to the right of the midline (f). In this case tomography must be considered determinant for the diagnosis

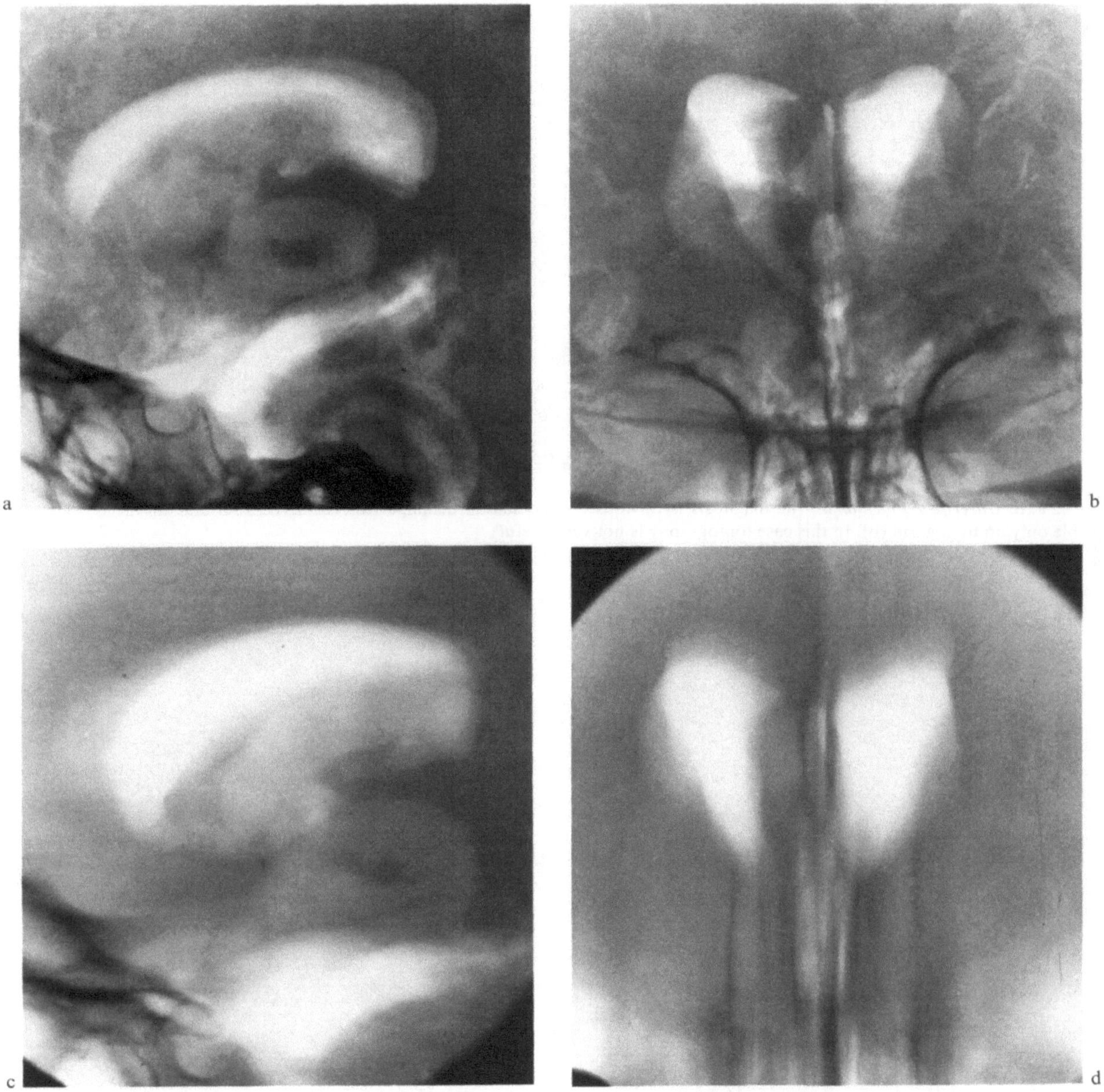

Fig. 1.41 a–d. *Intraventricular Tumor Invading the Anterior Part of the Right Ventricle.* Unquestionable diagnosis also on the standard images (a, b). In the lateral view the irregular borders of the filling defect are perhaps better visible on tomogram (c); on the contrary the slight interruption of the profile of the roof of the left ventricle, which is clear on the standard radiograph (b), is not visible on tomogram (d), passing 1.5 cm in front of the external auditory meatus. In this case tomography is of little utility

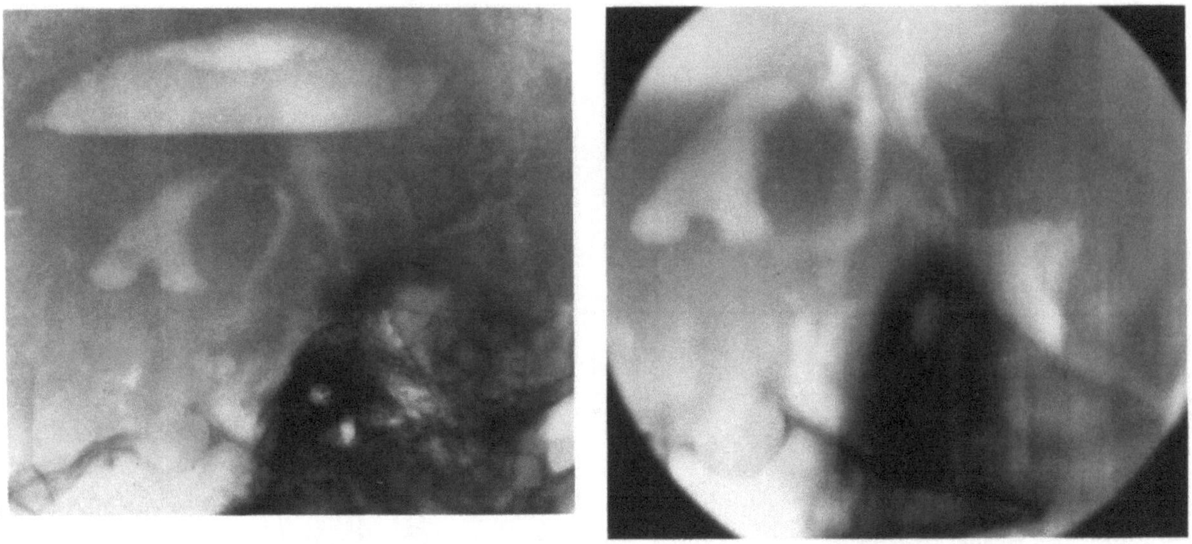

Fig. 1.42 a, b. *Unverified Pinealoma.* The diagnosis is obvious on the standard image (a). However, the aqueduct deformation is visible only on tomogram (b). In this case tomography is not very useful

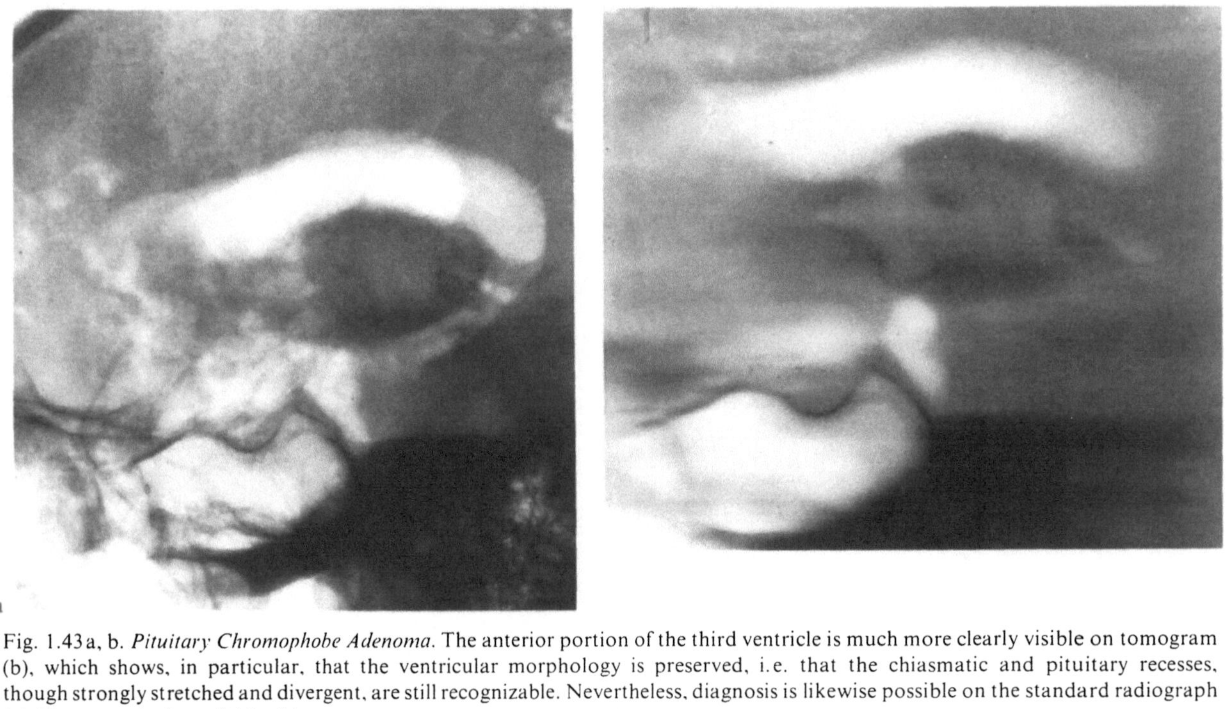

Fig. 1.43a, b. *Pituitary Chromophobe Adenoma.* The anterior portion of the third ventricle is much more clearly visible on tomogram (b), which shows, in particular, that the ventricular morphology is preserved, i.e. that the chiasmatic and pituitary recesses, though strongly stretched and divergent, are still recognizable. Nevertheless, diagnosis is likewise possible on the standard radiograph (a). Tomography is useful in this case

---

▷

Fig. 1.44a–f. *Deep Periventricular Right Frontal Glioma Infiltrating the Septum Pellucidum and Passing Extensively to the Opposite Side.* The vertical branch of the right Sylvian fissure is shifted backward; the right frontal horn is amputated; the left frontal horn is highly deformed; the anterior portion of the third ventricle is lowered; the septum pellucidum is broadened and deformed in its inferior portion, especially on the left side.

a–c) Standard radiographs. d) Midline tomography. e, f) Tomographies 1 cm to the right and left of the midline. The pathology is very well demonstrated by the standard X-rays (a–c); but the deformation of the third ventricle and the frontal horns is better visualized with tomography (d–f), thanks to the elimination of the superimposed image of the Sylvian fissures. Tomography is useful

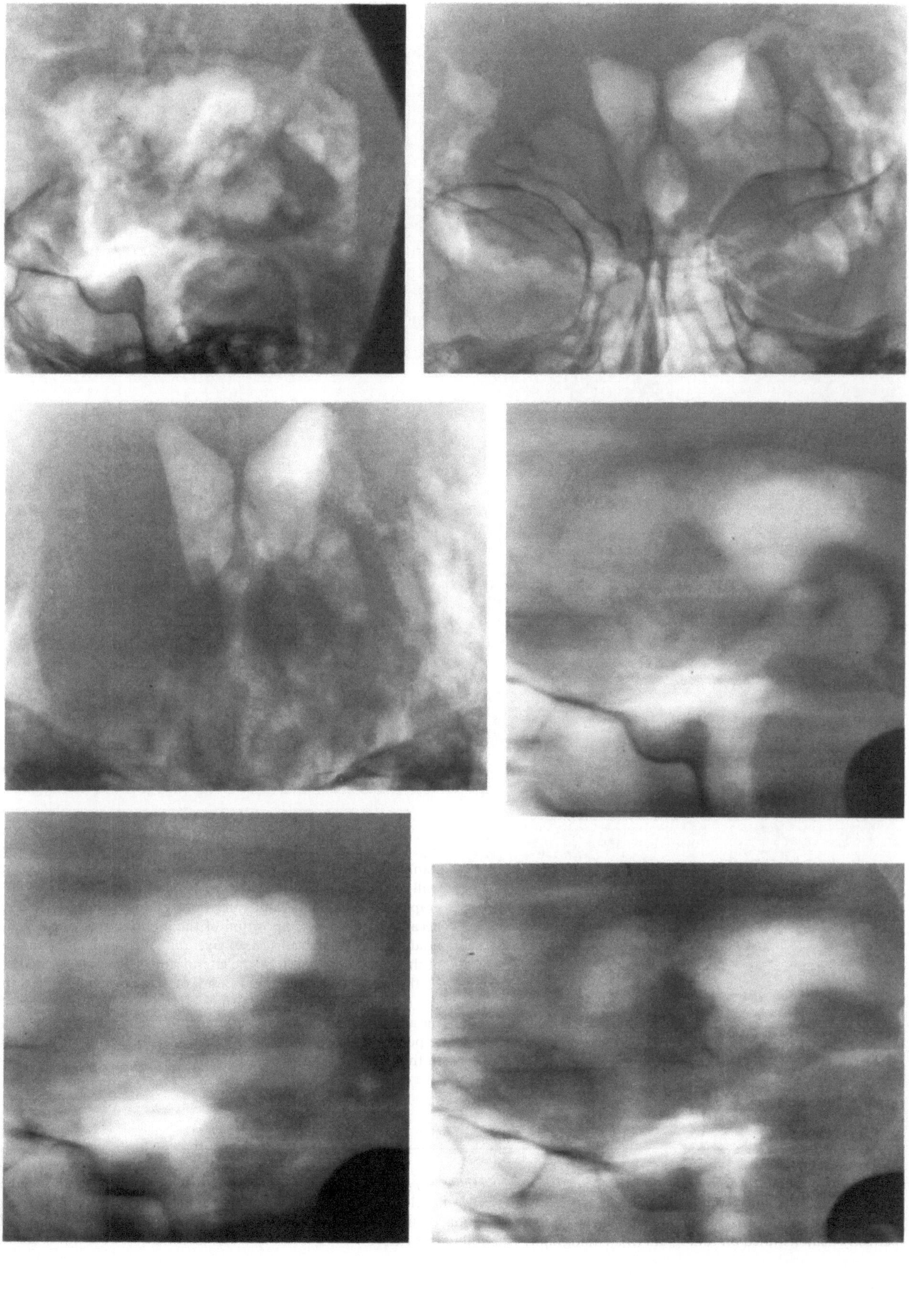

a b c d e f

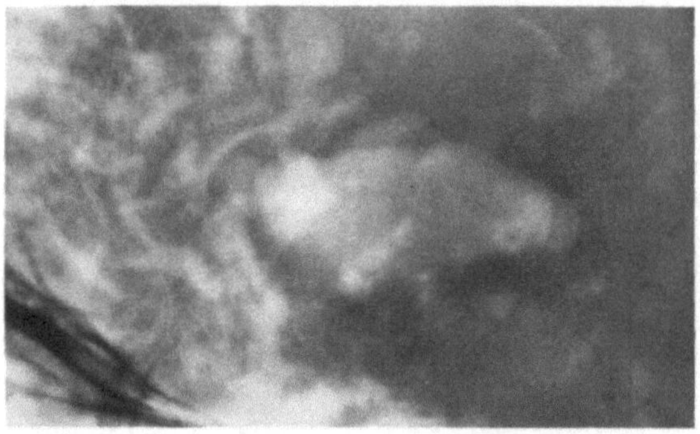
a

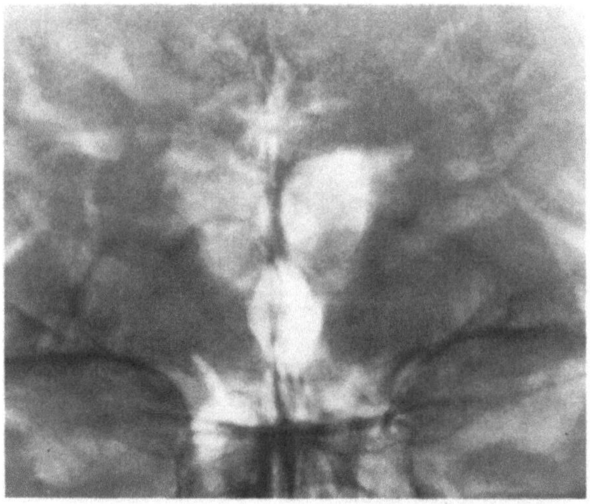
b

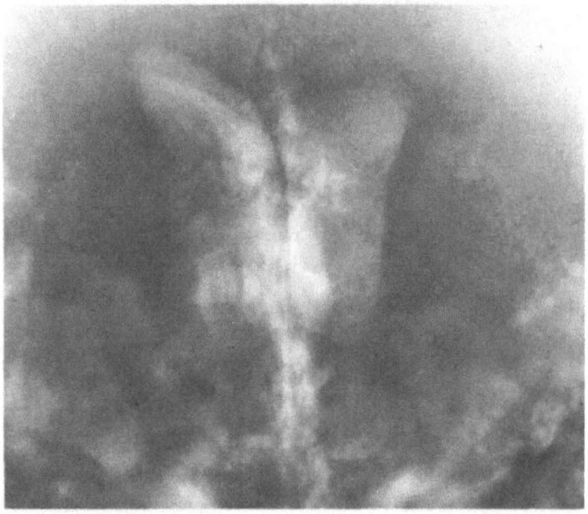
c

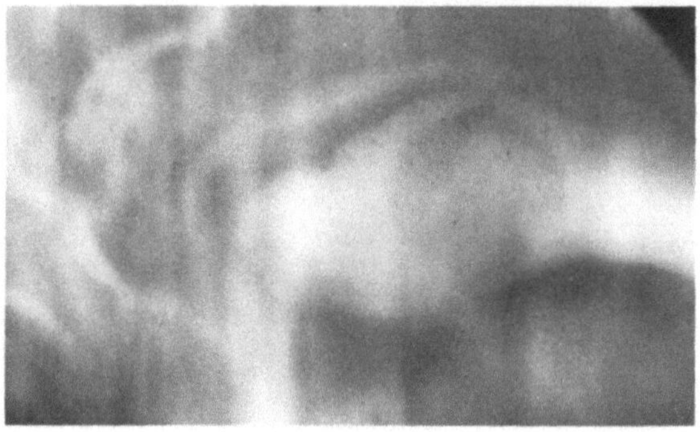
d

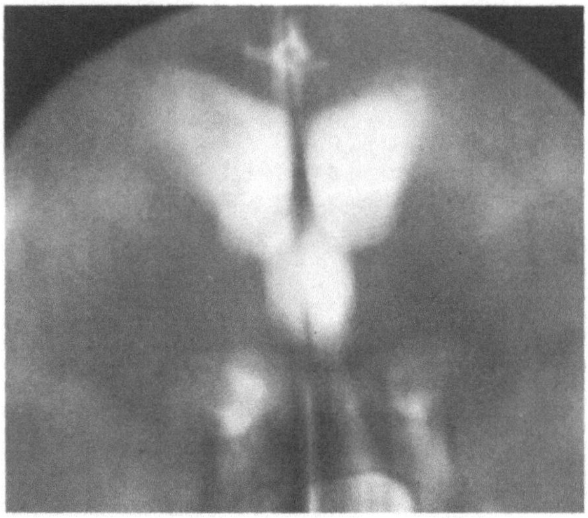
e

Fig. 1.45a–e. *Right Paraventricular Frontal Metastasis*. On the standard half-axial view (c) an impression is visible on the lateral wall of the right ventricle; this is not confirmed on the radiographs in the lateral (a) and antero-posterior (b) views, probably because of the superimposition of the highly dilated subarachnoid spaces. Tomograms (d, e) give quite a clear demonstration of the round impression on the lateral side of the anterior aspect of the right ventricular body and of the posterior aspect of the right frontal horn. In (e) note also the negative image of the anterior cerebral artery in the corpus callosum cistern, which appears less clearly on standard image (b). Tomography is useful in this case

---

▷

Fig. 1.47a, b. *Pituitary Chromophobe Adenoma with Considerable Suprasellar Development*. Standard radiograph (a) allows the diagnosis, but the antero-inferior deformed aspect of the third ventricle, and chiefly the air in the subarachnoid space bordering the superior pole of the tumor are hidden by the superposition of the contrast in the Sylvian fissures. The lesion is instead perfectly demonstrated on tomogram (b). Tomography is useful in this case

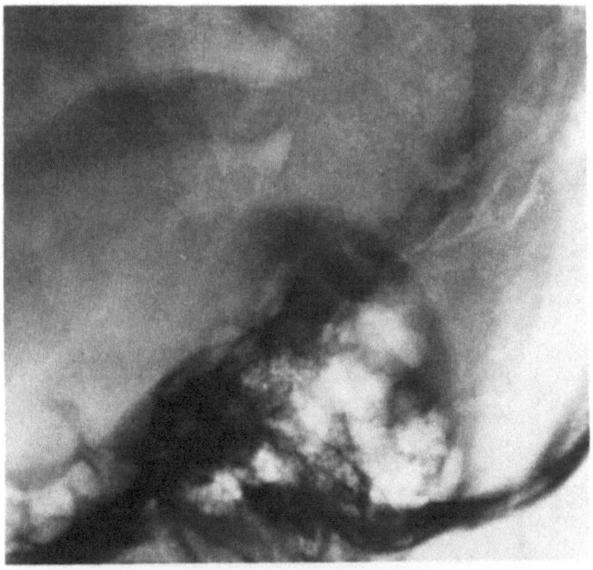

a

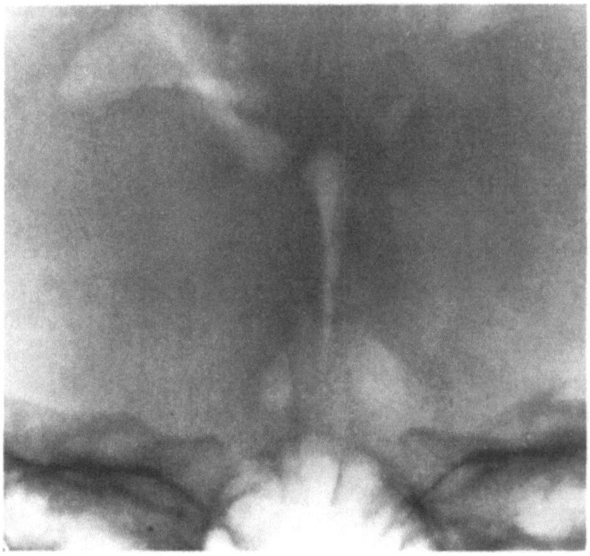

b

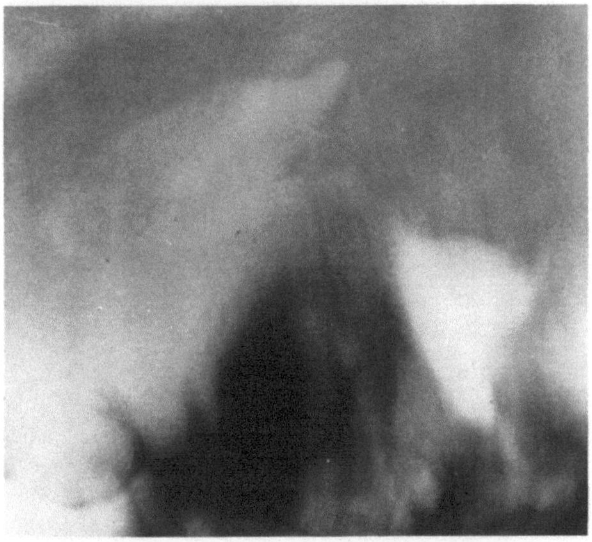

c

Fig. 1.46a–c. *Nonverified Multiple Metastases from Uterine Carcinoma.* The deformation of the right ventricle is easy visible on standard images (a, b); those of the third ventricle and the aqueduct are demonstrated on the standard image only in the postero-anterior projection, whereas in the lateral projection they are emphasized chiefly by tomogram (c). In this case tomography is rather useful

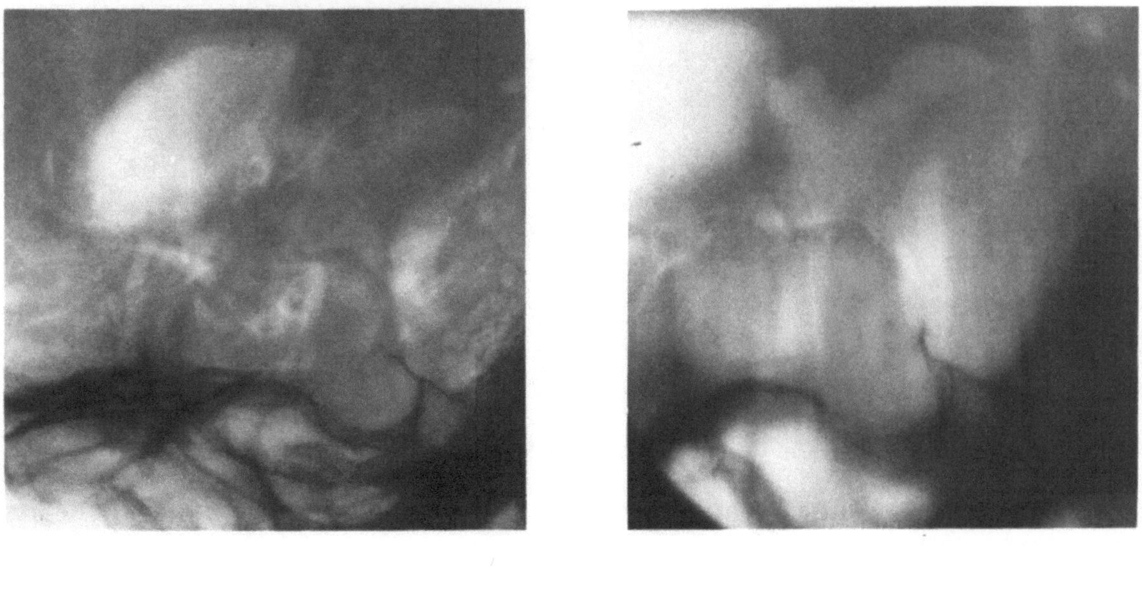

a b

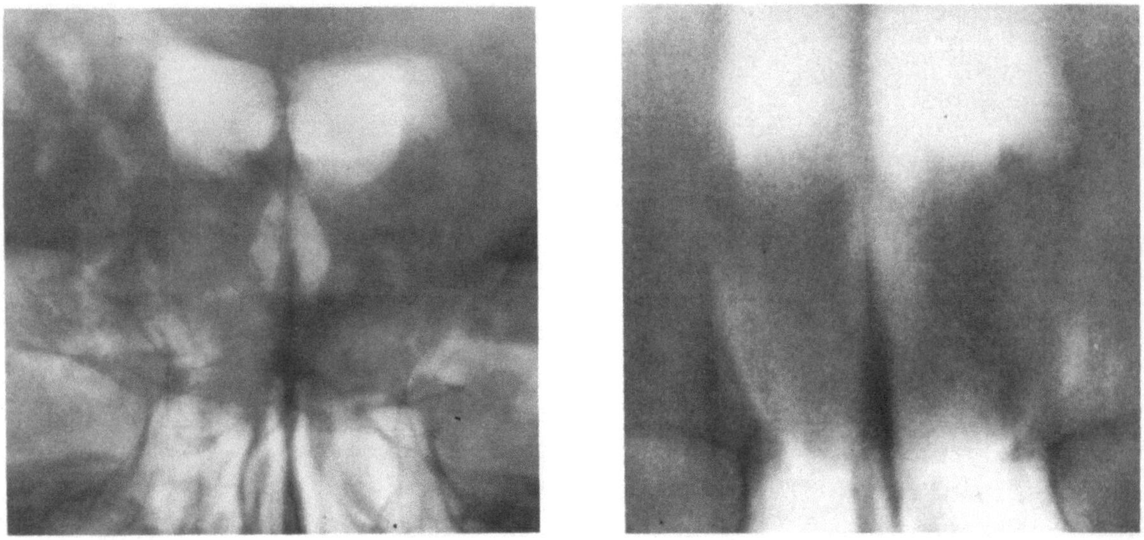

a b

Fig. 1.48 a, b. *Chromophobe Adenoma*. The standard radiograph in lateral projection allows a diagnosis. However, in antero-posterior projection, the tomogram (b) better outlines the lateral and lower limits of the tumor by the thin air layer in the subarachnoid space. In this case tomography is to be considered useful

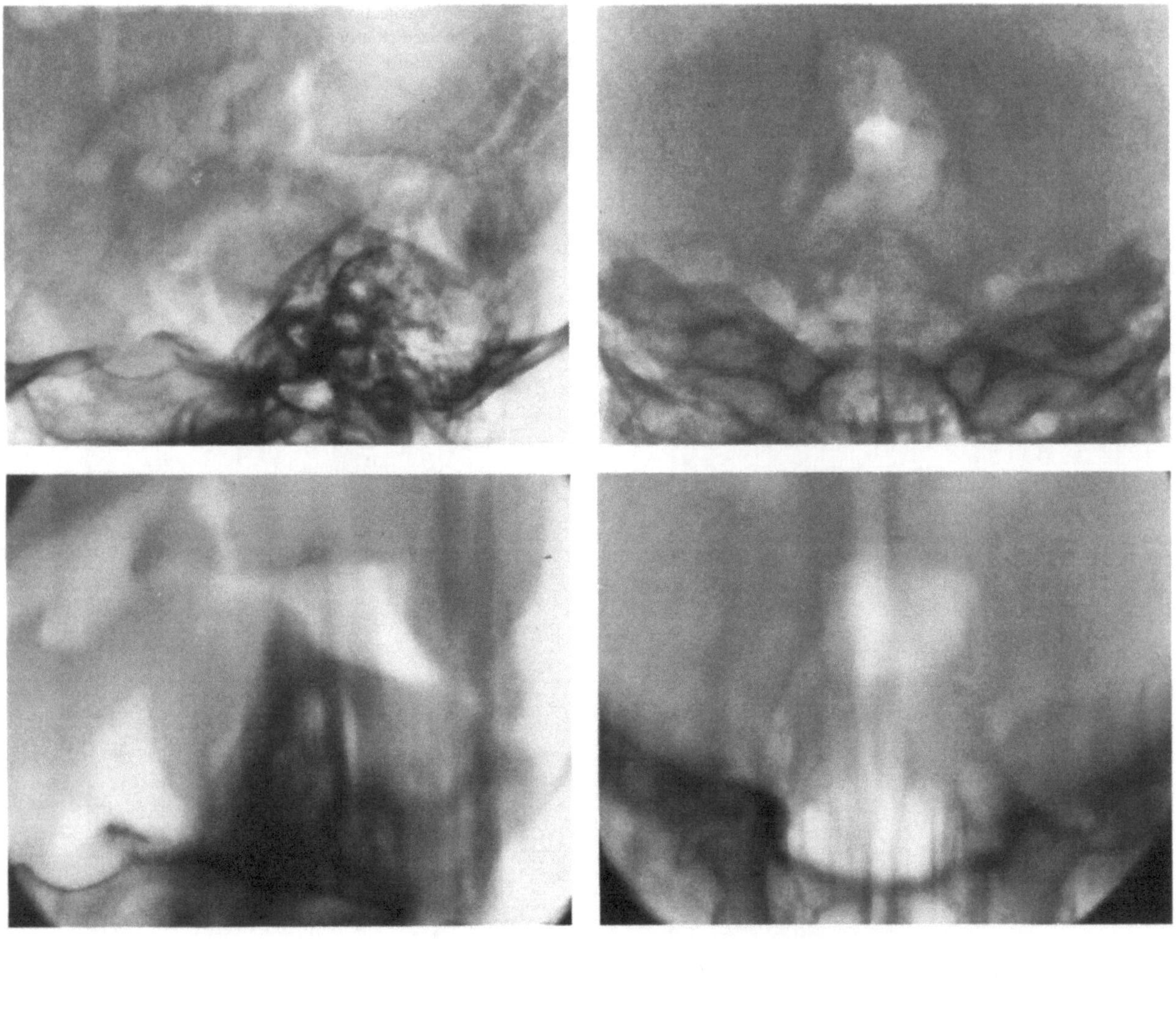

a b c d

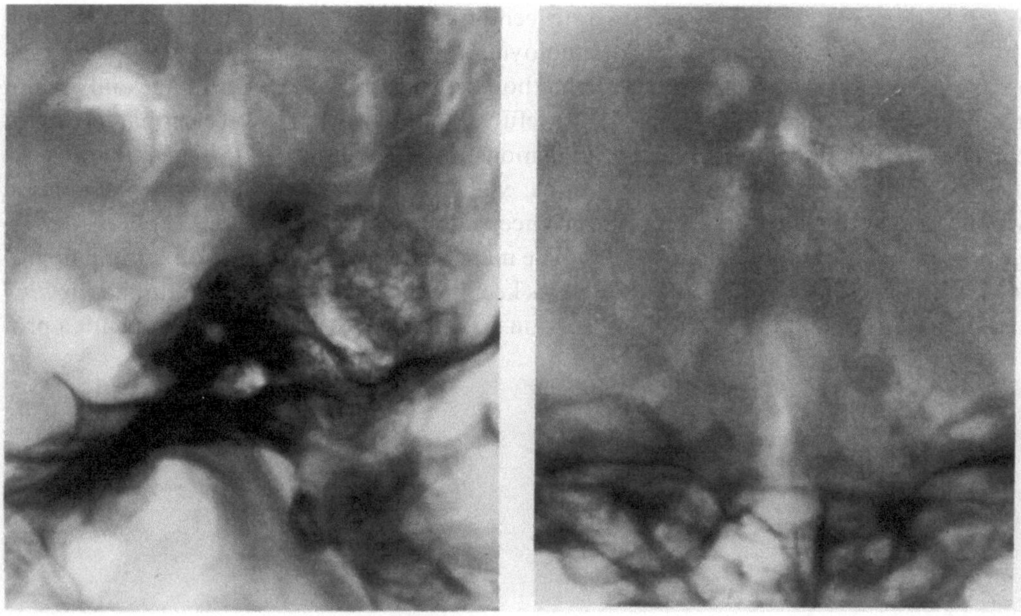

a b

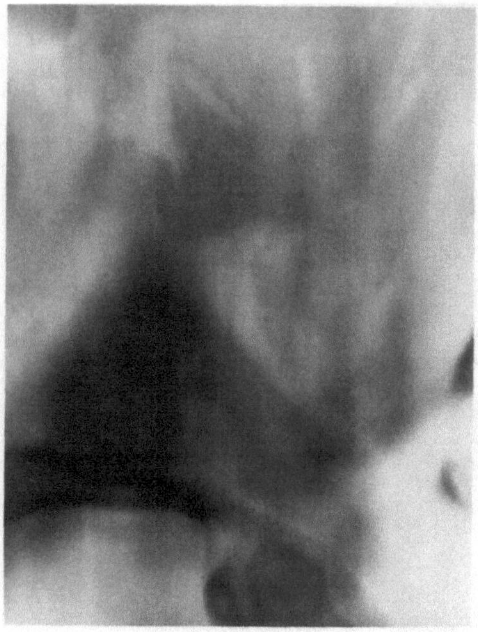

c

Fig. 1.50a–c. *Aqueduct Stenosis.* Diagnosis is possible on standard images (a, b): the fourth ventricle on the midline and the aqueduct are not visible, the brain stem (outlined by cisterns) is small, and the cerebellum is atrophic. On tomogram (c), however, the stenosed aqueduct is perfectly visualized. In this case tomography is very useful

◁
Fig. 1.49a–d. *Unverified Pontine Expansive Process.* Encephalography (a, b) shows a probable deformation of the floor of the fourth ventricle, the left border of which appears irregular in postero-anterior projection. Tomograms (c, d) specify that the left lateral recess is very poorly visualized, and also show the lesion in lateral projection. In this case tomography is very useful

11. Subtraction

In cerebral angiography the subtraction technique enjoys an almost universal consensus. The same is not true of encephalography. As a matter of fact, after the few samples shown by ZIEDSES DES PLANTES [484] in 1935, it was necessary to wait thirty years for the next subtraction encephalographic pictures. In 1966 RUGGIERO [383) suggested a rudimentary technique based on an attempt to obtain very accurate centering in the conventional way, without employing any special equipment. Obviously such a method depends too much on chance and cannot be useful in routine work. However, it had the merit of demonstrating the utility of the subtraction technique, which RUGGIERO considers an advance in the encephalographic technique.

The main difficulty in subtraction encephalography is keeping the head perfectly immobile. In 1967 RUGGIERO and MAZZACURATI [389–391] built a pro-

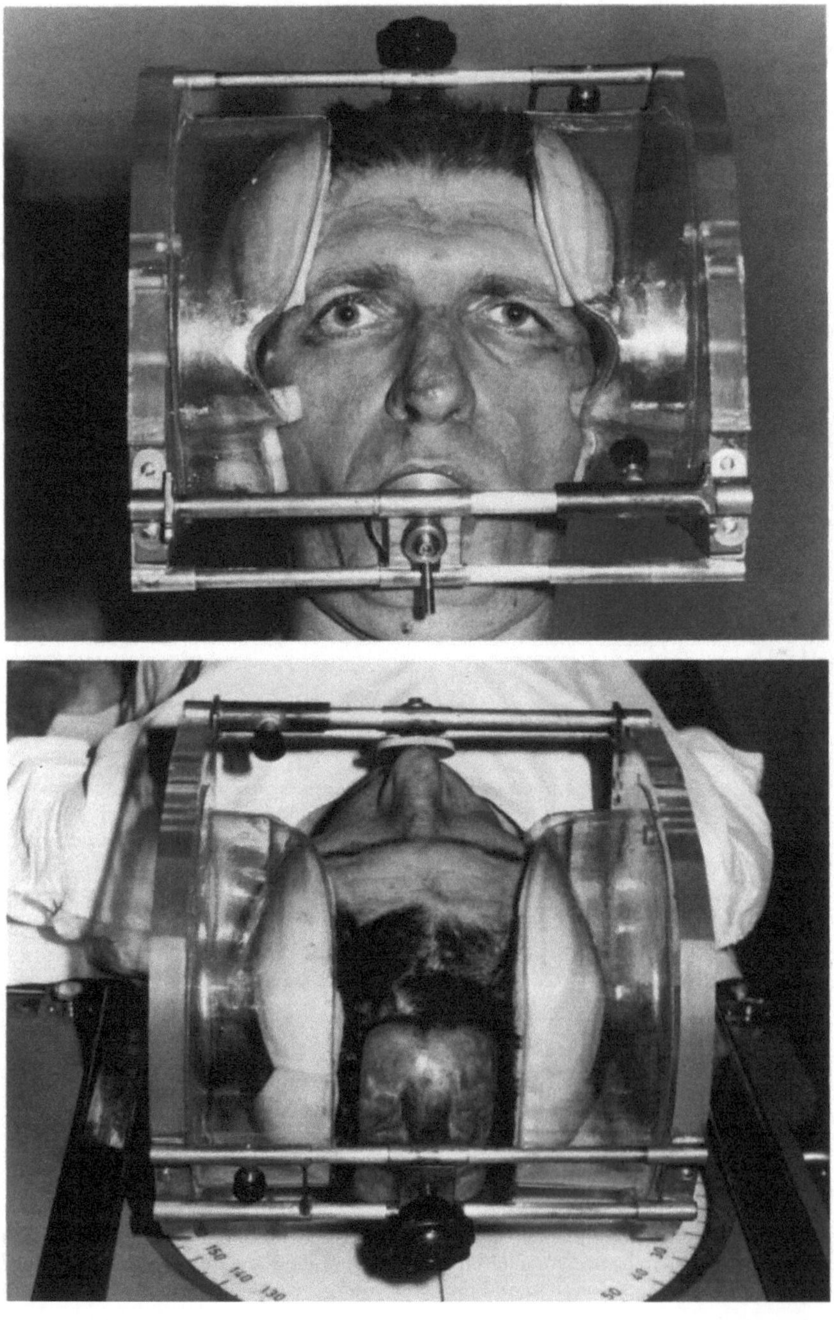

a
b

Fig. 1.51 a, b. *Subtraction*. RUGGIERO and MAZZACURATI's second apparatus fitted on the patient's head in the sitting (a) and supine (b) positions

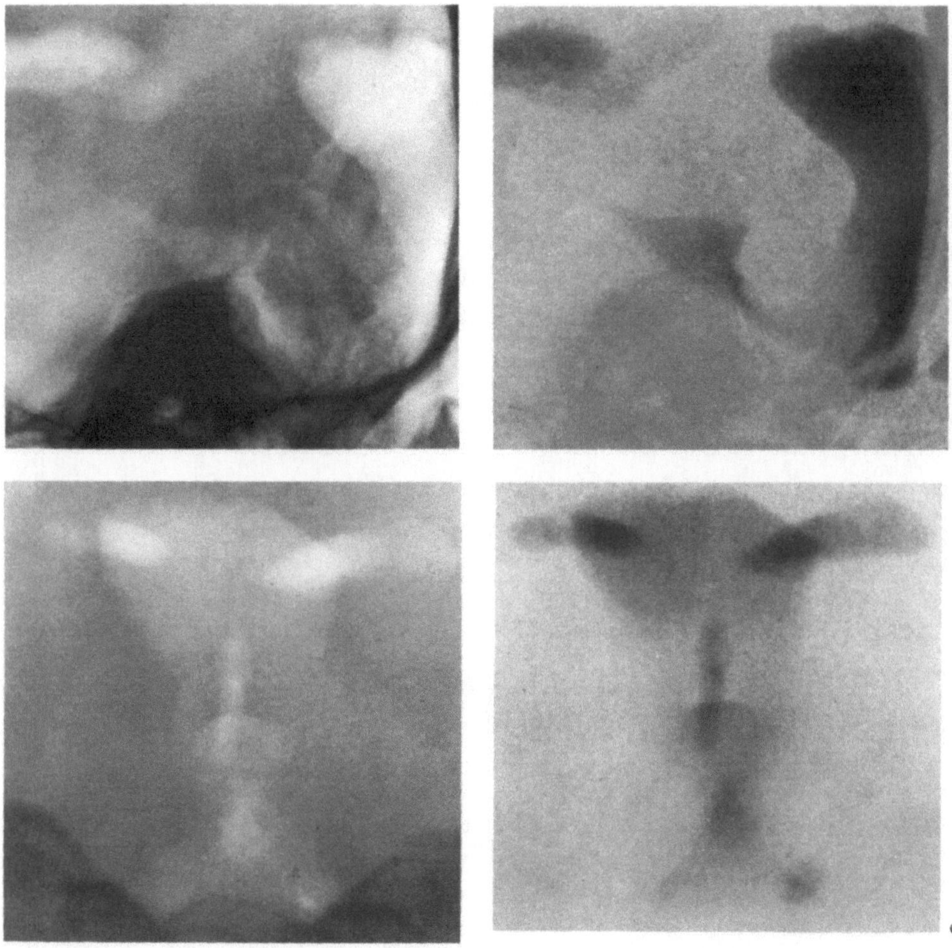

Fig. 1.52a–d. In the lateral projection the inferior portion of the fourth ventricle is not visualized in a good standard radiograph; it is perfectly shown on the subtraction (b) as well as the recessus of the third and fourth ventricle. Also, the negative image of the cerebellar tonsils and the inferior vermis are visible only on subtraction films. In the corresponding postero-anterior view the air–fluid level is demonstrated only by subtraction which also shows more clearly the vallecula and the walls of the third ventricle

totype based on the principle of having the patient's head fixed between two rigid hemicaps. There are symmetrical points on both hemicaps where the central beam can be focused for the different projections. The quality of standard images and subtractions made by this apparatus was fair; but it is now no longer used because of its considerable size, which made it difficult to set the patient in the required position. As a result the examination took considerably longer.

They therefore built a second, more sophisticated apparatus [390] consisting of two pieces, one for fixing the patient's head and the other for connecting the first piece to the Mimer (Fig. 1.51). With this apparatus X-ray pictures are available for subtraction more easily and rapidly; the quality of the subtracted images is usually fair, but that of the standard radiographs is poor because of the superimposition on the patient's head of the thick plexiglass arms attaching the head holder to the Mimer.

Since the first draft of this chapter was written four years have passed and the technique unfortunately has not made much progress. We have not yet solved the problem of achieving perfect immobility of the patient's head without using cumbersome materials. We have tried hollow caps in plastic material, rubber, etc., but the results have been rather poor.

Small movements of the head can produce differences between the mask and the picture to be subtracted. These differences can to some extent be avoided by reducing the field of the X-ray beam,

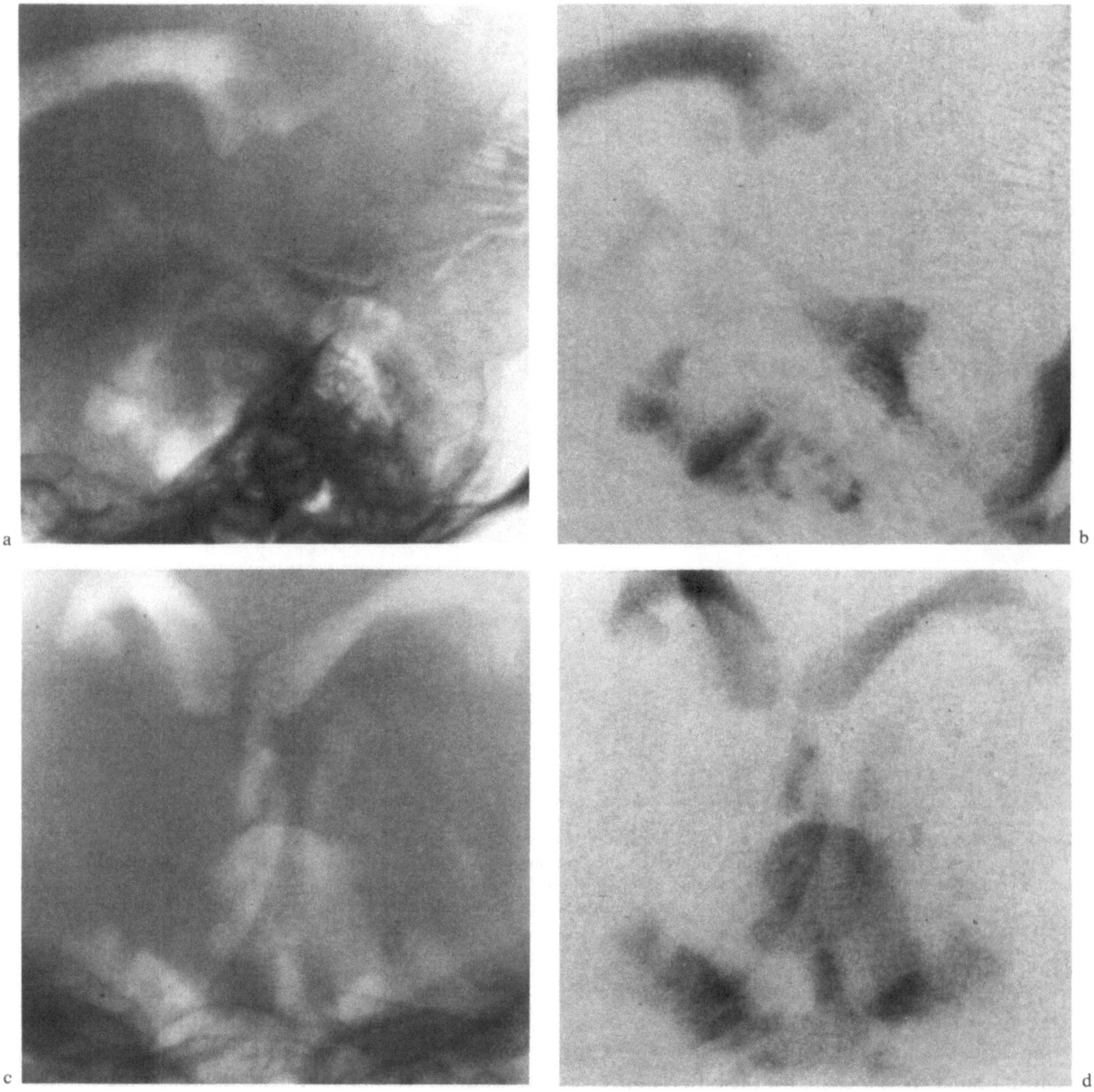

Fig. 1.53a, b. Subtraction of lateral and antero-posterior simultaneous views performed with a rapid seriograph. The quality of the pictures is inferior to the quality of nonsimultaneous radiographs, but the information given by subtraction is still considerable. Note in the lateral projection (b) the aspect of the cerebello-pontine angle cisterns

i.e. by accurate centering. Moreover, the structures that one most often wants to subtract usually lie on the midline: third ventricle, aqueduct, fourth ventricle.

Ruggiero and Trevisan [394] recently obtained excellent subtractions in two projections by taking, before injecting air, lateral and postero-anterior pictures in quick succession, and repeating them in the same way immediately after the air injection (Fig. 1.52).

These authors have also tried rapid encephalography, using AOT seriography for cerebral angiography during the air injection (Fig. 1.53).

The Neurocentrix (see Fig. 1.5) will probably allow us to make a further advance. This apparatus is equipped with a seriograph, which may be useful in studying at least the posterior fossa. The seriograph may be started a few seconds before the air injection, in order to obtain a series of radiographs including one or two pictures without contrast. Thus encephalography would be performed in the same conditions as an angiographic seriography. With these methods, obviously only subtraction of the posterior fossa can be achieved. We are now

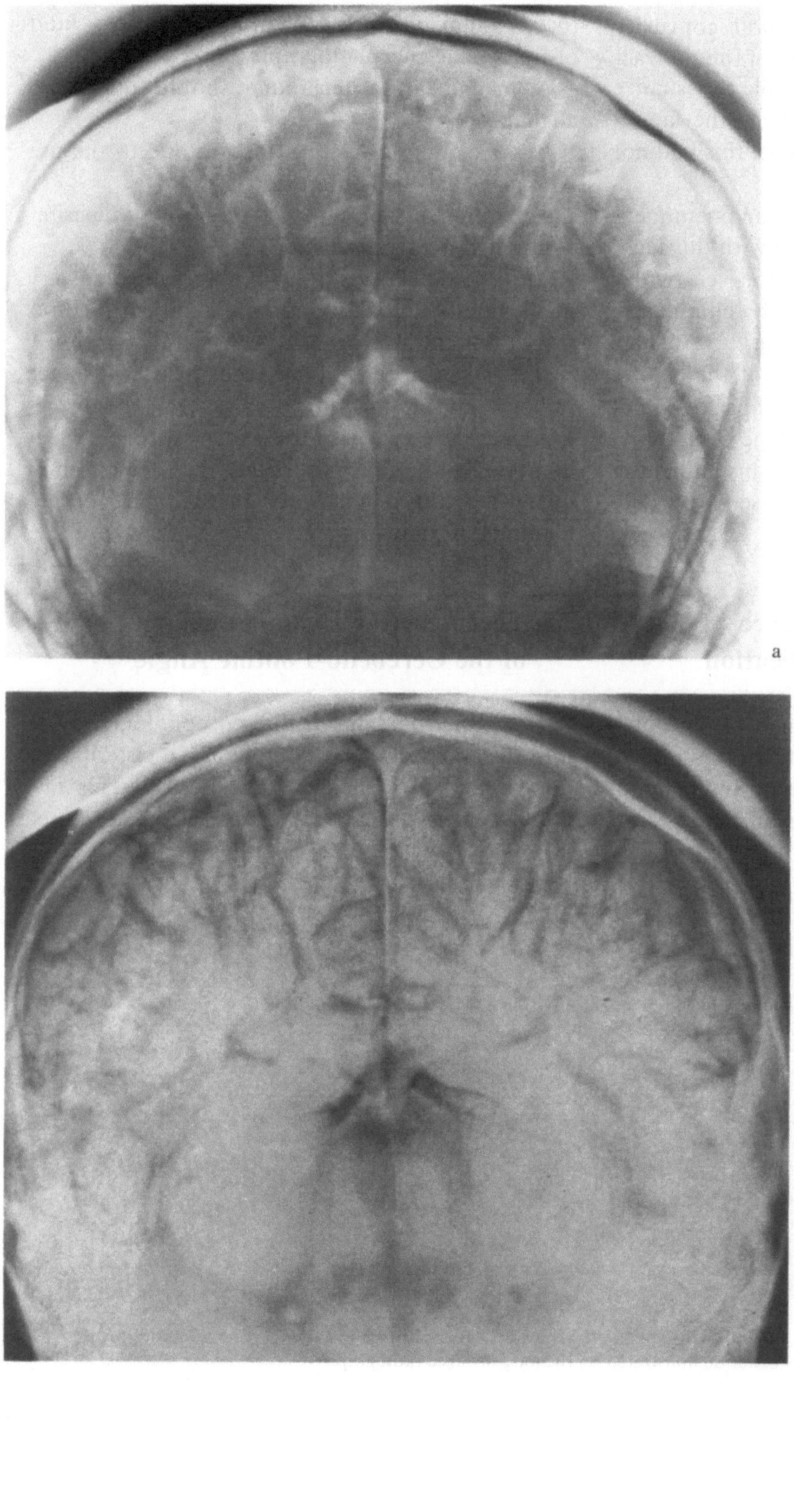

a

b

Fig. 1.54a, b. Subtraction of the subarachnoid sulci of the convexity working to further improve the technique of subtraction encephalography, and we hope that our research will serve as a basis for other doctors who wish to continue in this field. According to RUGGIERO and TREVISAN [394], the main indications for subtraction are the same as those for tomography, plus the examination of the cerebral convexity (Fig. 1.54). In addition, with the help of the subtraction technique, these authors were able to visualize the cerebello-pontine angle cisterns in the lateral view (Fig. 1.53b). To their knowledge, this had not been done before.

We believe subtraction has a future in pneumoencephalography. In fact, it is possible with this technique to obtain clearer images of the ventricular system and the subarachnoid space by eliminating the superimposed bony structures (Fig. 1.52). Thus, the subtraction technique has some of the advantages of the plain film and some of those of tomography, with the additional advantage over tomography that it can be carried out at any time after the examination, which is not the case with tomography.

12. Long Focus-to-Film Distance Radiography and Magnification

Discussing the recent refinements of encephalographic technique, RUGGIERO and TREVISAN [394] suggested long focus-film radiography and magnification. By comparing radiographs of the posterior fossa taken with a distance of 1 m or 3.30 m between focus and film, they were able to demonstrate that the longer distance is more suitable for outlining the structures, especially the fourth ventricle (Fig. 1.55). These authors also feel that further improvement could be obtained by increasing the focus-to-film distance to 5 m to produce a kind of stereotaxic encephalography.

A magnification technique should offer two advantages:

1. better definition of the structure due to the use of a smaller focus (Fig. 1.56).
2. separation of superimposed or partially superimposed structures.

RUGGIERO and TREVISAN [394] obtained some very good results by subtracting magnified pictures (Fig. 1.57).

In conclusion, both long focus-to-film distance radiography and magnification (as well as subtraction) must be considered to be still in an experimental stage, but it is easy to foresee that these techniques will occupy a remarkable place in the encephalography of tomorrow.

13. Technique for Examination of the Cerebello-Pontine Angle

It is not unusual, during the encephalography to find that one cerebello-pontine angle cistern does not visualize or visualizes only poorly. This fact is not very significant when the lesion is located

a 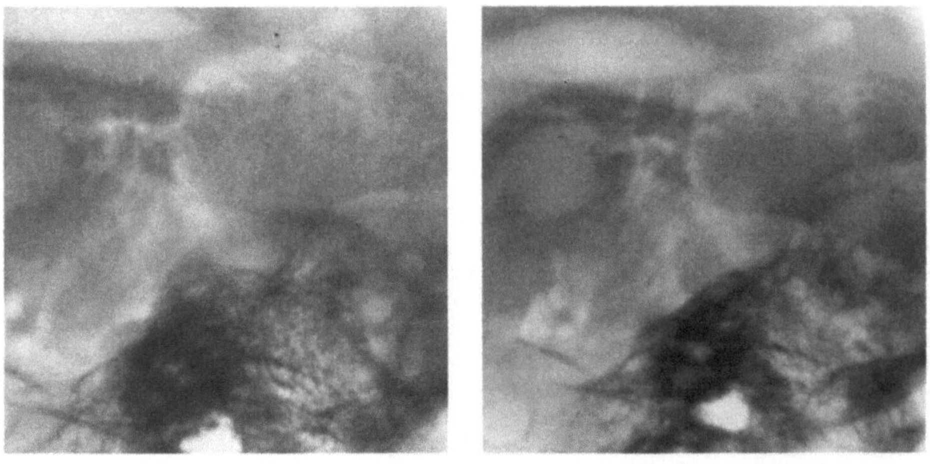 b

Fig. 1.55a,b. *Long-Distance Radiography.* (a) and (b) are pictures taken with a focus-to-film distance of 1 and 3.30 m, respectively. The fourth ventricle, especially its floor, is better demonstrated on the long-distance radiograph

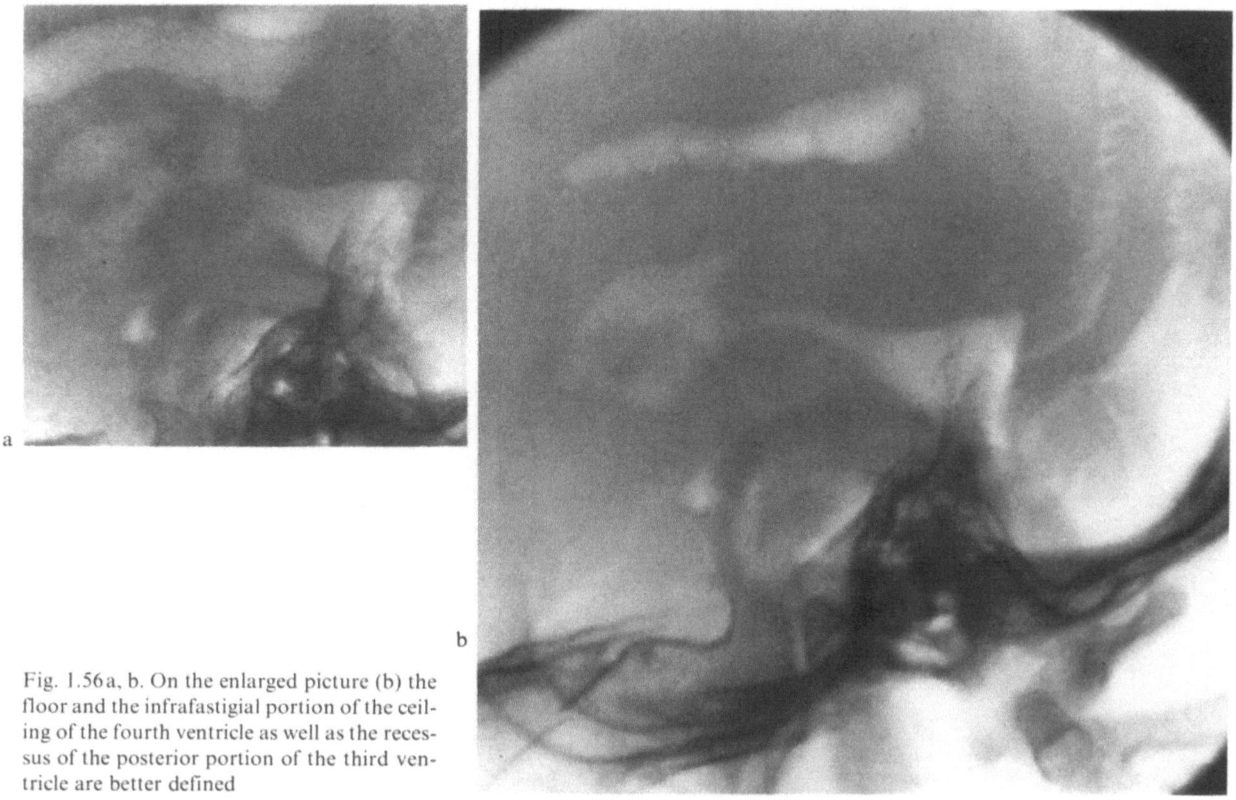

Fig. 1.56a, b. On the enlarged picture (b) the floor and the infrafastigial portion of the ceiling of the fourth ventricle as well as the recessus of the posterior portion of the third ventricle are better defined

far from the posterior fossa, but it might be important in subtentorial lesions. In cases of arachnoiditis of the cerebello-pontine angle, the nonfilling of the cistern is the major diagnostic finding, if not the only one; it is therefore fundamental, in such cases, to make sure that the nonvisualization of the cistern is not due to some technical reason. For this a special maneuver is suitable: the patient's head is extended and inclined toward the site opposite the cistern to be examined (Fig. 1.58), which consequently lies higher. Five ml of air is injected in this position; then the head is straightened and flexed somewhat more than for the usual position in order to fill the aqueduct and the fourth ventricle. With this maneuver the air will necessarily collect—and remain—in the cerebello-pontine angle cistern; failure to fill can thus be considered proof that the cistern is obstructed. However, the maneuver is difficult; it is therefore advisable to repeat it when a first attempt is unsuccessful. It might even be better to repeat the encephalography if failure of one cistern to fill is the only positive finding in a case of suspected cerebello-pontine angle lesion.

Recently ISHERWOOD [219] reported the results of 100 cases, of which 24 were acoustic neurinomas. Linear tomography was used and the head was positioned so as to obtain transverse sections of the petrous portion of the temporal bone.

14. Encephalographic Technique for the Examination of the Sellar Region

The encephalographic study of the sellar region is based essentially on the aspect of the antero-inferior portion of the third ventricle, the chiasmatic cistern, and the anterior part of the interpeduncular cistern. The temporal horns as well as the medial portion of the horizontal branch of the Sylvian fissure may also be involved.

When the symptoms give reason to suspect a lesion in the sellar region—either a tumor or arachnoiditis—the subarachnoid space has to be examined with particular care.

One must make sure that both the pontine and interpeduncular cisterns are well filled with air,

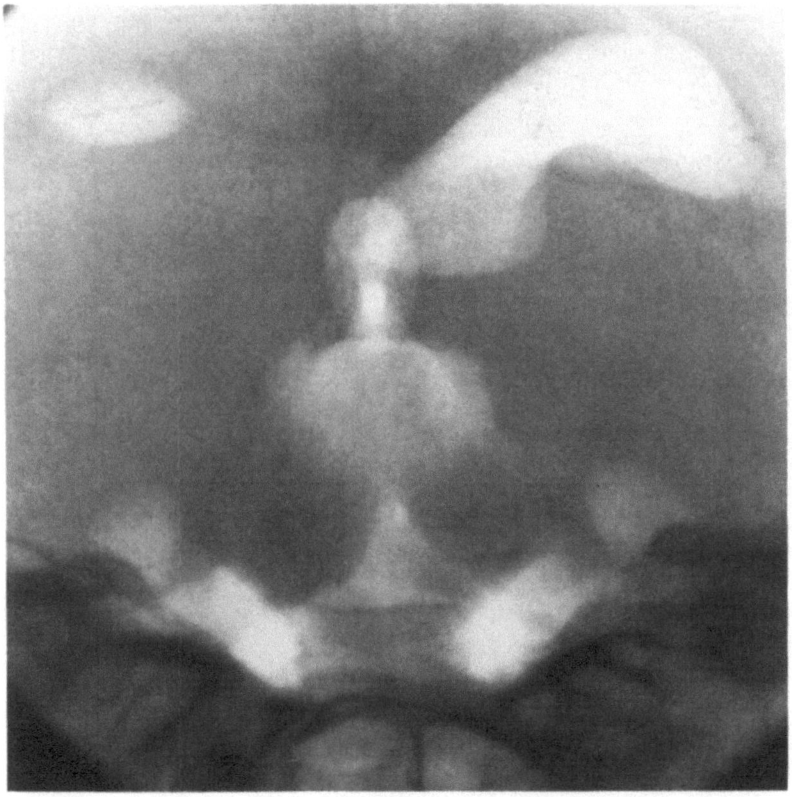

a

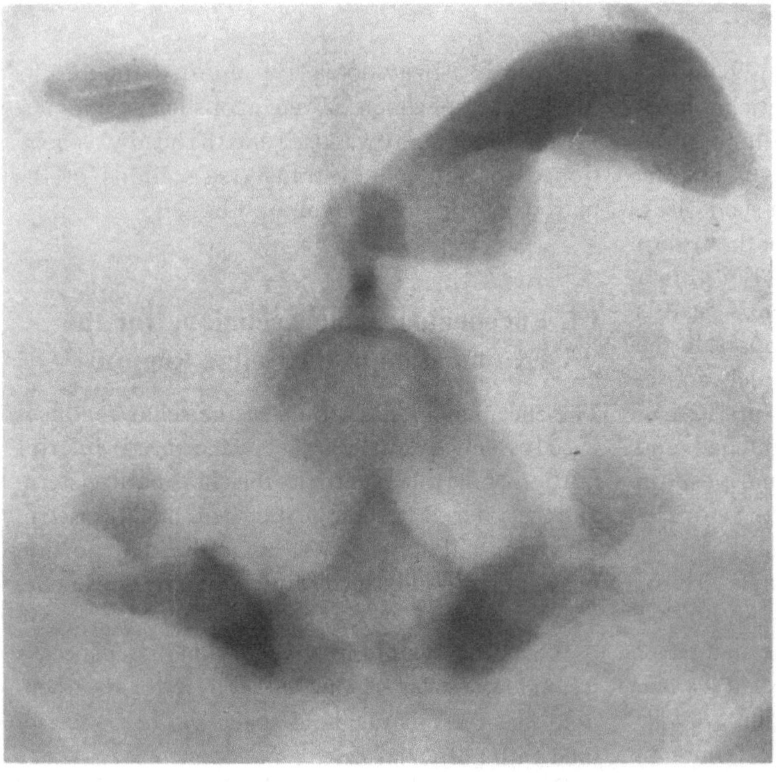

b

Fig. 1.57a, b. On the subtraction (b) of the magnified picture (a) the lateral recessus of the fourth ventricle are demonstrated more clearly

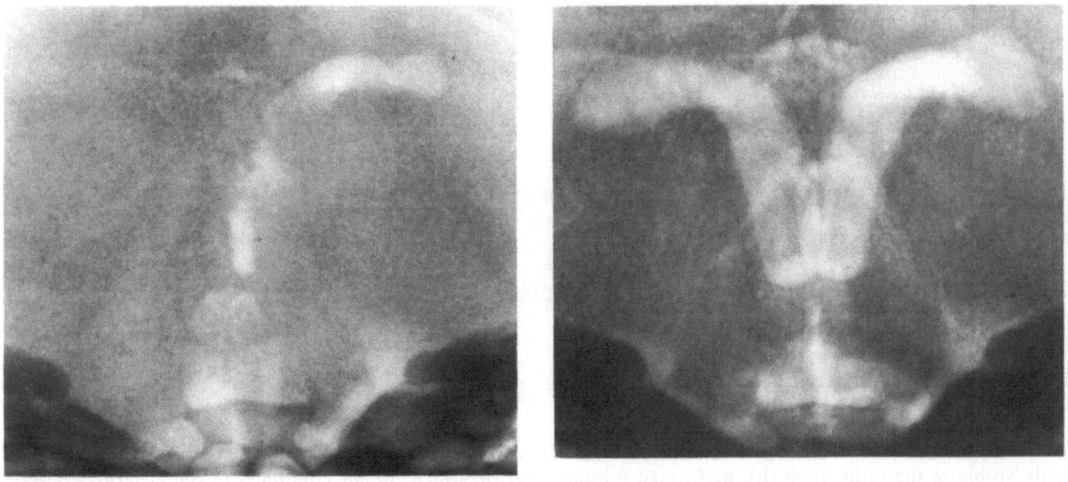

Fig. 1.58a, b. Selective filling of the left and right cerebello-pontine angle cisterns, with the technique illustrated in the text, p. 55

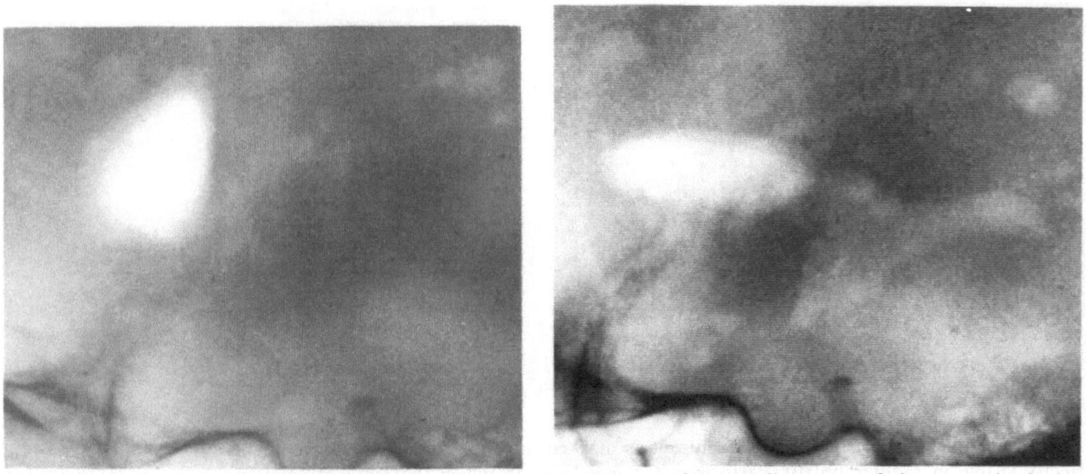

Fig. 1.59a, b. *Special Maneuver for Filling the Third Ventricle*. Because of the small amount of air present in the lateral ventricles, in the supine position the air-fluid level does not reach the foramen of Monroe, and consequently the gas does not enter the third ventricle. This appears, however, perfectly visualized after the deflexion of the head (b)

while the patient is still in the sitting position and before removing the needle. When the patient is moved from the sitting to the supine position, the air present in the interpeduncular cistern moves toward the basal-frontal subarachnoid space through the chiasmatic cistern. If only the interpeduncular cistern is filled, the air may pass through so quickly that it is impossible to radiograph the chiasmatic cistern. This cannot happen if the pontine cistern is also well filled because, while the patient is changing his position from sitting to supine, the air present in the pontine cistern collects in the previously emptied interpeduncular cistern. The best visualization of the chiasmatic cistern is obtained in lateral projection (Figs. 1.34a, b). The antero-posterior projection is useful only, but not always, on tomograms (Fig. 1.34d) showing the lateral extension of the cistern and its relationship with the Sylvian cisterns. On the other hand, tomography can also be useful in lateral projection to dissociate the chiasmatic cistern from the superimposed Sylvian cistern and/or the subarachnoid spaces of the convexity. The aspect of the anterior part of the third ventricle is also indispensable for the differential diagnosis of lesions of the sellar region. It must therefore be examined very carefully with the help, if necessary, of tomography (Fig. 1.31) and/or a special projection with the head hyperextended (Fig. 1.59). The late radiographic control can also be useful since the image of the

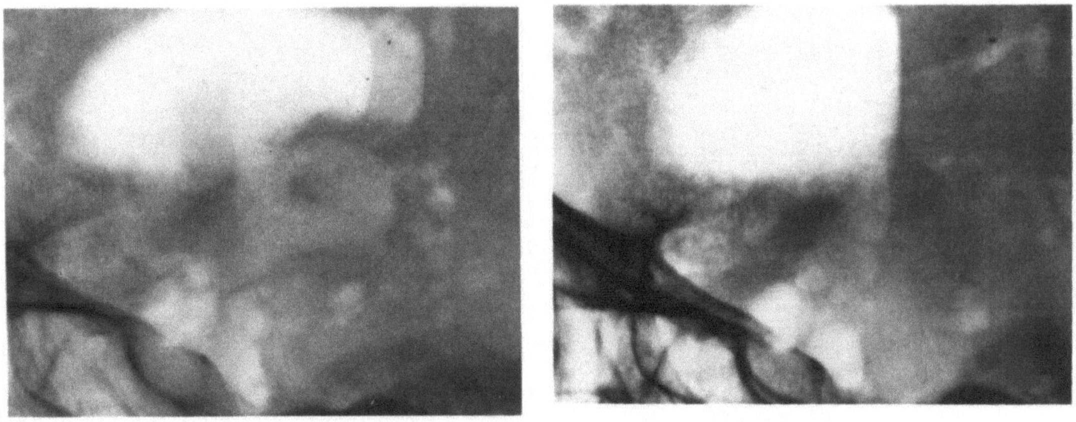

Fig. 1.60a, b. The antero-inferior part of the third ventricle is masked, on the standard radiograph, by air in the subarachnoid space; it is perfectly visible in the radiograph (b), performed 6 hours later, in which the air contained in the cisterns has been reabsorbed

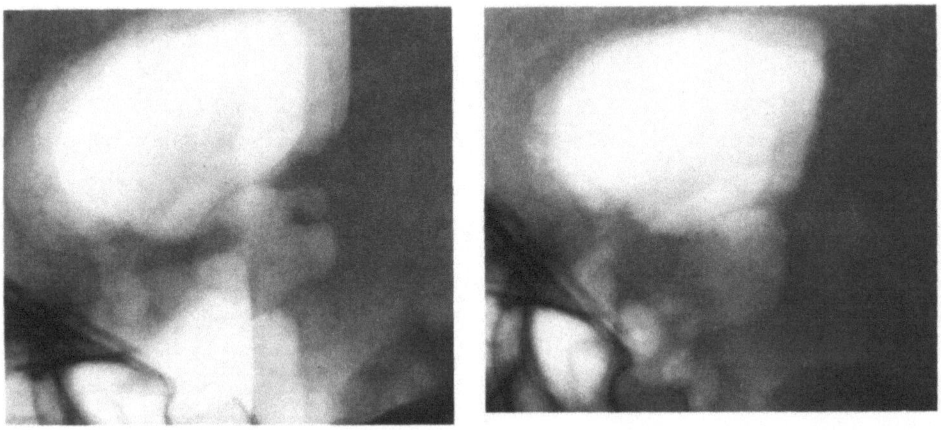

Fig. 1.61a, b. The antero-inferior part of the third ventricle is masked, on the standard radiograph, by air in dilated temporal horn; it is perfectly visible in radiograph (b), performed 6 hours later, in which the air contained in the temporal horn has been reabsorbed

third ventricle appears free from the superimposition of the air contained in the cisterns (Fig. 1.60) or in other structures (Fig. 1.61). Some difficulty may be encountered when the motorized rotating chair is used in radiography where the patient's head is extended—at least with the Princeps, where the tube and cassette cannot be moved down far enough. With these chairs, when the head is down the feet are necessarily up, and there is consequent compression over the diaphragm; this may cause trouble with the pulmonary ventilation, even if the time necessary to take the radiograph is not long. In the majority of cases it is better to release the patient from the head holder and do the radiography in the supine position with the head extended, according to the classical technique.

GAIST and MARTELLI [159] point out that a lumbar puncture often causes syncope in patients with opto-chiasmatic arachnoiditis. They suggest, when a lesion of this type is suspected, that air injection and radiography of the subarachnoid space be carried out first, so that the encephalography is usable even when a syncope prevents its continuation. This problem, however, is now less important because TV monitoring makes the examination much faster. A "functional" cisternography, namely the recording of the time the air takes to progress into the subarachnoid space, has been suggested by BELLONI [33, 34], who wrote valuable papers on the air study of the sellar region. Such a time recording, however, is also afforded by encephalography, which also allows the indispensable examination of the third

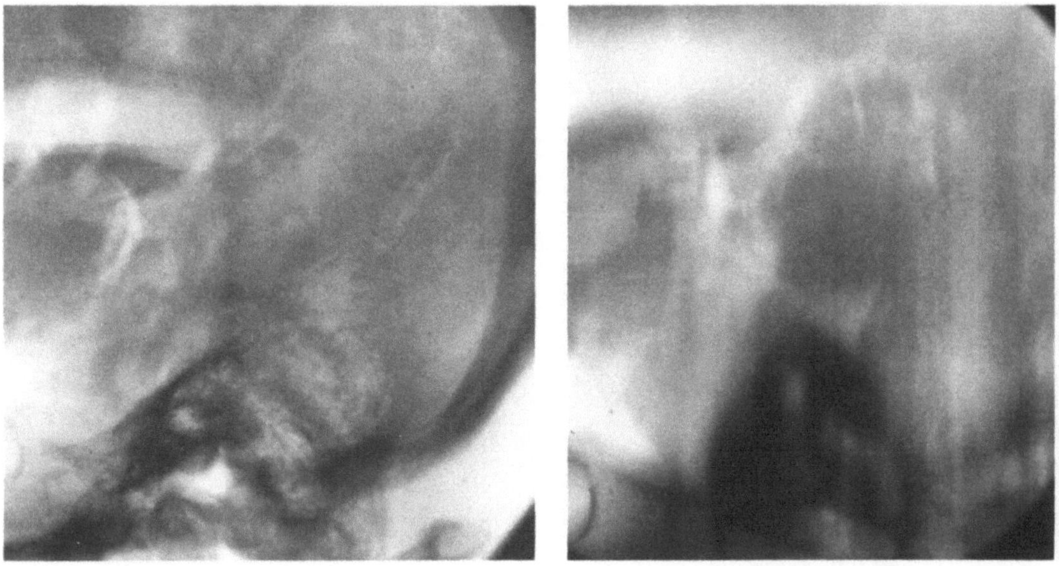

a b

Fig. 1.62a, b. Sulci of the cerebellar vermis are very poorly visible on the standard radiograph (a), while they are rather clearly demonstrated by the tomogram (b)

ventricle together with the cisterns. It is indeed for this reason that fractional encephalography must always be preferred to cisternography.

METZGER [301], SALAMON *et al.* [395] and WACKENHEIM *et al.* [471] have placed particular emphasis on the utility of tomography for the examination of the parasellar cisterns. The last group of authors suggest performing tomography with the head hyperextended and the cutting planes on the midline and 5 to 10 mm to either side. This technique enables both the internal and the external portions of the pericarotid cistern to be studied.

15. Encephalographic Technique in Cases of Atrophy

Cerebellar Atrophy

In normal conditions it is possible to visualize the sulci of the vermian cortex (Fig. 1.62a). The radiological demonstration of such structures is facilitated by tomography (Fig. 1.62b). The encephalographic diagnosis of cerebellar atrophy is based on the dilatation of these subarachnoid sulci (Fig. 1.63), whether associated or not with fourth ventricle dilatation. Even this finding is usually better demonstrated by tomography (Fig. 1.64). Some authors suggest special techniques. LINDGREN [255] increases the head flexion to inject additional air (5–10 ml) while the patient is still in the sitting position and after the study of fourth ventricle, aqueduct, and pontine cistern. With the patient in this position the air passes behind the cerebellum to fill the great cistern and the upper cerebellar cistern. To show a good filling, the radiographs must be taken during or immediately after the introduction of air, since the air tends to reach the cerebral convexity through the cistern of Galeno.

ROBERTSON [371] too, insisted on the importance of a very marked flexion of the head: in the postero-anterior view the central beam forms an angle of 50° with the orbitomeatal plane.

THIÉBAUT, WACKENHEIM, and co-workers [455, 457] described a technique for the visualization of the prevermian cisterns essentially based on lateral midline tomograms. After an injection of 7 ml of air to visualize the fourth ventricle, the aqueduct, and the posterior part of the third ventricle, the head is flexed as much as possible and a further 10 ml of air is rapidly injected; after that the head is kept in this position for another 10 seconds. Then the head is partially drawn back (the central beam and the orbito-meatal plane form an angle of 20–30°) and is kept in this position for 10 seconds. Finally, the head is moved to the initial position and another rapid injection of 5 ml of air is given. For the lateral projection the central beam is directed on the midpoint of a line joining

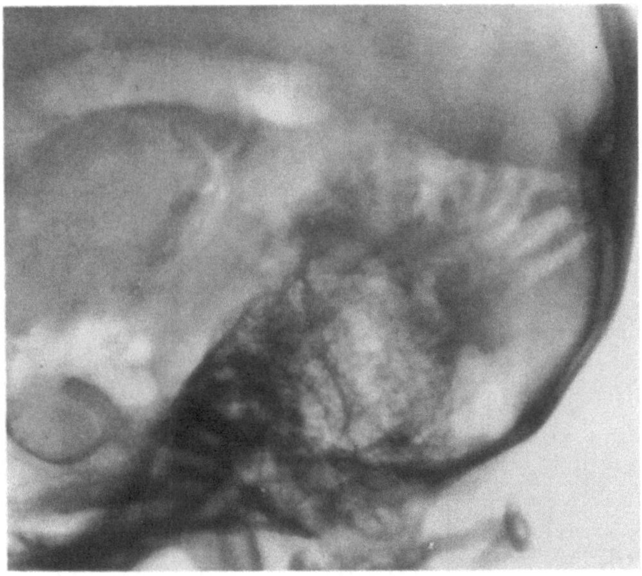

Fig. 1.63. *Cerebellar Atrophy*. Note the dilated vermian sulci

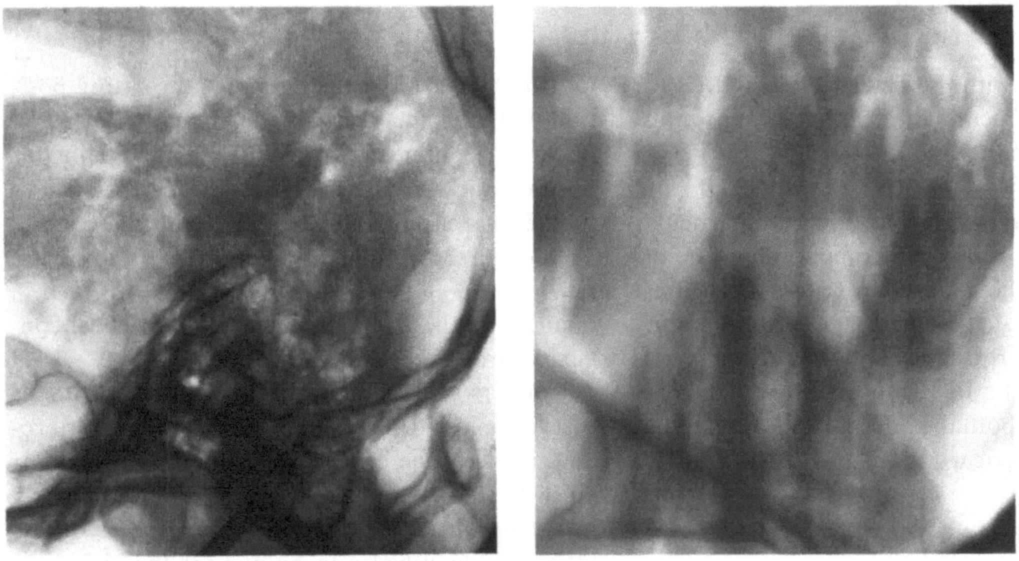

Fig. 1.64a, b. The cerebellar sulci are rather easily visible on the standard radiograph (a); however they are better demonstrated on the tomogram (b)

the external occipital protuberance to the external auditory meatus. If the prevermian cistern is not visualized, the second and third stages of the technique are repeated. In cases of marked cerebellar atrophy, 15 ml of air may be insufficient and further injections may be necessary.

With THIÉBAUT and WACKENHEIM's technique [455, 457] only the median sagittal plane is explored, and we have no reliable information on the cerebellar hemispheres; SUBIRANA and VROUSOS [442] in 1964 therefore suggested making tomograms of the posterior fossa in the postero-anterior view. These are performed after the lateral tomograms and after a further injection of 10 ml of air, always with the head hyperflexed. Four to six tomographies are performed in this way in order to give a better visualization of the air collected over the cerebellar convexity. The first tomogram is taken at the level of the external auditory meatus, the others at distances from 0.5 to 1 cm apart. The tomographic visualization of the subarachnoid space over the cerebellum may be spoiled by the shadows of the facial bones

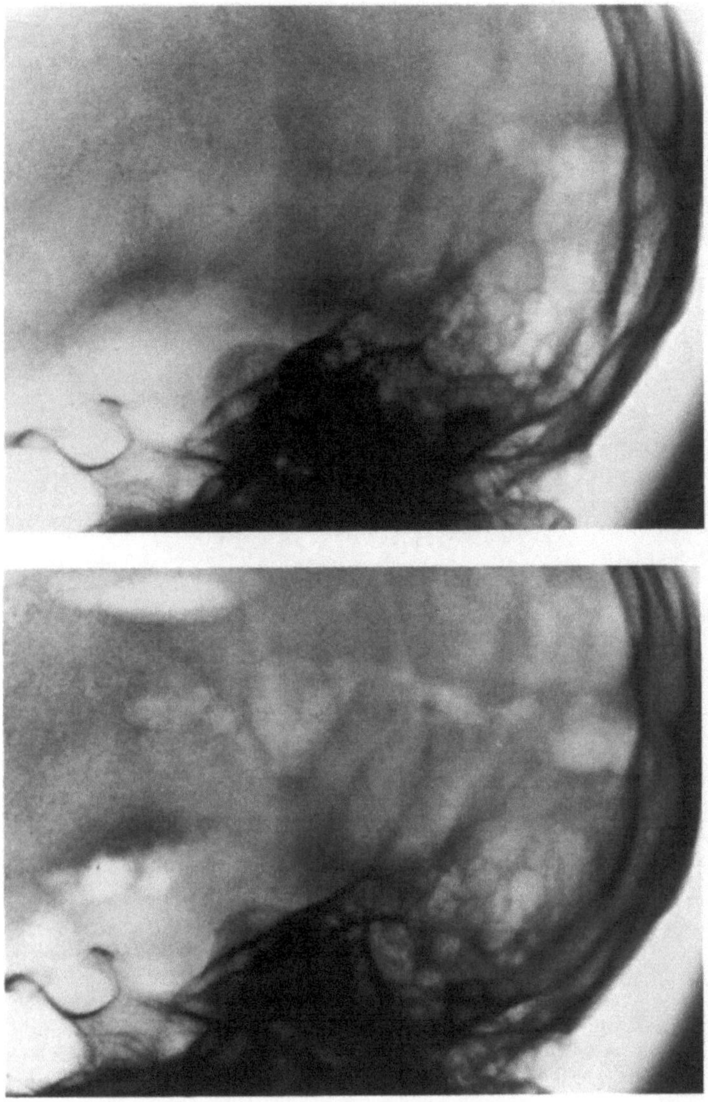

a

b

Fig. 1.65a, b. The head is positioned for filling the ventricular system. After two 10-ml injections the air collects in the great cistern (a). The head has been hyperextended and then flexed again. The air fills partially the ventricular system and partially the vermian sulci (b), which it reaches by the anterior way; in fact, a small amount of contrast is still present in the upper portion of the interpeduncular cistern, while the amount of air in the great cistern has considerably decreased

and by the air in lateral ventricles. In this case one must reduce the head flexion so that the orbitomeatal line forms an angle of 25° with the horizontal plane (through which the central beam passes).

To be honest, we do not think that one should speak about special techniques when studying cerebellar atrophy. Tomography is a complementary detail in the encephalographic technique, which must be employed, when necessary, in cases of atrophy in the same way as with the study of other lesions. Also, we are not convinced of the necessity of injecting large amounts of air to "force" the filling-up of the great cistern, but we do favor the passage of air into the vermian cistern. On the other hand, we think that the subarachnoid space above the cerebellum is more easily filled through the anterior route, namely through the cistern of Galeno. In our opinion a marked flexion of the head facilitates the visualization of the vermian sulci (Figs. 1.65, 1.66) because such a flexion brings the upper part of the brain stem to a lower level than the upper pole of the vermis.

Cerebral Atrophy

The encephalographic diagnosis of cerebral atrophy is based on two signs: dilatation of the lateral ventricles and/or of the third ventricle (atrophy of the white matter) and dilatation of the subarachnoid space of the convexity (cortical atrophy). These two

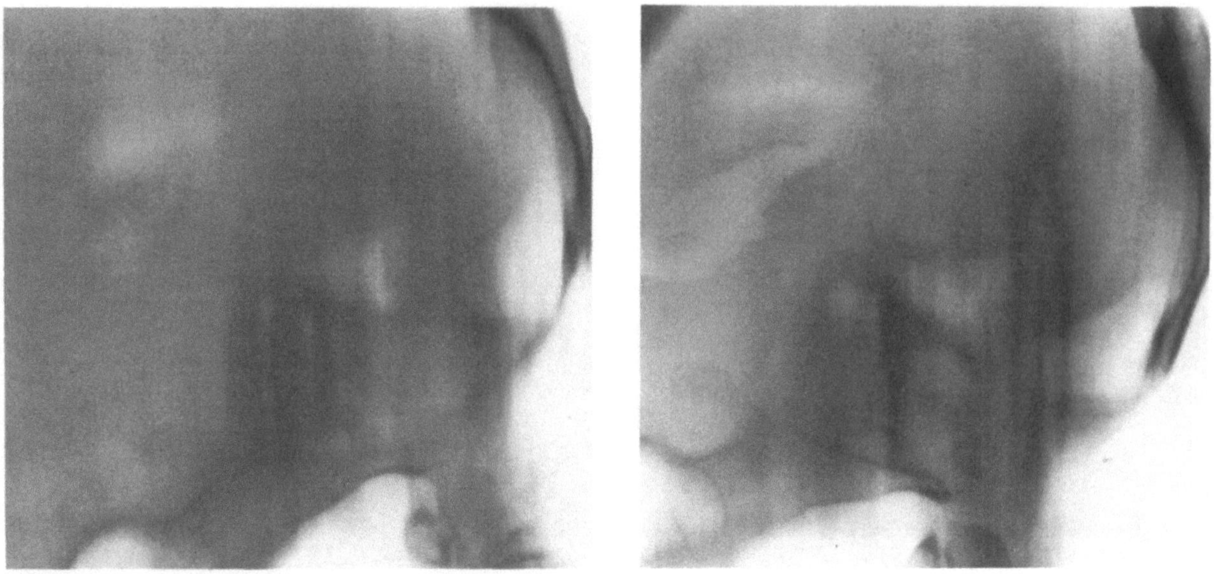

a

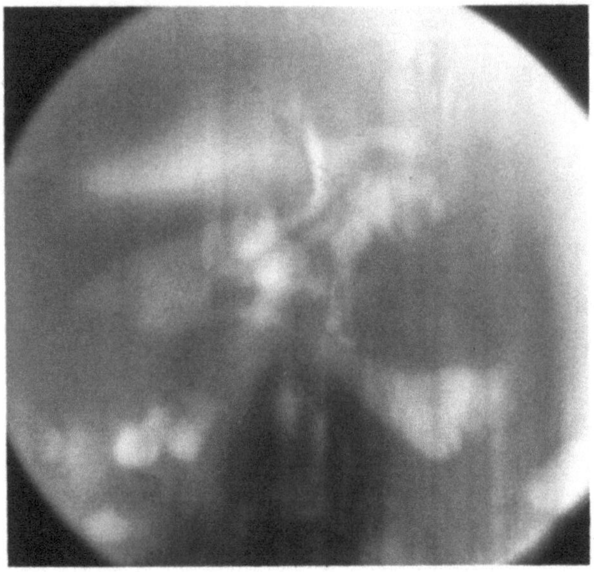

c

Fig. 1.66a–c. *Influence of Head Position for Filling of the Superior Vermis Sulci.* a) The examination begins. The head is flexed. The great cistern, the fourth ventricle, the aqueduct, and the posterior part of the third ventricle are visualized. b) The head is hyperflexed (radiograph is performed immediately after a). The cerebellar sulci are not visualized, but some air contained in the third ventricle re-enters the fourth ventricle. c) After the head has been extended to fill the basal cisterns, the head is flexed again. Interpeduncular and Galen's cisterns are visualized. No additional air was injected between a) and c)

forms can be either diffuse or localized and can co-exist.

Ventricular dilatations of small extent must be evaluated with caution. Various factors should be considered: age, sex, relationship between ventricular and cranial morphology; normal variations in the size and shape of the ventricles; and technical factors like the focus-to-film distance and the amount of air injected.

The focus-to-film distance is important since the structures appear smaller on radiographs taken at a greater distance. This problem, however, does not arise with modern craniographs where the focus-to-film distance is usually constant. The amount of air injected must be carefully evaluated to avoid insufficient and/or asymmetric filling of the lateral ventricles, which might make it difficult or even impossible to diagnose localized cerebral atrophy.

In 1951 LINDGREN [256] emphasized that the quick filling of the subarachnoid space is a sign of cortical atrophy. His opinion was confirmed in 1957 by RUGGIERO [374], who thinks that when a structure appears on a radiograph on which it should not be visible, one must be aware of the probability of atrophy.

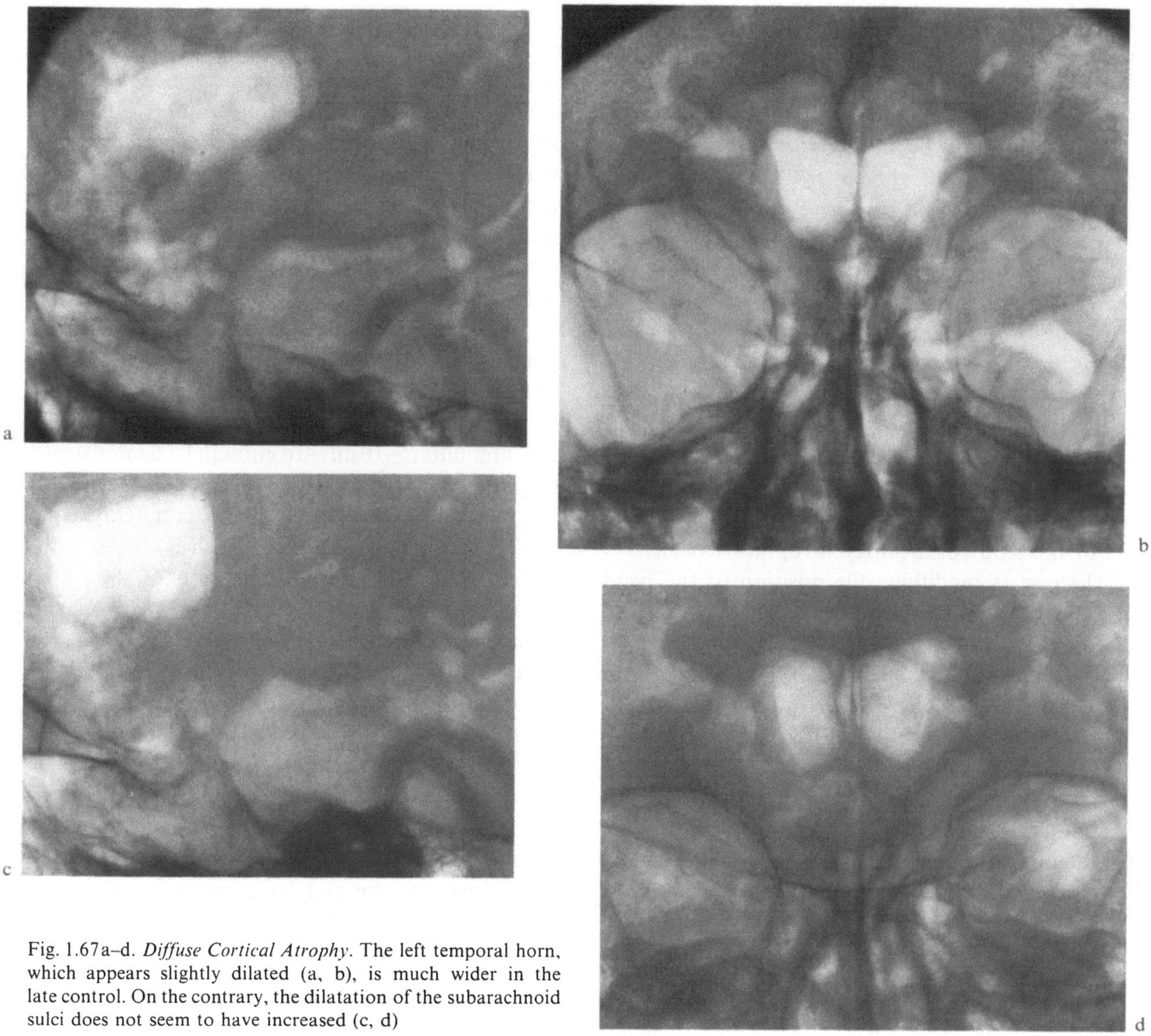

Fig. 1.67a–d. *Diffuse Cortical Atrophy*. The left temporal horn, which appears slightly dilated (a, b), is much wider in the late control. On the contrary, the dilatation of the subarachnoid sulci does not seem to have increased (c, d)

Marked asymmetrical filling of lateral ventricles may lead to diagnostic errors. LINDGREN [256] demonstrated that in cases of ventricular dilatation (and consequently of atrophy) the unequal distribution of air in the two ventricles may cause modification in the appearance of the septum pellucidum. Such modifications are variable: sometimes the septum pellucidum appears to bulge on the side opposite the better filled ventricle, and sometimes it is actually displaced. In LINDGREN'S [256] opinion diagnostic errors are easier in the latter case.

Late radiographic follow-up may also be useful, facilitating the distinction between some ventricular and subarachnoid structures which sometimes may appear superimposed at the moment of the examination. The trick of this method consists of exploiting the different times of air reabsorption at the level of the different structures. By this method, poroencephaly was demonstrated by PENDERGRASS and PERRYMAN [334], and by PENDERGRASS *et al.* [335]. RUGGIERO [375] showed asymmetries of the temporal horns (Fig. 1.67). None of these findings were present at the moment of encephalography.

The examination of the poroencephalic cavities must be very accurate in order to demonstrate their actual dimensions. Radiographs in frontal and lateral projections should be taken with the patient in supine and prone positions and also lying on either side.

When the subarachnoid space is dilated, a larger amount of air must be injected (and possibly more CSF withdrawn) with the patient's head extended.

Sometimes, in cases of severe cortical atrophy, air collects in the subarachnoid space at the very beginning of the examination, yet no air enters the ventricular system in spite of the correct position of the head. A technical trick, though it does not always help, can be used in such an event: the air is injected very slowly while the patient's head is kept flexed as far as possible; after that the head is gradually extended. With such a technique the contrast is first accumulated in the great cistern; then it is "accompanied" into the fourth ventricle.

For the study of localized atrophies ROBERTSON [371] suggests modifying the position of the head in different ways, according to the site of the lesion. He states that, once the pontine and interpeduncular cisterns are filled, the air can be directed from these structures in one of four different directions by giving the patient's head different positions:

1. *Head Flexed.* The air moves through the circumpeduncular cisterns, toward the cistern of Galeno, and from the latter it spreads chiefly into the parieto-occipital and calcarine fissures.
2. *Head and Neck Extended.* The air moves toward the chiasmatic cistern and later toward the cisterna terminalis, corpus callosum, and cingulate sulcus.
3. *Head Straight.* The air moves through the suprasellar cistern toward both the Sylvian cisterns to spread, finally, into the frontal and parietal sulci. If the head is inclined to one side, there will be an elective filling of the contralateral structures.

For the particular study of the frontal region ROBERTSON [371] advises extending the head with the patient still in the sitting position, after having completed the injection of the ventricles and the subarachnoid space. Radiographs should be taken in postero-anterior, oblique projection with the cassette inclined about 120 and the central beam directed perpendicular to it. On the other hand, for the study of the occipital sulci, the head should be flexed and the projection inverted.

The manner of the air injection and the position of the patient's head play an important role in the correct filling of the subarachnoid space. We have already seen that rapid air injection is advisable to ensure a good visualization of the basal cisterns, since it prevents the air from proceeding toward the convexity. Now, in the case of cortical atrophy, the air should be injected slowly, and consequently the patient's head has to be kept extended for a longer time, as also suggested by ROBERTSON [371]. Of course, such a maneuver has to be performed after the study of the basal cisterns.

The various authors do not agree on the amount of air to be injected. LINDGREN [256] thinks that small amounts (5–10 ml) are enough to demonstrate atrophy if the subarachnoid space is not obstructed and if it is filled with CSF. The air is quickly aspirated in the atrophic region, which is more easily studied without the superimposition of the other structures. SHAPIRO and ROBINSON [418], on the contrary, consider a small amount of air inadequate, especially in the case of diffuse atrophy. In our opinion the truth is somewhere between: there is no doubt that the elective and rapid filling of an area of cortical atrophy by a small amount of air is pathognomonic; but it is also true that in some cases larger amounts are necessary: for example, when the atrophic area is too limited (insufficient to aspirate the air), or conversely, when the atrophic process is diffuse and small amounts of gas can reveal only part of it. We must remember that, in contrast to what happens in the ventricles, the air does not move easily in the subarachnoid space.

16. Encephalography with Urea

Introduction and Literature

JAVID and SETTLAGE [236, 237] in 1956 suggested the use of urea to reduce the cerebral edema. The method spread immediately to both neurological and neurosurgical practice; see references 29, 54, 76, 83, 178, 184, 194, 225, 234, 235, 247, 277, 278, o10, 441, 473, 480. The use of urea in encephalography was prooposed between 1961 and 1962, by

ENGESET and HAUGE [140] and by RUGGIERO and PACIFICO [392], working independently, and two different techniques were developed.

ENGESET and HAUGE [140] injected intravenously a 30% solution in a 5% glucoside at the speed of about 60 drops a minute, following JEPPSSON and JÄRPE's technique [240]. The total amount of urea injected is 1.5 g/kg body weight. The encephalography is performed from a few hours to 24–48 hours afterward.

The technique proposed by RUGGIERO and PACIFICO [392], to be described in the next section, is based on the principle of using urea *during* the encephalography and *only* when necessary; the amount injected never exceeds 40 g.

A report based on 33 cases was published. Later on, RUGGIERO [379] presented at the National Hospital in London an analysis of 67 urea encephalographies; the value of this technique was then confirmed at the Seventh Symposium Neuroradiologicum in New York [383].

In 1964 BACIOCCO and CHIAPPETTA [20], unaware of RUGGIERO's work, published their experience of 50 cases of "intracranial hypertension syndrome and clinical signs of posterior fossa tumors" verified anatomically (by operation and/or autopsy). In none of these cases had the encephalography led to a correct diagnosis, even though a generic diagnosis of posterior fossa tumor was possible in many of them. The examination was repeated "after injection of a 30% solution of urea in 10% invertine": in 30 cases the subtentorial part of the ventricular system was visualized, allowing a definite diagnosis; in 11 cases only the cisterns were visible, leading to the diagnosis of an expansive process in the posterior fossa; in the remaining 9 cases air did not enter the skull, but the diagnosis was suggested by the signs of herniation of the cerebellar tonsils and of "cervical overfilling" (DI BIAGIO and SASSAROLI [115]).

BACIOCCO and CHIAPPETTA [20], as well as ENGESET and HAUGE [140], limited their study to the tumors of the posterior fossa, while RUGGIERO and his co-workers [378, 387, 388, 392] insisted on the utility of the urea technique for supratentorial tumors as well. RUGGIERO and his co-workers feel that, in contrast to what happens in posterior fossa tumors, the correct encephalographic localization of a supratentorial lesion can very seldom be obtained without visualization of the ventricular system.

In 1963 DILENGE *et al.* [132] suggested diluting the urea in mannitol instead of in glucose. The "rebound" action of urea, inducing a new stage of cerebral edema following the cellular dehydration, would thus be reduced or even avoided. This technique has also been used in our department. Although no comparative systematic research was made, our results seem to confirm those of DILENGE *et al.* [132]. These authors do not refer to the mechanism of the combined action of urea and mannitol, and we have been unable to find any explanation in the neuroradiological literature. For this reason, and because of our great interest in this technique, we deem it useful to give a short résumé of what we were able to understand about this problem with the help of some anesthesist colleagues.

Mechanism of Action of Urea and Mannitol

The osmotic activity of a substance is directly proportional to the number of particles present in a certain amount of solute.

Osmotic diuresis is the increase in the urine flow caused by the excretion of the particles carrying water. Therefore, a fundamental element of osmotic diuresis is the presence in the injected diuretic solution of a large number of solute molecules, without any direct relationship with their molecular weight. Obviously, the diuretic effect is more active if the solute is only partially absorbed by the nephron (urea) or not absorbed at all (mannitol).

The dehydrating effect of osmotic diuretics is essentially due to two factors: increased loss of water by the tissues and loss of electrolytes, especially sodium. The natriuric effect depends on three factors: 1. reduced tubular reabsorption of sodium due to the creation of a transtubular sodium gradient (the transtubular gradient of an electrolyte is the expression of the difference in ion concentration between the wall of the renal tubule and the urine present in the tubular lumen); 2. the washing effect on the tubules exerted by high urine flow; 3. passive diffusion of the electrolyte.

The ideal osmotic diuretic must have the following fundamental properties:

1. low molecular weight (mol.wt.). This allows a high concentration, and consequently an increased osmotic action.
2. It should not be metabolized, so its effect is constant and intense.
3. It should not diffuse in the cells to ensure that there will be no rebound.
4. There should be no secondary effects and toxicity, especially for the kidneys.

From the analysis of the above-mentioned factors, it is clear that the relationship between the molecular weight and the concentration of the particles favors urea. Hence urea (mol.wt. 60) can be used in a higher concentration (30%) than mannitol (mol.wt. 182.17). Furthermore, urea is not metabolized, while mannitol is partially metabolized, even if 80% of the given dose is eliminated by normal subjects in the urine within 24 hours. However, the high diffusivity of the urea, both in the cells and in the interstitial tissue, causes cellular hyperhydration (rebound effect) following the initial cellular dehydration that exists when the diuretic substance is present chiefly in the plasma. This happens because water is bound to the urea and they both move together from one milieu to another; this movement stops when osmotic equilibrium is established between the particles present in the circulating fluid and the urea molecules present in the cells on the one hand, and the interstitial tissue on the other.

Mannitol has almost no rebound effect. In fact, because of its higher molecular weight, it seems to diffuse only in the extracellular space. First there is a water flux from the extracellular space toward the vessels; then, as the drug spreads in the extracellular space, there is a water flux from the intracellu-

a

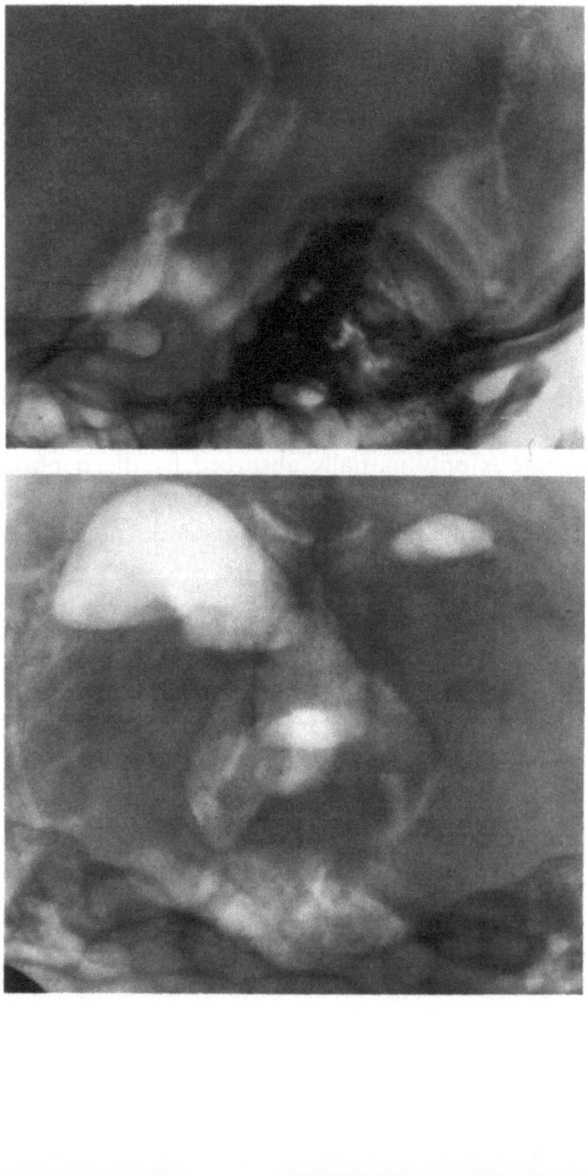

c

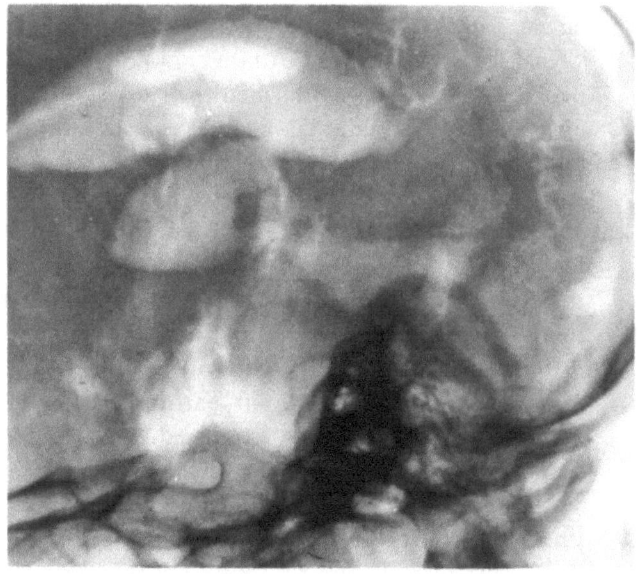

b

Fig. 1.68a–c. *Urea Technique. Medulloblastoma of the Fourth Ventricle.* The air does not fill the ventricular system (a); the aspect of the subarachnoid space indicates the presence of a tumor in the posterior portion of the posterior fossa. After injection of 20 g urea (b, c), the visualization of the fourth ventricle is excellent and diagnosis is unquestionable lar space to the extracellular space. The absence of tubular reabsorption, and consequently the total elimination of the drug by the kidney, still further reduces the possibility of a rebound effect.

The low diffusivity of urea in the cerebral tissue (especially a sick one) produces an increase of osmotic pressure in the brain, and consequently flows toward it. In other words, in the first stage the high concentration of the urea in the circulating fluid creates an osmotic gradient between the vessels and the system cerebral tissue–CSF, which is extremely favorable from a therapeutic viewpoint. The diffusion of urea toward the cerebral tissue and CSF proceeds slowly; thus the osmolarity of these structures increases progressively until osmotic equilibrium is achieved. During this time CSF pressure decreases very quickly (i.e. urea acts more rapidly on CSF than on the nerve cells). Later on, the particles present in the blood decrease as a result of the elimination of the urea via the kidneys. Since the osmolarity of the brain decreases more slowly, there will be a favorable gradient to the brain, with consequent reflux of water toward the nerve cells. This explains the mechanism of the rebound phenomenon.

Brain dehydration is at its maximum about 20–30 minutes after urea administration; it returns to normal values in 1 to 6 hours. With the highest doses of urea used by us in encephalography (40 g in an adult subject) the fluid displacement from the cerebral to the plasmatic sector was about 250 ml. The effect of urea is observed only at the level of the CSF, as proved by tests made with radioactive urea. With a mannitol solution of the same density, the displacement of the fluid in the first 2–4 hours is about 200 ml; the total displacement of the fluid requires 5–8 hours and is about 500 ml. Urea has therefore a more rapid, but less actively dehydrating effect on the brain than mannitol.

The urea rebound effect seems to reach its maximum 12–18 hours after the administration of the drug and to disappear 24 hours later when it diffuses from the tissues into the blood. Naturally, this explanation is only schematic; in reality, the phenomena of dehydration and rebound continuously alternate until the drug is completely eliminated in the urine.

The above is the most generally accepted theory to explain the urea rebound effect. It does not, however, explain why urea does not have the same effect on the cerebral cells and the CSF pressure.

To conclude, urea seems to be the most suitable hyperosmotic agent for the neuroradiologist's purpose because of its rapid action, especially on CSF pressure. Mannitol could be used instead of glucose as the solvent for urea since it increases the latter's dehydrating effect, yet delays or even abolishes its rebound effect.

Technique

If, during an encephalography, the filling of the ventricular system is poor or absent, urea administration is started: 40 g of urea crystals dissolved in 110 ml of 10% mannitol solution is given as an intravenous drip, at the rate of 60 drops a minute. The effect of the urea is monitored on TV. If it is working well, administration is stopped; otherwise, the entire amount of solution is injected. To prepare the solution and set up the transfusion requires at least 5 minutes. This might be too long in cases of severe intracranial hypertension where the safety of the examination often depends on its speed. It is advisable, therefore, to prepare the solution before starting the encephalography; it is better to waste the solution than to prolong the examination in the sitting position.

The maximum amount of urea injected is—we repeat—40 g. Rarely, however, is the whole dose necessary, since the effect of the urea is usually seen after 15–20 g (Fig. 1.68). The injection should not be stopped too soon. Fig. 1.69 illustrates a case in which the examination was repeated with the injection of an increased amount of urea, giving a much better result.

It would be a mistake to limit the use of the urea technique to cases in which increased intracranial pressure is demonstrated by manometric control of the lumbar CSF. In some supratentorial tumors there can be severe edema, usually with temporal herniation. This may cause such severe compression of the brain stem that the cisterns and/or the aqueduct can be occluded. In such cases there is no longer any communication between the supra- and intra-tentorial CSF circulation, so that the pressure measured is actually the pressure of the spinal subarachnoid space, and this can be normal or even below normal (Fig. 1.70).

Complications

After urea administration the patient's reaction is constantly observed by means of cardio-circulatory, respiratory, and renal monitoring.

During the examination cardiac rhythm, blood pressure, and respiration are checked every 10 min. A slight increase in blood pressure (10–20 mm Hg) is usually observed, while a slightly increased heart rate (about 20 beats per min) and respiration rate (5–10 inspirations per min) is observed in about 20% of the patients.

On the morning of the encephalography the urine and blood nitrogen are tested. These tests are repeated 1 hour after the examination and then every 8 hours until values are normal. Hyperazotemia is observed in nearly all cases at the end of the examination, very rarely exceeding 1 $g^0/_{00}$ and usually becoming normal after 48 hours. Proteinuria, hematuria, and sedimented cylinders are also occasionally noted.

Up to now about 300 urea encephalographies have been performed in our department, mostly for intracranial expansive processes. The technique can definitely be considered benign, the only contraindication being severe renal and/or hepatic insufficiency.

Results

In this chapter we emphasize points from some of our previous works [378, 379, 383, 387, 388, 392] and from the paper which Dettori *et al.* [114] recently presented at the Annual Meeting of the European Society of Neuroradiology in Bologna.

First of all, it is necessary to define what we mean by a useful examination. We feel that the urea technique must be regarded as useful because it frequently permits better visualization of the ventricular system and the subarachnoid space which were previously not visible or only poorly visible. In other words, urea is useful when its administration favorably influences the diagnosis.

Dettori *et al.* [114] include 179 cases from the Neuroradiological Department of the Ospedale Maggiore in Bologna. Their conclusions are as follows:

1. Urea gives better results in supratentorial tumors than in infratentorial ones.
2. Urea gives better results in hemispheric tumors than in midline and paramedian ones.
3. Urea gives better results in extracerebral tumors than in intracerebral ones.
4. Better results are obtained for hemispheric and/or extracerebral tumors, regardless of whether the lesion is infratentorial or supratentorial.

In some cases the urea technique is unsuccessful. Why? In the presence of a tumor the CSF pathways can be reduced to a virtual cavity, either by the tumor itself or by the nervous structures adjacent to the tumor, which are often edematous. It is obvious that in the first case the CSF pathways can "reopen" as a result of the action of urea, which reduces the edema, whereas no such effect can take place in the case of direct tumor invasion.

Concerning tumors in the posterior fossa, there is one important statistical consideration: when urea has no effect it is very likely that the tumor occupies the midline. Moreover, recent progress in

a

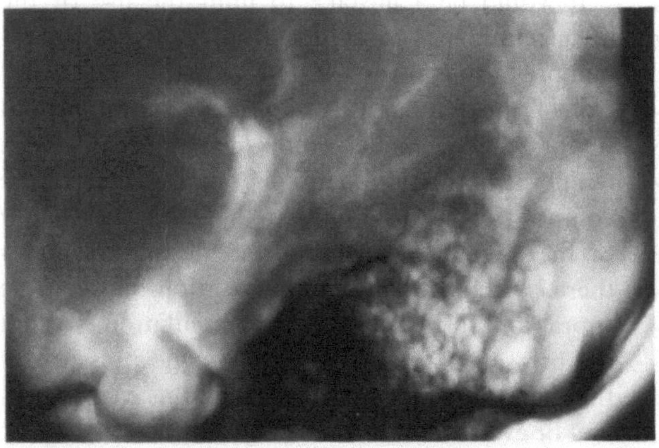

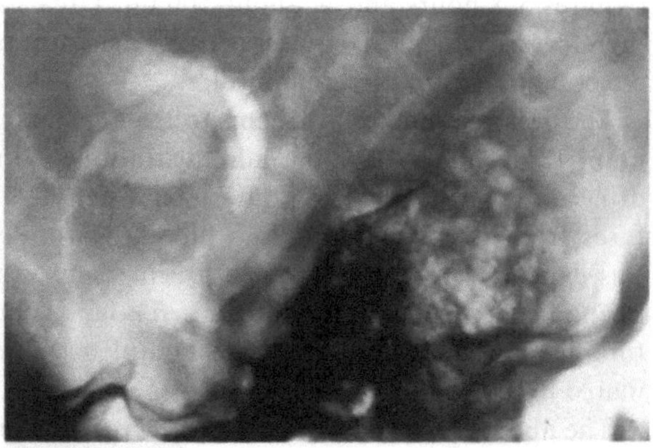

b

Fig. 1.69a and b

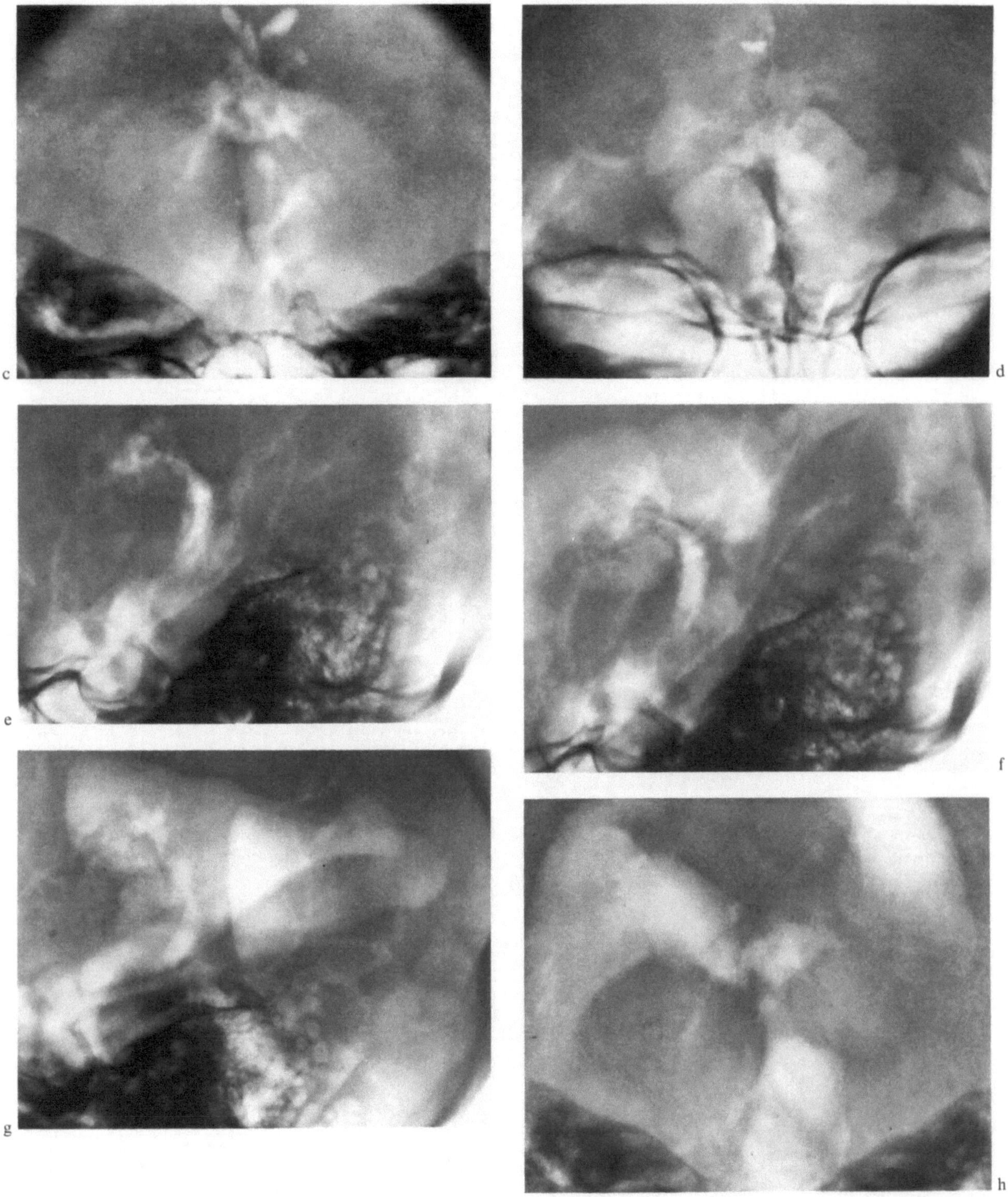

Fig. 1.69 a–h. *Urea Technique. Tentorium Meningioma with Both Supra- and Infratentorial Development.* The ventricular system is not filled (a). The fourth ventricle, aqueduct, and posterior portion of the third ventricle are visualized after urea injection (b, c). This was stopped after 34 g, and more air was injected only a very small amount of which entered the ventricles; this was insufficient for a complete study (d). Encephalography was repeated two weeks later. Again the air did not enter the ventricular system (e) and a further administration of urea was carried out: after 40 g, the air entered the ventricles easily (f), showing the deformation of the right trygone and occipital horn (g, h). The dilatation of the aqueduct and fourth ventricle also shows that the edema had disappeared

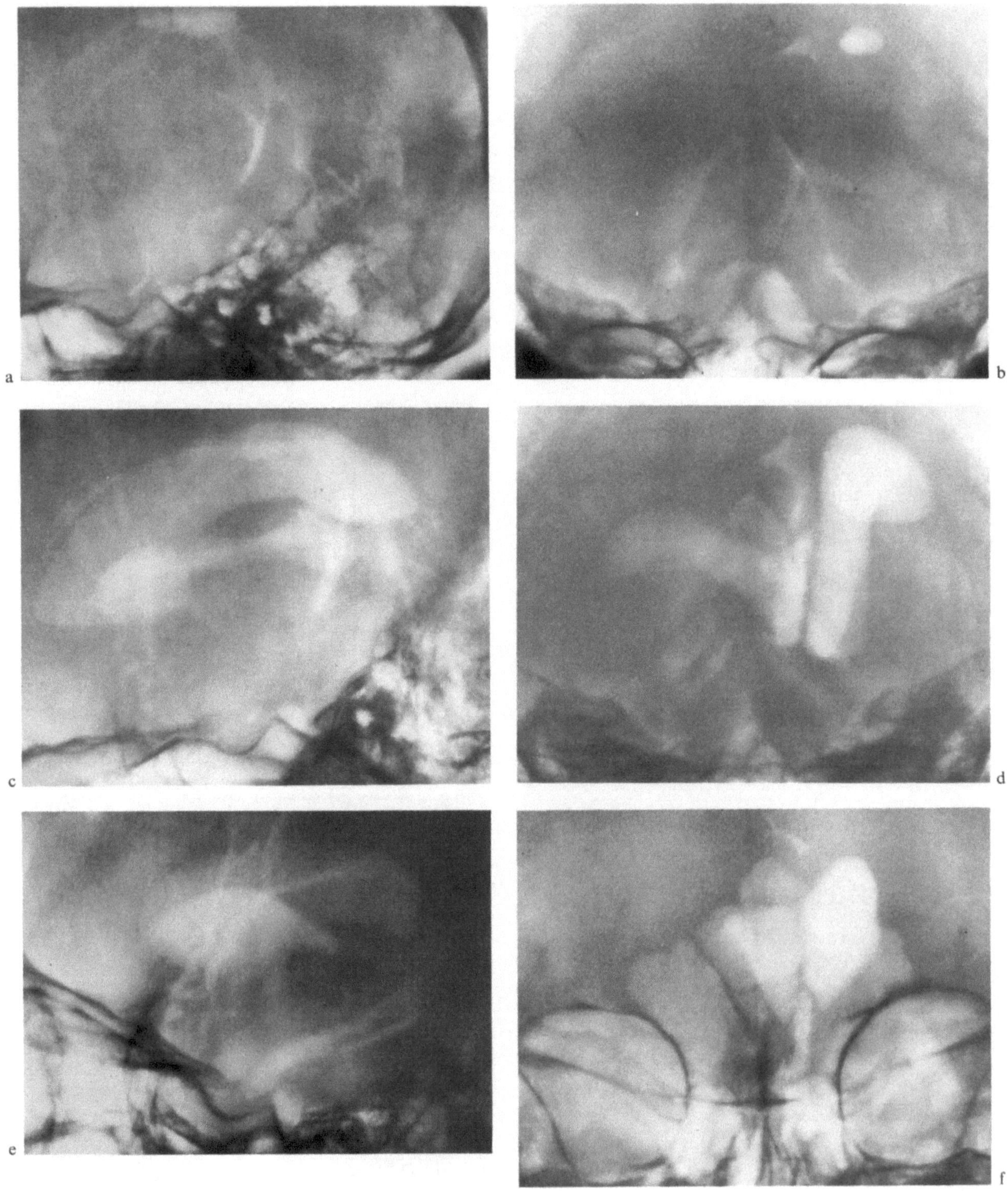

Fig. 1.70a–f. *Right Parasagittal Meningioma.* The initial CSF pressure is 22. The air practically does not pass above the tentorium (a, b). After injection of 30 g of urea, the lateral ventricles are perfectly visualized (c–f)

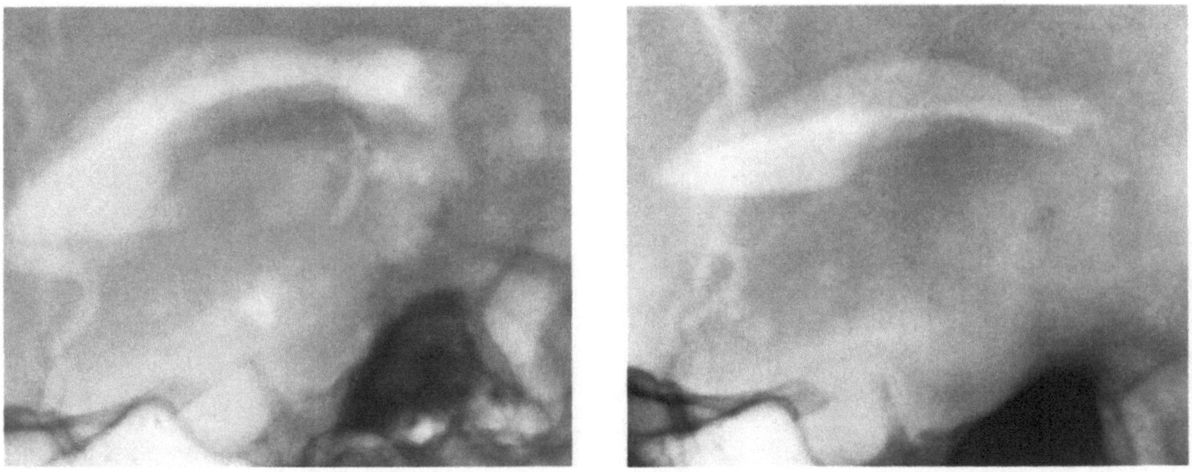
a b

Fig. 1.71 a, b. *Left Fronto-Parietal Arteriovenous Aneurysm.* In the late control (b) the downward displacement of the left ventricle seems to be increased

the examination and interpretation of the cisterns, and the use of tomography, which can increase the diagnostic value of an unsatisfactory ventricular filling, means that good visualization of the aqueduct and fourth ventricle today is less essential for the diagnosis of posterior fossa tumors than it used to be.

Finally, we should mention that urea can also influence the filling of the subarachnoid space. However, we do not wish to express a final opinion on this point at present. As a matter of fact, it has not been shown that easier filling of the cisterns (as a result of reduced edema of the adjacent structures) necessarily means diagnostic improvement, because our diagnosis is based solely on the cisterns. In conclusion, there are still many unsolved points. There is no doubt, however, that the urea technique is useful for the diagnosis of cerebral tumors and that it should be regarded as a definite advance of the encephalographic technique.

17. Encephalography with Pulmonary Hyperventilation

Bernini *et al.* [39] performed pulmonary hyperventilation "with both positive and negative pressure" in 25 cases (10 normal subjects, 10 with infratentorial tumors, 5 with supratentorial tumors) in which the ventricular system was not visualized at encephalography. These authors used a mixture of equal parts of oxygen, nitrous oxide, and atmospheric air. They obtained good visualization of both the ventricular system and the subarachnoid space in all cases. They claimed that this favorable result was a result of the reduction of the cerebral mass, secondary to the diminution of the arteriolar lumen and increased venous outflow. The technique was well tolerated in all cases and no rebound phenomena were observed.

18. Late Radiographic Follow-up

In 1960 Ruggiero and Smaltino [376] demonstrated the diagnostic usefulness of a radiological re-examination of the ventricular system 24 hours after encephalography. They showed that this technique was particularly useful in patients with tumors. Prior to this the matter had been referred to in papers dealing with the volumetric modifications of the ventricles [62, 145, 241, 249, 404, 437], the aspect of the subdural space [177, 293, 329], and occasionally the study of atrophy [333, 399].

The utility of late radiographic follow-up was recently confirmed by Ruggiero *et al.* [393], who reviewed a large number of examinations. The technique works for two reasons: 1. the deformation of the ventricular system can increase with time; 2. some structures—either normal or pathological—that were not visualized or poorly visualized at the time of encephalography can be satisfactorily shown in later checks. To explain these findings,

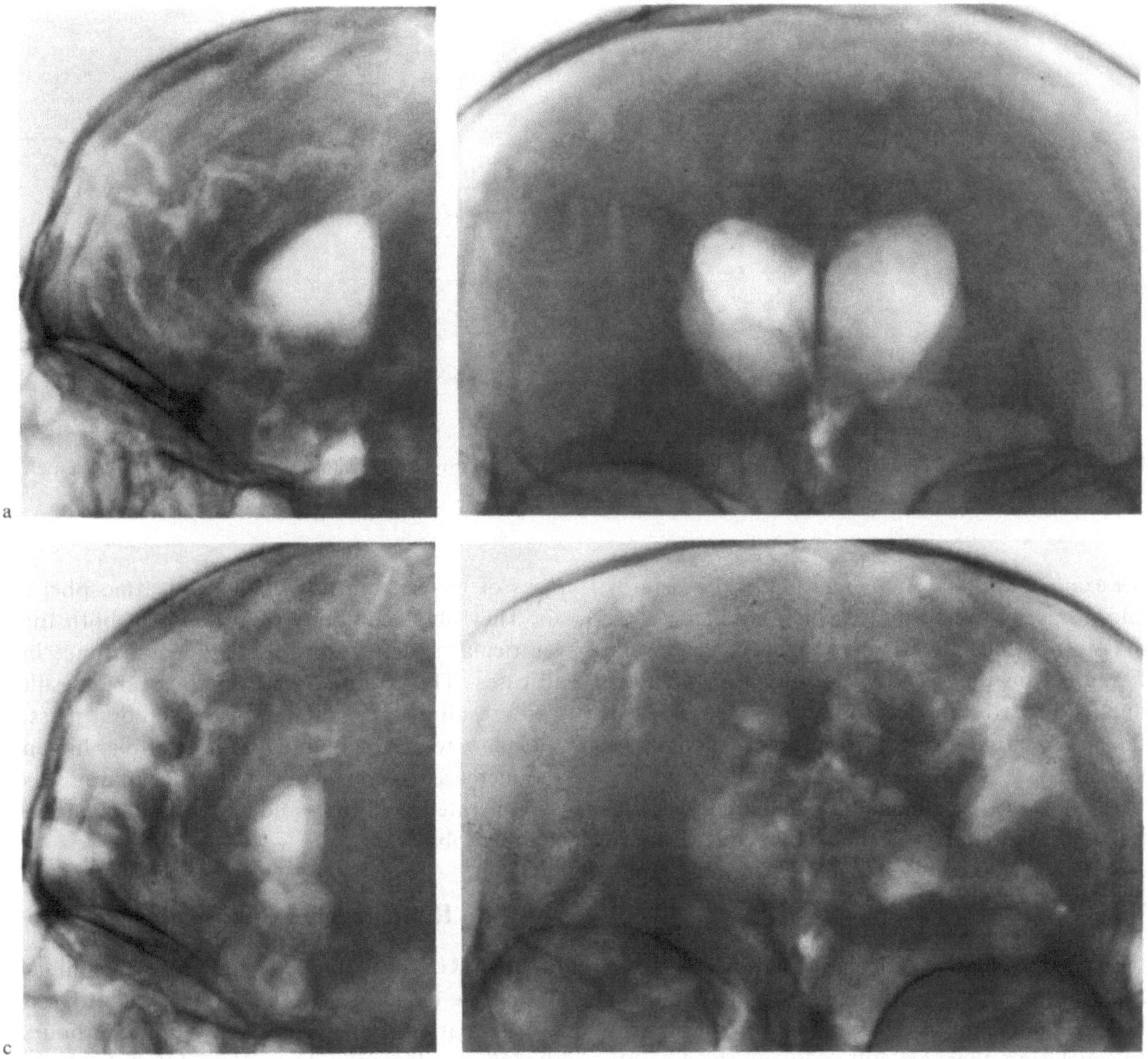

Fig. 1.72a–d. *Left Frontal Cortical Atrophy*. On the standard radiographs (a, b) the ventricles appear dilated, the subarachnoid space is not very well injected but it has a normal appearance, except for a slight dilatation of the frontal sulci. After 6 hours (c, d) these appear considerably dilated, especially on the left side, where the air is collected in a big pouch having a vague poroencephalic appearance

the authors [393] carried out a series of checks on 10 patients under particular technical conditions. Each patient was checked every hour for 6 hours. Their conclusions were as follows:

1. In normal conditions air reabsorption in the ventricles is rapid during the first hour; it becomes slower from the second to the sixth hour. The contrary is true for the subarachnoid space. After longer intervals (for example, 24 or 48 hours after the examination) the phenomenon is inverted: almost all the air present in the subarachnoid space is reabsorbed, while a certain amount of air still remains in the ventricles. Then the ventricular outline can be recognized more easily without the superimposition of the air in the subarachnoid space. In this way a sort of "ventriculography without ventricular puncture" can be obtained, offering the advantages of both encephalography and ventriculography. (Fig. 1.60, 1.61).

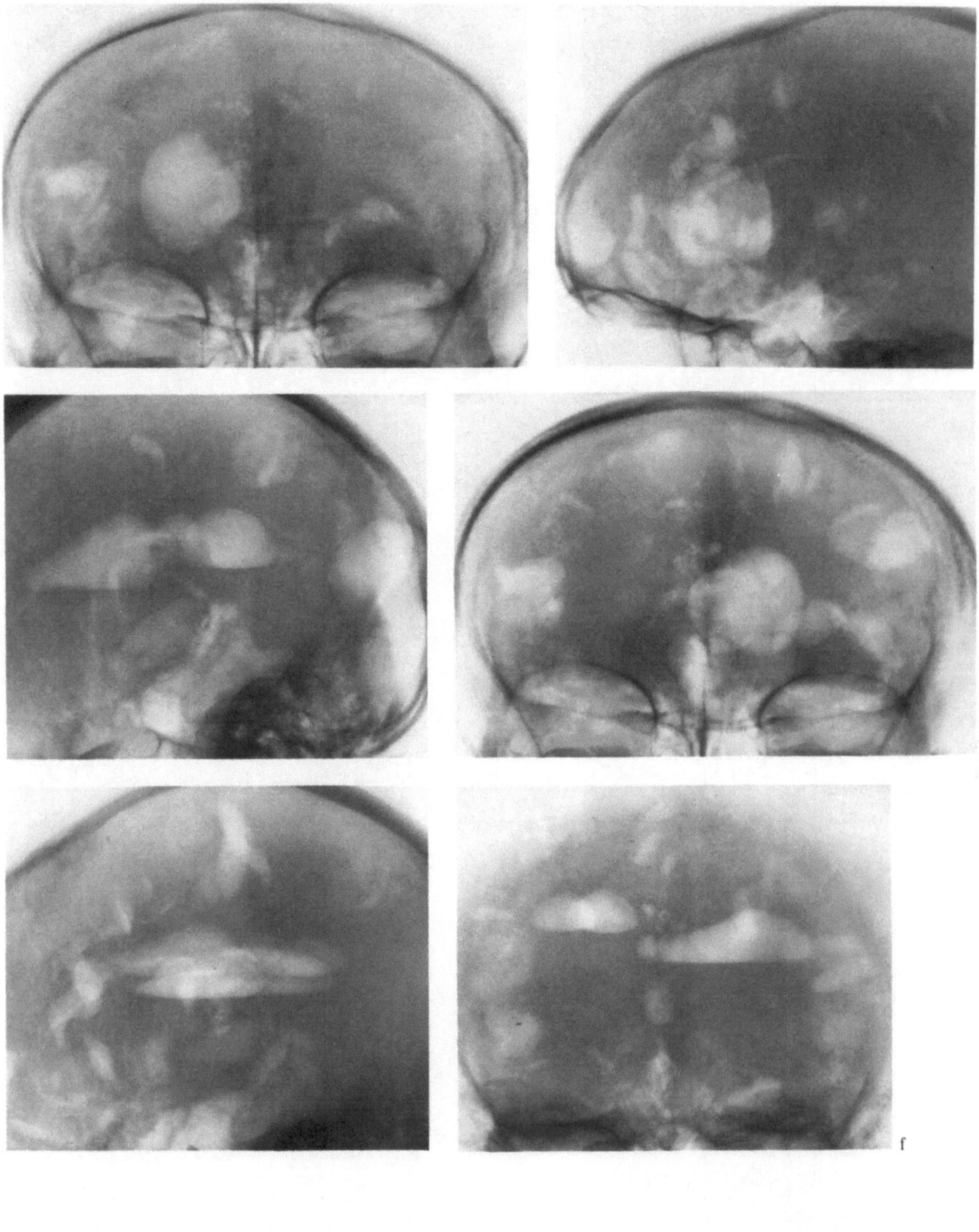

Fig. 1.73a–f. *Cerebral Cysticercosis.* a, b) In spite of urea injection the air fills only the right ventricle, the body of which is deformed. Note the „cystic" cavity on the convexity. c–f) After 6 hours the air moved to the left ventricle and in the sitting position both ventricles appear visualized. Note the „cystic" cavities in the left frontal periventricular region and on the convexity of the left cerebral hemisphere

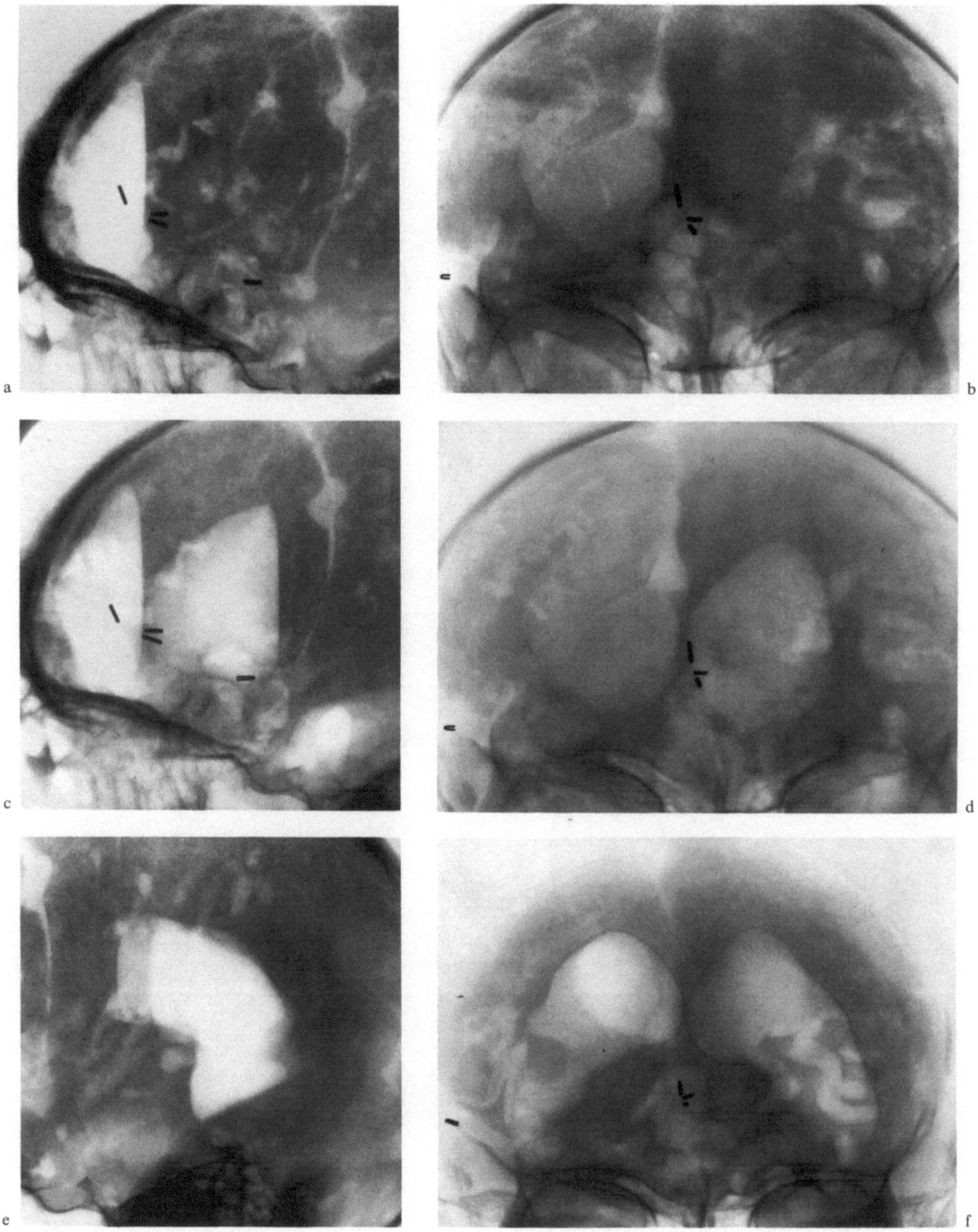

Fig. 1.74a–f. *Right Frontal Glioma Operated. Recurrence?* Only the right ventricle is visualized (a, b). The subarachnoid space is well injected. Six hours later there is good filling of both lateral ventricles and of the left temporal horn; the subarachnoid space is poorly injected. The air seems to have „shifted" within the ventricular system (c–f)

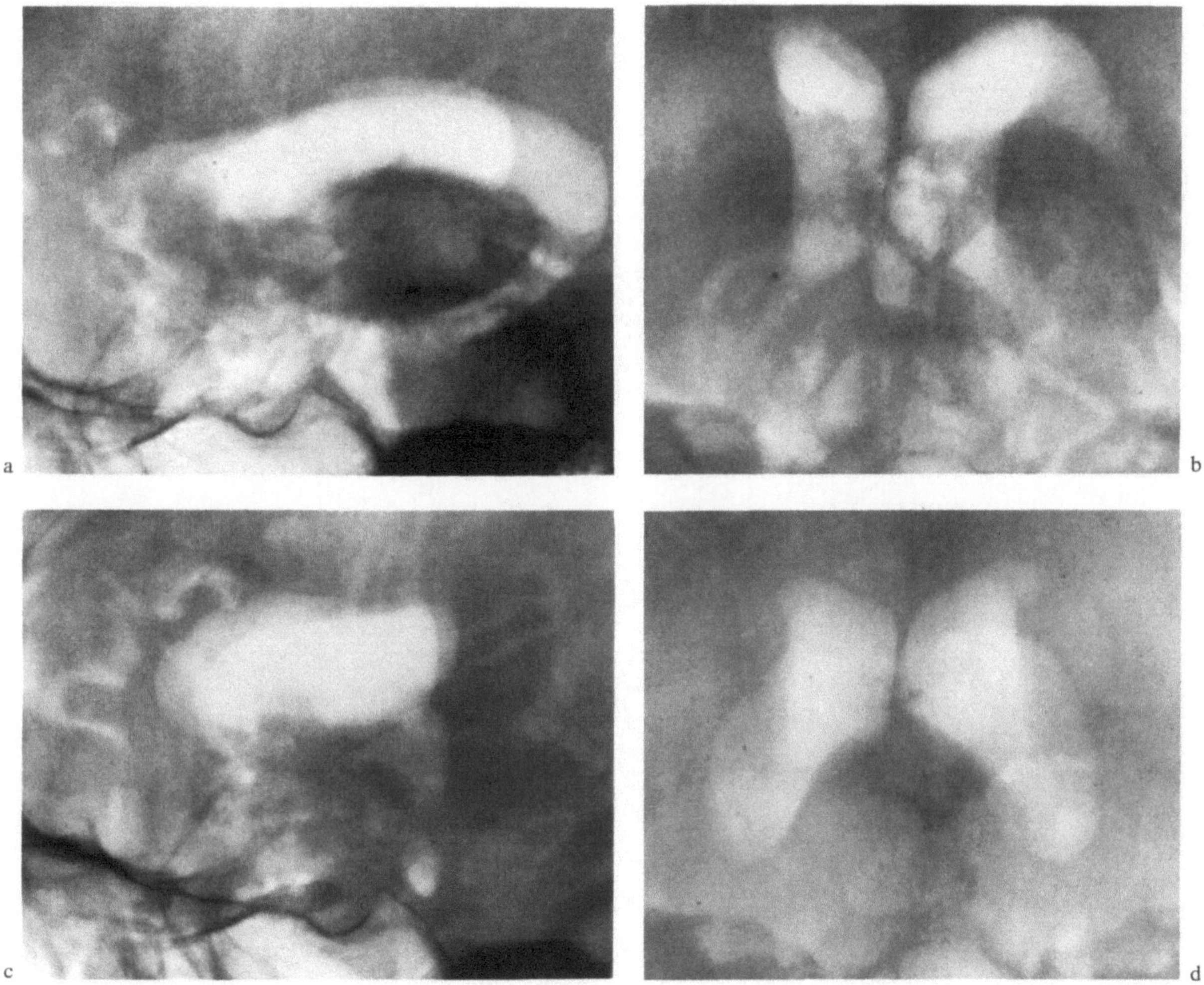

Fig. 1.75a–d. *Suprasellar Meningioma.* The border of the anterior part of the frontal horns is hardly visible (a, b), causing suspicion of an infiltrating lesion. After 6 hours (c, d) the frontal horns appear dilated and better visualized, as well as the anterior portion of the third ventricle, which is free from the superimposed air in the subarachnoid space. These features make the diagnosis of an extracerebral lesion easier

2. Air reabsorption in both the ventricular system and the subarachnoid space is faster when encephalography is performed under general anesthesia.
3. In cases of dilatation—either diffused or circumscribed—of the ventricles and/or the subarachnoid space, air reabsorption is slower.
4. In some cases of cortical atrophy it is possible to observe in the late checks an increase in the degree of dilatation of the subarachnoid space.
5. There is a possibility of communication between the subarachnoid and subdural spaces.
6. Some spontaneous moveement of air may take place within the ventricular system and subarachnoid space independently of the head movements. The distribution of air in the two lateral ventricles will become more uniform; consequently, it will be easier to compare them.
7. Some modifications in the aspect and size of the ventricular system may take place. For example, the frontal or temporal horns, which look normal and symmetrical at the time of the encephalography, become asymmetrical; or the asymmetry and the dilatation of the frontal and temporal horns observed at the moment of the encephalography appear increased in the follow-up.
8. Figs. 1.71 through 1.78 illustrate some aspects of the above findings.

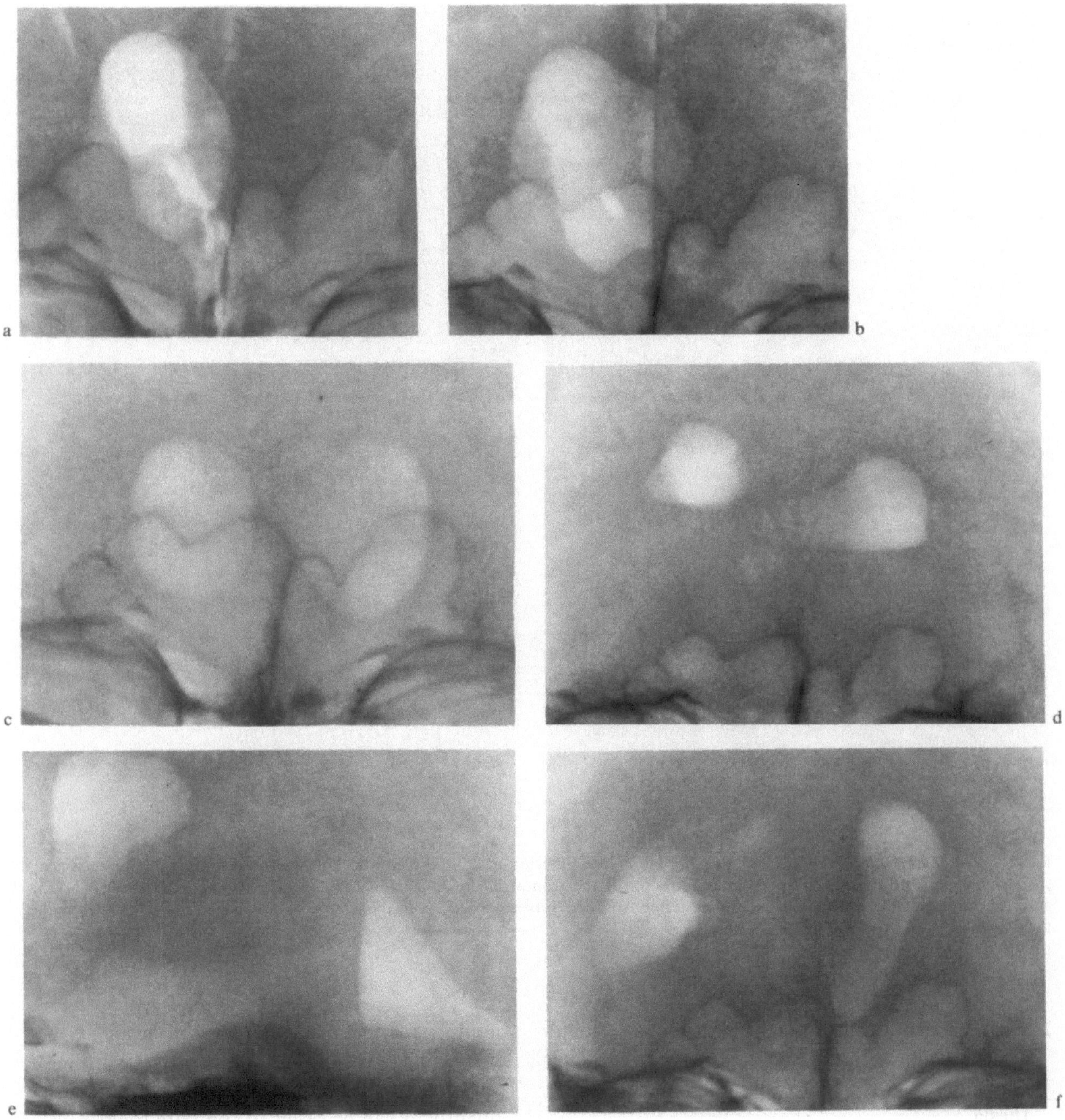

Fig. 1.76a–f. *Intracerebral Posterior Frontal Expanding Process Invading Midline Structures.* a) After urea injection only the right ventricle is visualized. b) After 6 hours the picture is unchanged. c–f) After 72 hours both ventricles are visualized; there is a typical deformation of the left ventricle

Finally a word of caution is necessary: these late follow-ups must not be left to technicians but must be carried out by the neuroradiologist himself, as an exact selection of those films considered important at the moment of the examination is mandatory.

Concerning the duration of the interval, our experience has shown that the 24-hour period, as previously proposed by Ruggiero and Smaltino [376], is usually too long. At the present time a radiographic follow-up is routinely performed in our department about 6 hours after the encephalog-

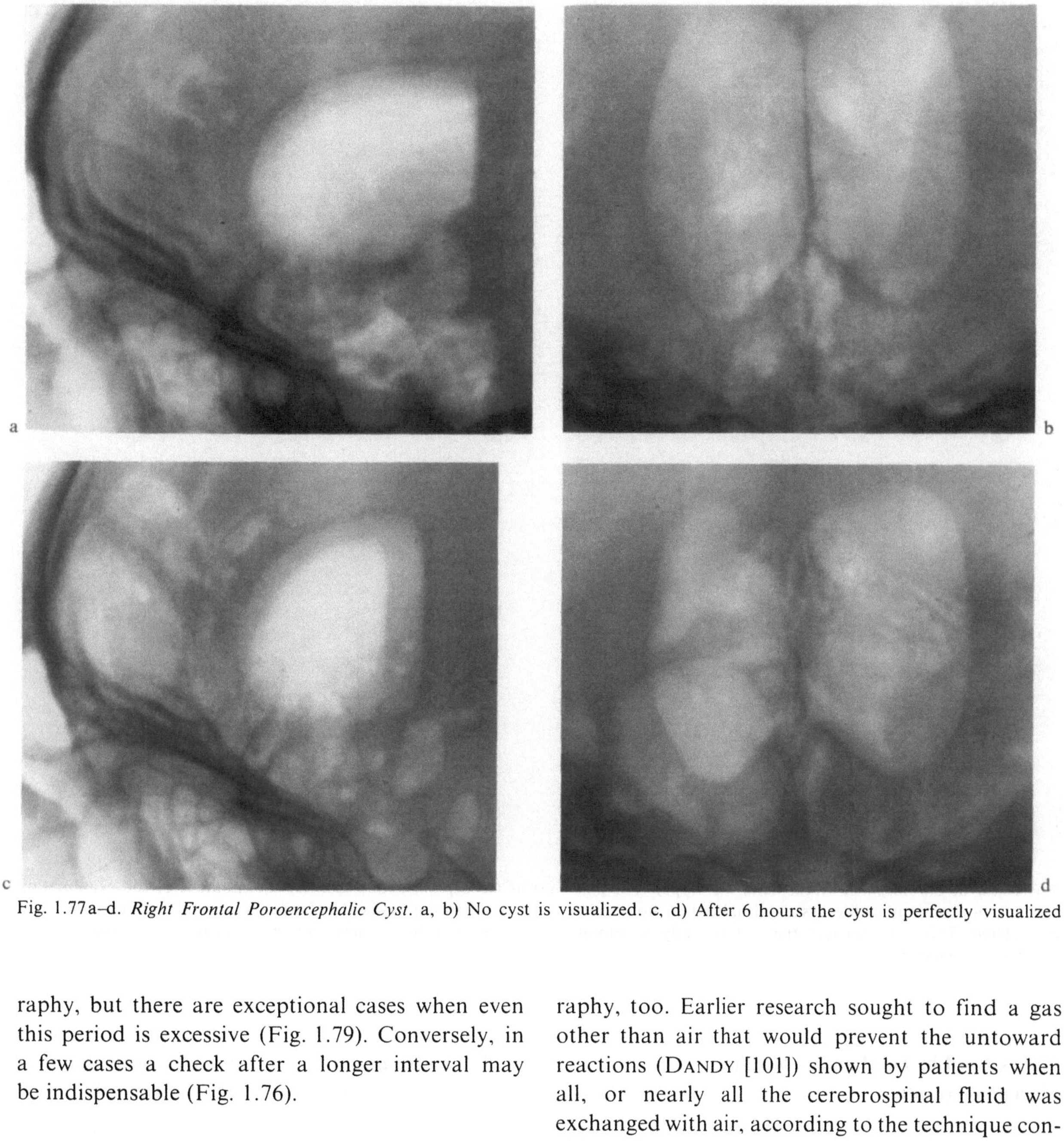

Fig. 1.77a–d. *Right Frontal Poroencephalic Cyst.* a, b) No cyst is visualized. c, d) After 6 hours the cyst is perfectly visualized

raphy, but there are exceptional cases when even this period is excessive (Fig. 1.79). Conversely, in a few cases a check after a longer interval may be indispensable (Fig. 1.76).

19. Gaseous Contrast Media

Introduction

Most papers concerned with the comparative study of the different gases injected during pneumoencephalography are based on reports of total encephalographies. Quite recently this subject has been reviewed in connection with fractional encephalography, too. Earlier research sought to find a gas other than air that would prevent the untoward reactions (DANDY [101]) shown by patients when all, or nearly all the cerebrospinal fluid was exchanged with air, according to the technique considered indispensable at that time (GRANT [180]). The results were of dubious value, as in most cases the reaction of the patient (and therefore the results of the examination) proved to be influenced rather more by the quantity of gas injected than by its nature. However, this early work is still valuable, even if we only consider the experience supplied for modern techniques; therefore, the first part of this chapter is devoted to early work on gaseous contrast media.

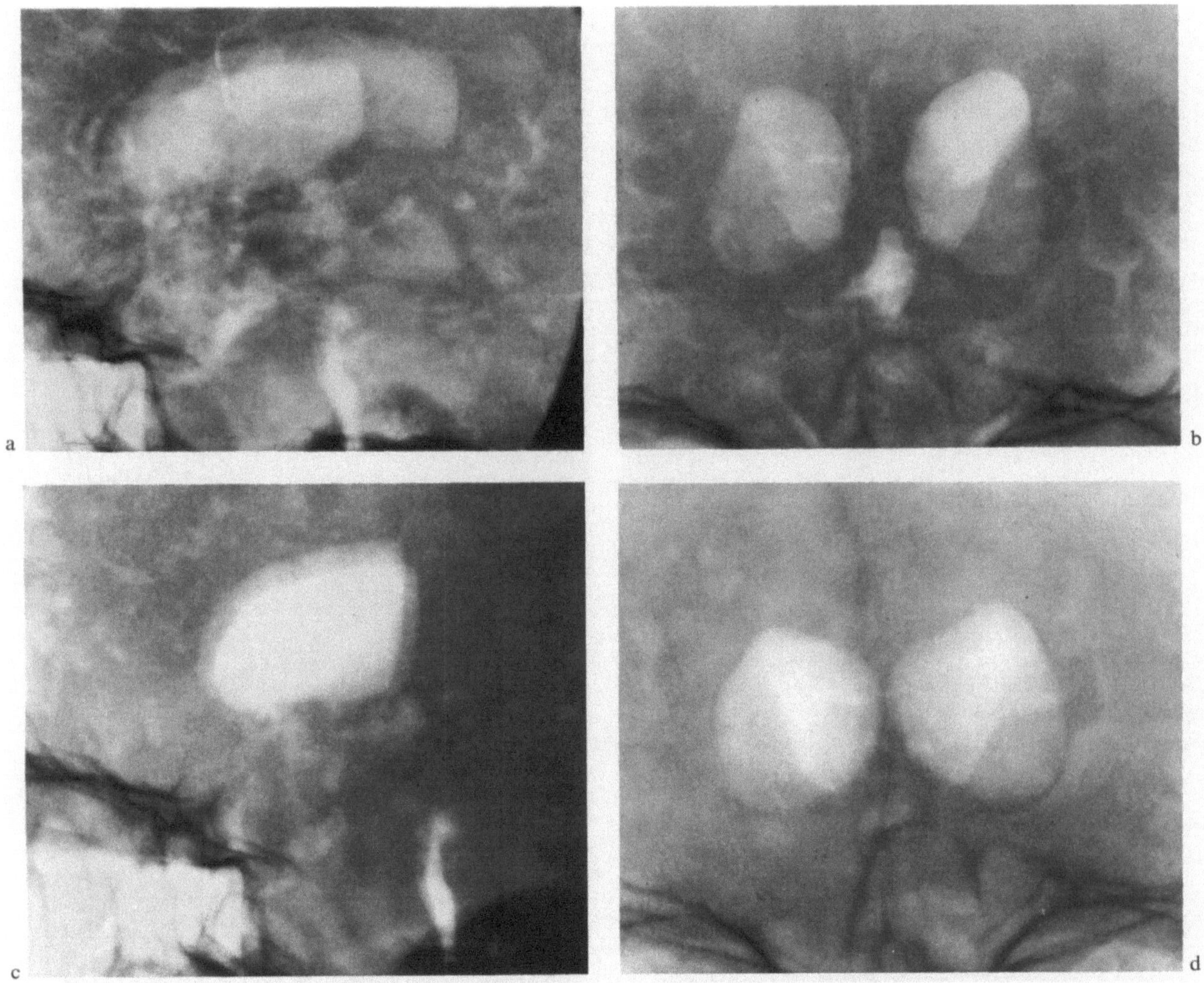

Fig. 1.78 a–d. *Chromophobe Adenoma of the Hypophysis and Cyst of the Septum Pellucidum.* At the moment of the examination (a, b) a noncommunicating cyst is visualized; 6 hours later (c, d) the septum pellucidum appears normal and the ventricles are dilated. This indicates that the cyst is really a communicating one which becomes noncommunicating probably because of a valve mechanism

Gases Used in Total and Subtotal Encephalography

The following gases have been used in total and subtotal encephalography: atmospheric air, ozone, oxygen, carbon dioxide, nitrogen, helium, xenon, and anesthetic gases (acetylene, ethylene, nitrous oxide).

Atmospheric Air

Atmospheric air consists of oxygen (20.9%), nitrogen (78%), water (1%), carbon dioxide (0.20%), rare gases (0.01%), and a variable quantity of elements in suspension (dust and germs).

Experimental Work

The consequences of complete air-fluid exchange have been studied in the dog by AIRD [4]. The experiment was performed under general anesthesia with sodium amytal, which is a sufficiently mild agent to preserve reactions to painful stimulation. The animal's cardiac and respiratory rate were recorded,

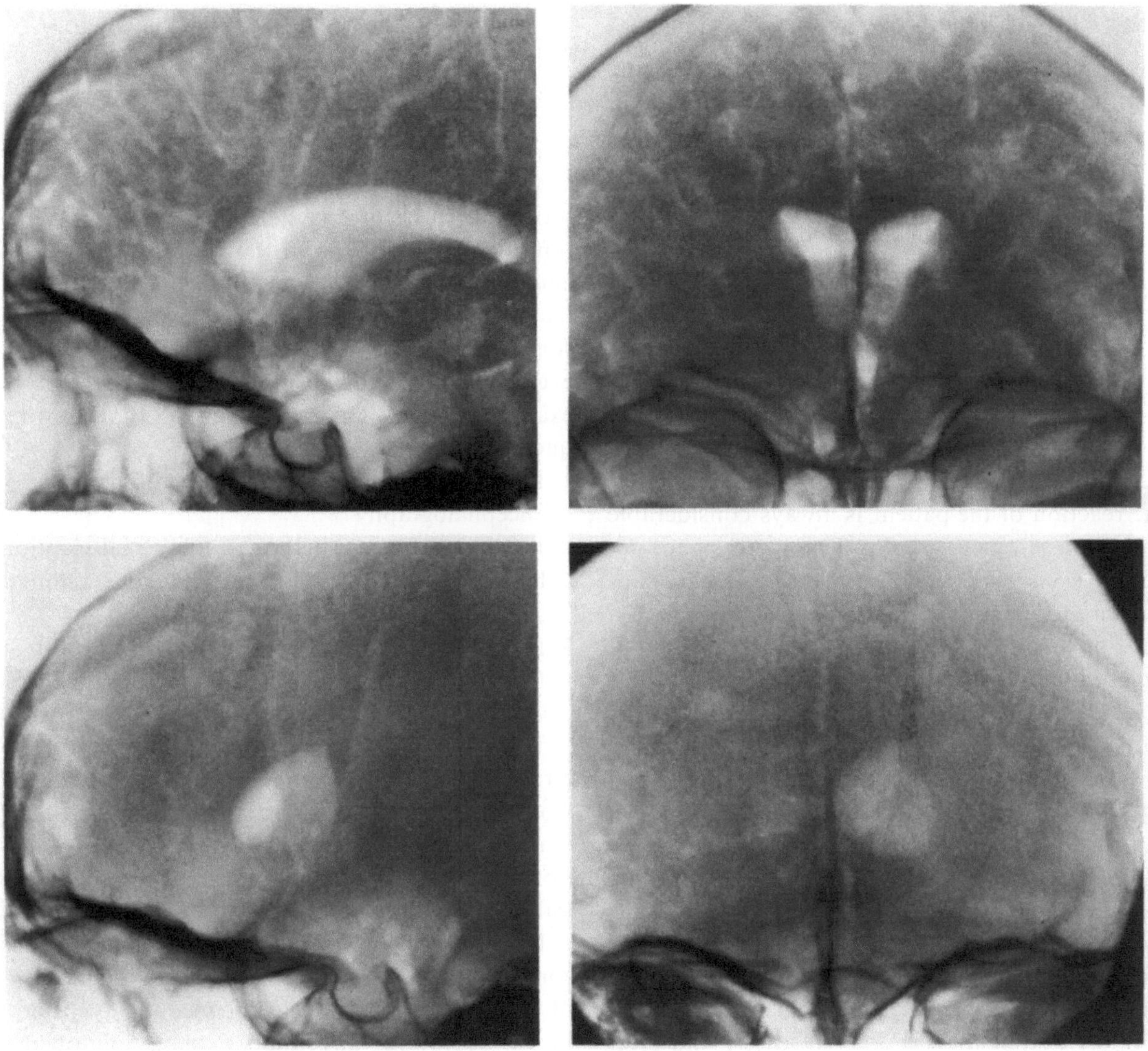

Fig. 1.79a–d. *Epilepsy*. a, b) Standard radiographs showing excellent filling of the ventricular system. After 6 hours (c, d), the air has nearly disappeared from both the ventricles and the subarachnoid space

together with color changes, reflexes, and muscular tension. Immediately after the replacement of CSF by air, the dog showed an acute reaction, followed by a prostration state lasting from 1 to 3 days (on an average, it takes 7 days for the air to be reabsorbed). CSF pleocytosis followed (on average, 1200 elements per ml), with a prevalence of elements of leukocytic type at the beginning and of mononuclear type on the 7th day. No significant modifications of the fluid pressure were observed in the days following the examination, and autopsy showed no alterations of either medulla or meninges.

CSF changes were also studied by KASHARA *et al.* [224]: immediately after the introduction of air, an increase was observed in the number of cells, reaching its peak from the 3rd to the 6th hour. The increase diminished progressively, disappearing after 72 hours, and occasionally after one week.

When small quantities of air were injected, lymphocytes predominated; with large amounts, polynucleates were prevalent. No modifications of the protein concentration or of the albumin-globulin ratio are observed; cellular modifications of the CSF are therefore a function of the quantity of air injected.

Manner of Injection

The original technique of DANDY [101] consisted in withdrawing the CSF in small quantities and replacing it progressively by air. Subsequently, other procedures have been proposed: simultaneous exchange under constant pressure, or even bubbling the air through a solution capable of precipitating the elements in suspension. In the early days 150–200 ml of air was injected; later, in 1932, DAVIDOFF and DYKE [103] demonstrated that 50–70 ml could be sufficient when the ventricular system was not dilated.

Reaction of the Patient

The reaction of the patient is always considerable with total encephalography. The acute symptomatology is characterized by violent headache, nausea, vertigo, emesis, and profuse sweating, with a more or less marked state of shock. These symptoms gradually subside but do not disappear before the 2nd or 3rd day. More severe complications, with an occasional fatal outcome, are reported in cases of cerebral tumors. During subtotal encephalography the headache generally appears after injection of 20 ml of air, whereas sweating, lowered pulse rate, lowered arterial pressure, nausea, vomiting, and sometimes syncope usually appear only at the end of the examination. However, the symptoms run a different course with the two techniques: with subtotal encephalography, they disappear 24 hours after the examination in 25% of cases, and after 3 days only 30% of patients still show symptoms, depending not only on the quantity of gas injected but also on the size of the ventricles and the nature of the disease.

Air Reabsorption

DAVIDOFF and DYKE [103] have studied air reabsorption by means of a series of radiographs taken in the sitting position 24, 48, 72, and 96 hours after encephalographies carried out by injecting different amounts (20, 40, 60, and 80 ml) of air. Their conclusion was that the air in the subarachnoid space is reabsorbed earlier—usually 48 hours after the examination—than the air in the ventricles, where, at the same time, about one-third of the contrast medium injected is still present.

When we first started work on this subject, we were making radiographic checks 24 hours after the encephalography [374], but we later reduced the interval to 6 hours, since with our technique of fractional encephalography the amount of air present in the ventricular system after 24 hours was usually too small to be of any help in diagnosis. At the time this chapter was written our experience included more than 100 cases, and we were definitely inclined to believe that the mechanism of air reabsorption does not follow any constant rule. However, we wanted to make a final check. We therefore examined 100 cases in order to answer the following questions:

1. Is the ventricular volume modified 6 hours after encephalography?
2. Is there a difference in the rate of air reabsorption between the ventricles and the subarachnoid space?
3. Does the air move—and in what proportion — from the subarachnoid to the subdural space?

Our results are as follows:

To check any possible modifications of ventricular size, we measure the maximum diameter of the frontal horns in antero-posterior projection. After 6 hours this diameter was increased but the variations were always very small, not exceeding a few millimeters.

In 11 cases there was found in the subdural space some air which was not present in it at the moment of the examination. To our knowledge there is not, in the literature, any valid explanation of this phenomenon, which we are presently investigating.

In cases of obstructive hydrocephalus (FOERSTER [149]) reabsorption of the air may last 2 or 3 weeks.

Cytochemistry of CSF

All authors except WEIGELDT [474] describe an increase in the number of cells, especially polynucleates. Figures vary from 20 (ELEY and VOGT [137]) to 19500 cells (FRIEDMAN [156]) as does time of highest concentration: 12 hours for CESTAN and RISER [77], and 24 or 48 hours for TSCHUGUNOFF [459]. NEWMAN [314], on samples drawn 24 hours after the examination, found an average of 1200–1400 leukocytes per mm^3. An increase in protein concentration has been described by CESTAN and RISER [77] and TSCHUGUNOFF [459].

CSF Pressure

According to ELSBERG and SOUTHERLAND [138] there was a CSF pressure drop of 2 to 12 cm of water, whereas TSCHUGUNOFF [459], reporting on 32 cases, observed an increase in CSF pressure in 82% of patients. From a practical viewpoint, both hypertension and hypotension of the CSF are considered important complications of the encephalography, especially in cases of increased intracranial pressure. ADSON [2] ascribes some fatal outcomes to CSF.

Ozone

In 1959 DESCUNS *et al.* [112], performed subtotal encephalography by injecting 120 ml of air drawn at the outlet from an ozonegenerating device. According to the authors, such a mixture of air and ozone is reabsorbed six times faster than pure atmospheric air; there were no particular reactions, but for CHECAN [78] this was due to the small quantity delivered by the apparatus. Ozone is a very irritant gas, as our experience also shows, and it would be very dangerous to inject pure ozone.

Oxygen

Oxygen is a pure gas. Its molecular weight is 32. Its density is 1.05, compared with that of air taken as 1. At 37° C and at 760 mm Hg its solubility in water is 2.4 vol%.

Experimental Work

AIRD [4] repeated in the dog with oxygen the experiment already made with air. After the examination, the animal showed acute reactions followed by a prostration state lasting 24–48 hours. Reabsorption was complete after 24 hours. The modification of CSF cells and pressure were the same as observed with the injection of air.

Clinical Work

JÜNGLING [242], in 1922, and DENK [111], in 1923, performing total encephalography with oxygen, observed that the patient's reactions were somewhat less severe than with air. However, the comparative study of the two techniques performed by these authors is not very satisfactory, since their main purpose was to demonstrate the danger of air encephalography due to embolism. According to CLEVELAND and END [81], the duration of postencephalographic symptoms is slightly less when the examination is done with air. There is no difference between the two techniques as far as modifications of the CSF are concerned.

Carbon Dioxide

The molecular weight of carbon dioxide is 44. It is heavier than air: 1.54:1. Its solubility in water, at 36.5° C, is 54.5 vol%. It combines with water to produce carbonic acid (H_2CO_3).

We are not aware of any experimental work. In 1933 LIBERSON [252] tried to inject carbon dioxide into the subarachnoid space of man, but concluded that it was not useful because reabsorption was too rapid and might perhaps also be dangerous because it produces an alteration in the pH of the CSF.

Nitrogen

Nitrogen is an inert gas, molecular weight 28, a little lighter than air: 0.967:1. It is weakly soluble in water: 1.28 vol% at 37° C and 760 mm Hg.

In 1933 LIBERSON [252] utilized nitrogen in 40 encephalographies with the same results as with air.

Helium

Helium is an inert gas, molecular weight 4, lighter than air: 0.17:1. It is very weakly soluble in water: 0.87% (at 37° C and 760 mm Hg), very diffusible, and devoid of toxicity.

In 1933 LIBERSON [252] tested helium in 12 patients subjected to total encephalography: the examinations were tolerated better than those made with air. In 1942 CLEVELAND and END [81] injected this gas during encephalographies made under general anesthesia with Pentothal or Avertin; the duration of secondary symptoms was about 20 hours, therefore considerably shorter than those observed with air or oxygen.

Xenon

Xenon is an inert, colorless, odorless, tasteless gas, and not explosive. It is present in infinitesimal quantity in the atmospheric air.

PITTINGER *et al.* [352] in 1956 utilized it in 10 encephalographies. Their work is important, and we analyze it in detail. After administration of barbiturates and atropine, the gas is injected at a low pressure, under manometric control, 10 ml at a time, while an equal quantity of CSF is withdrawn simultaneously with another needle. The total amount of gas injected varies from 65 to 200 ml, and radiographs are performed 15 minutes after the end of the injection.

During the examination headache almost always occurs, with or without emesis; it persists for 24 hours, thus less time than is generally observed when the examination is carried out with air, whereas the acute reaction is similar with the two techniques. The course of reabsorption has been studied in 5 patients: 2 hours after the examination an appreciable quantity of gas is already reabsorbed; the reabsorption rate then gradually diminishes, being very slow at the fourth hour.

The gas has not shown analgesic or narcotic effects, nor any depression of the respiratory centers; the authors have checked possible changes in the chemistry or pressure of the CSF. From the radiographic viewpoint, the results were as good as those obtained with air; however, their work has not encouraged them to continue encephalographies with xenon.

Acetylene

In 1937 AIRD [5] considered using anesthetic gases as contrast media in encephalography. His research led him to select three: acetylene, ethylene, and nitrous oxide. The formula of acetylene is C_2H_2; it is lighter than air (0.92 : 1) and explosive; therefore it cannot be used in the X-ray room and must be injected in another room. According to AIRD [4], the injection of acetylene into the subarachnoid space of the dog produces excellent and rapid narcosis; reabsorption is very quick, and the gas does not produce irritation of the central nervous system; in man acetylene has never been used in encephalography. ZELLER [482] has injected this gas intrathecally for the therapy of meningitis.

Ethylene

Ethylene, C_2H_4, molecular weight 28, is lighter than air (0.97 : 1); like acetylene it is explosive and cannot be injected in the X-ray room; generally it is contaminated by other gases, including carbon monoxide.

Again according to AIRD [4], in the dog, after total CSF replacement by ethylene, the gas is completely reabsorbed in two hours. A sedative effect is almost always observed, but neither an acute reaction nor a protracted depressive state follows the examination. CSF changes are analogous to those observed with air. Brain, spinal cord, and meninges do not show lesions.

Following this research, AIRD [4] utilized ethylene in human subjects; he injected up to 200 ml, simultaneously withdrawing CSF, so that the initial pressure was kept constant. It is surprising that he performed encephalography under general anesthesia, since in his experimental work on the dog AIRD noted the sedative, and even analgesic effect of ethylene injected intrathecally. The author does not mention the patient's reaction.

NEWMAN [314] also utilized ethylene in human subjects in 30 cases of encephalography that he compared with 189 examinations made with air. The injections technique is the same. From the radiologic viewpoint the results are the same: in 24 cases treated with ethylene the visualization of the subarachnoid space and the ventricular system was perfect; in one case it was insufficient, but even with air the result was not better. The author emphasizes the necessity of performing the examination rapidly, since 15 minutes after the injection much of the ethylene is already reabsorbed. In the acute phase the secondary symptoms of the examination made with air appear, but they disappear after 3 to 4 hours. The cellular reactions of the CSF are identical to those that occur when air is used: when examined 24 hours after encephalography, the CSF shows pleocytosis of the order of 1200–1400 leukocytes per mm^3. The advantages of ethylene are ascribed by NEWMAN [314] to its diffusibility (and not to its anesthetic properties): radiographic control showed that half of the gas present in the ventricles was reabsorbed after 3 hours and that after 24 hours only a small amount remained visible. However, there are also some disadvantages. In one case CSF pressure was studied by leaving in situ the Babcock's needle connected to an aneroid manometer: immediately after the examination the pressure was +35 cm of water; an hour later it had dropped to −13 to increase progressively again, reaching 0 after 1 hour, and +15 after 5 hours. NEWMAN [314] ascribes these striking variations to the difference between the rates of ethylene reabsorption and CSF renewal; under normal conditions the latter is about 20 ml/h, while the CSF is completely renewed every 6 hours. For these reasons NEWMAN [314] abandoned the method, though he never observed any complications.

Nitrous Oxide

The molecular weight of N_2O is 44; it is heavier than air (1.53:1); its solubility in water at 37° C is 44 vol%; solubility in fats is 144 vol%.

Nitrous oxide was used in man by NEWMAN [314]. If CSF is completely replaced by this gas, regardless of the initial pressure, the volume of the injected gas can exceed by 40% that of the CSF extracted. With this technique the author performed 8 encephalographies, with satisfactory radiologic results in only 3 cases. Generally, a fairly good filling of the ventricular system is obtained; but because reabsorption is too quick, the visualization of the subarachnoid space is insufficient.

Summary

From the papers analyzed above it appears that:

1. Of the gases utilized for total and subtotal encephalography, good results have been obtained with air, oxygen, nitrogen, helium, and xenon whereas carbon dioxide, acetylene, ethylene, and nitrous oxide proved unsatisfactory.
2. Whichever gas is used, the patient shows an acute reaction, more or less comparable to a state of shock, and a secondary reaction chiefly characterized by headache and sometimes vomiting. This secondary reaction seems to last about the same time with nitrogen and air, less with oxygen, and still less with helium or xenon. The symptoms are in proportion to the quantity of gas injected and its rate of reabsorption, which seems to be slower when the ventricular system is dilated and is also influenced by the nature of the disease. A few instances of cardiac arrest caused by too rapid gas reabsorption have also been described [82].
3. Again regardless of the type of gas, an increase of cells is observed after the examination, with a prevalence of polynucleates in the first stage and mononucleates in the second stage. CSF pressure generally does not change with the injection of air but shows a considerable drop when more diffusible gases are used.

Gases Used in Fractional Encephalography

Air and Oxygen

In fractional encephalography 30–35 ml of gas is generally sufficient for the study of the nondilated subarachnoid space and the ventricular system.

During the examination, the patient may feel some discomfort; most authors ascribe this to the penetration of the gas into the subarachnoid space. No acute reactions occur, such as after a total encephalography, and complications are generally minor. According to ROBERTSON [371], these drawbacks are independent of the gas used, and the choice between air and oxygen must be based on clinical criteria. When there are good reasons to think that the ventricles are greatly dilated, oxygen is more suitable, whereas for normal ventricles and subarachnoid space, air is preferred. Always, according to ROBERTSON [371], the rate of gas reabsorption is a function of the ventricular volume as already emphasized by DAVIDOFF and DYKE [103] relative to subtotal encephalography. In any case, oxygen is always reabsorbed more rapidly than air. CSF modifications have been very well studied by MURRACK, MARKS, and COUCH [311] in 85 fractional encephalographies done under local anesthesia, with a maximum injection of 40 ml of air and a maximum examination time of 45 minutes. Two CSF samples were taken: the first (2–3 ml) immediately after the lumbar puncture; the second (generally more than 10 ml) whole fluid extracted during the examination. Cellular elements and the concentration of glucose and protein were studied in both samples. The results of MURRACK, MARKS, and COUCH [311] are indicated in Fig. 3 of their work; they show that in the second sample the cells—a particular type of mononucleate called type M—are more numerous and that the protein concentration is inferior, while the glucose is unchanged. The authors note that, if no air is injected, successive samples of CSF have a lower protein content, and also fewer cells (FREMONT-SMITH and PUTMAN [155]). They explain the variations between the two samples of CSF as due to the fact that the first sample is purely subarachnoid, while the second consists of CSF from both subarachnoid space and ventricles. The concentration of proteins is usually lower in the ventricular CSF so that in our opinion the increase in the number of cells is the only modification of the CSF produced by encephalography.

This was confirmed by STOJANOVIC [439], who observed an increase of cells in 33 out of 60 patients when encephalography was carried out with quantities of air varying from 30 to 50 ml; the pleocytosis may already appear on the first sample of CSF withdrawn after the injection of 5 ml of air. STOJANOVIC thinks the phenomenon is not inflammatory but he does not suggest any hypothesis concerning its origin. We believe it may be due to local cellular desquamation produced by the puncture.

As far as we know, there is no work in which, as has been done for total encephalography, CSF changes in the hours and days following fractional encephalography have been studied systematically. ROBERTSON [371] examined in 10 patients the CSF withdrawn by the lumbar route 24 hours after the examination: the number of cells per mm^3 varied from a minimum of 7 lymphocytes and 36 mononucleates to a maximum of 150 lymphocytes, 310 polynucleates, and 30 large monocytes.

According to TAVERAS and WOOD [453], some changes of an inflammatory type (increase in sugar and albumin concentration, leukocytic pleocytosis) occur after encephalography, with highest intensity after 12 hours. Under normal circumstances the CSF resumes its normal composition 36 or 48 hours after encephalography.

It appears from the literature that the modifications of CSF pressure during or after fractional encephalography are few and independent of the gas employed, whether air or oxygen. According to SHAPIRO and ROBINSON [417], with the patient in the sitting position, pressure increases by, on average, 9 cm H_2O (from 3 to 17) after the injection of 5–8 ml of air. SHEALY and NEW [420] studied the behavior of CSF pressure in 73 patients in whom encephalography was performed without any CSF withdrawal. In 8 of them a slight decrease was observed; in all the others, there was a slight increase, not accompanied by symptoms. Their observations are similar to those made by one of us (A. T.): the injection, for two times, of 5 ml of air, produces an increase in pressure that does not exceed 10–15 cm H_2O. CRONQUIST *et al.* [96] studied the behavior of the intraventricular pressure during fractional encephalography performed with oxygen in patients with intracranial hypertension: immediately after the injection of gas, a slight increase in pressure occurs; in some cases this gradually decreases, but often a second rise occurs which, after a variable interval, is followed by a pressure drop. It would seem to be a vasomotor reflex following the first pressure rise; this reflex would produce dilatation of the cerebral arterioles and hence an increase in cerebral blood volume. This phenomenon recalls the spontaneous fluctuation of the intraventricular pressure observed by GUILLAUME and JANNY [193] and LUNDBERG [266] in cases of intracranial hypertension where rapid rises occur (up to 50–100 mm Hg) that persist for 5–20 minutes and coincide with the appearance of headache, face flushing, loss of consciousness, hyperpnea, nausea, vomiting, and convulsive movements, followed by stiffness of the limbs. These symptoms, though variable, have been observed also when CSF pressure rises during the encephalography. GANGLBERGER [160] considered they might be relieved by injecting aminophylline and ephedrine.

Summary

1. Air and oxygen are the gases most frequently used in fractional encephalography.
2. Oxygen is reabsorbed more rapidly than air, especially at the level of the subarachnoid spaces, for the study of which it therefore is unfit. The rate of reabsorption decreases if the ventricles are dilated.
3. The patient shows a mild and transient malaise at the moment of the injection, usually when the gas enters the subarachnoid space. Complications are generally minor.

4. *During the examination* the CSF may show a pleocytosis of monocytic type, not exceeding 30 elements per mm^3, and it is accompanied by a slight drop in protein concentration, whereas glucose remains constant. These modifications of the CSF are not of the inflammatory type observed *after the examination*, where there is leukocytic pleocytosis and a slight increase in protein and glucose concentrations.
5. At the end of the examination, CSF pressure is approximately the same as the initial pressure.
6. During encephalography it is possible to observe a "diphasic" rise in the intraventricular pressure; the second rise is more important in cases of intracranial hypertension.

Points (3) through (6) refer to examinations performed with both air and oxygen.

Note. The statements in this chapter are essentially the result of an analysis of the literature. Further confirmation is necessary, especially in regard to the paragraph on CSF pressure changes, a subject to which one of us (G. R.) has devoted special attention for years. We are convinced that these modifications are variable and depend on a number of factors. This problem deserves to be investigated under perfect technical conditions, which we are still hoping to achieve.

Helium

In 1960 FOURNIER [150] reported the results of 100 fractional encephalographies performed with helium: the total quantity of gas seldom exceeds 25 ml; radiographic results are good, in spite of the extreme diffusibility of the gas. The author stresses the harmlessness of the examination, though the patient sometimes shows a mild malaise, as happens with air.

Carbon Dioxide

In 1967 REARDON *et al.* [363] reported a technique of fractional encephalography with carbon dioxide that they have employed 15 times for the study of the posterior fossa and 5 times for a complete examination. The gas is drawn into a syringe, through a filter, from a bottle provided with a pressure regulator and gasometer. Samples of CSF are drawn before and after the introduction of the gas in order to evaluate the pH and the partial pressure of CO_2. The total amount of CO_2 injected is between 100 and 150 ml. A rotating chair is necessary, since the needle must be left *in situ* until the end of the examination; because of its great diffusibility, the gas must be injected several times.

As a result of its quick reabsorption, only 50–80% of the gas injected reaches the structures to be examined, and after 20 minutes 90% of it is reabsorbed.

Five minutes after the injection of 20 ml of carbon dioxide by the lumbar route, the pH of CSF goes from 7.34 to 6.9, then back to 7.5, 15 minutes after the injection.

Encephalography is very well tolerated: during the examination the patient complains of mild headache, but half an hour later he can sit up, and within 2 hours he is able to eat. Another advantage is the considerable increase in cerebral blood flow produced by carbon dioxide; this would make the technique particularly advantageous in cerebrovascular disease where encephalography with air or oxygen seems to produce a fall in arterial pressure.

The technique is interesting and we are awaiting the results of further experience. However, a few reservations seem justified: in the report of REARDON *et al.* [363] there are only 5 cases in which the examination was complete; it is not clear how the CSF was extracted and how much; apparently CSF pressure was not measured; finally, and above all, the quality of the radiological pictures is inferior to the average standard achieved in a department of neuroradiology.

Nitrous Oxide

We have seen that, according to AIRD [4], nitrous oxide would be the ideal contrast medium but that unfortunately it cannot be used because it is reabsorbed too quickly. It seems that this drawback might be avoided, at least when the examination is performed under anesthesia (PHILIPPART and THIBAUT [345, 346], BERGSTRÖM *et al.* [36]): if the patient breathes N_2O, the contrast is retained in the cerebral ventricles and in the subarachnoid space throughout the examination yet is eliminated very rapidly when the patient wakes up.

With the original technique of THIBAUT and PHILIPPART [345, 346] the maintenance of anesthesia is assured by 75% nitrous oxide and 1% fluothane; once the blood is saturated with nitrous oxide (which takes about 10 minutes), encephalography starts, and it is performed with the same technique used with air. The N_2O is introduced into the subarachnoid space under sterile conditions at approximately room temperature (near the ambient temperature) and with the injection pressure about equal to the pressure of the CSF. Thirty-six patients were examined, 20 of whom were under 2 years of age. The average volume of gas injected was 30 ml (between 20 and 50), and the average quantity of CSF extracted was 33 ml. The examination lasted an average time of 45 minutes. From the radiologic viewpoint the results are analogous to those obtained with air. Gas reabsorption during the examination is not appreciable radiologically; half-an-hour after the patient's awakening 50% of the gas is already reabsorbed; an hour later it has disappeared. After the examination the CSF pressure remains practically constant (8% on an average, compared with the initial values). A short febrile reaction (up to 38°C) was present in 15 patients, generally occurring within the first 24 hours after the examination. Two patients suffered emesis, and 4 a mild headache.

In 6 cases the CSF was re-examined during the 24 hours following the examination, always with a negative result.

Indication of the Method

According to the authors the main indication of the method is represented by patients with increased intracranial pressure, in whom encephalography is performed under general anesthesia. Actually—as discussed in the chapter on anesthesia—gaseous exchanges occur between the intracranial air and the gases dissolved in the blood, producing a rise in the intracranial pressure; such a rise, however, does not occur when nitrous oxide is used as contrast medium.

Conclusions

When encephalography is performed with the patient awake, atmospheric air is again the best, most practical, and safest contrast medium. No argument advanced in favor of oxygen, helium, or xenon would stand up to serious criticism. Carbon dioxide seems to be well tolerated; but, apart from the fact that it is not useful for the study of the subarachnoid space, the fact that it is too quickly reabsorbed precludes the follow-up that sometimes can be useful for the diagnosis (see Chap. I, p. 71).

The problem is not as simple where the examination is performed under general anesthesia. The gas used as a contrast must have a composition as similar as possible to that of the gas or gases inhaled to maintain anesthesia; if one of these is nitrous oxide, it is dangerous to inject air into the skull, especially in the presence of intracranial hypertension.

20. Anesthesia in Fractional Encephalography

Introduction

We prefer to perform encephalography (as well as other neuroradiological examinations) without general anesthesia. However, this is not always possible, as in the case of emotional or uncooperative patients.

Until some time ago anesthesia was almost exclusively induced by the inhalation of fluothane and nitrous oxide (N_2O); this technique, as we have seen, may lead to complications in encephalography, probably on account of the increase in intracranial pressure secondary to the depressed respiration induced by fluothane. For this reason γ-hydroxybutyric acid has been tested; it has no depressant effect on respiration. Finally, in cases where general anesthesia was advisable only because of the patient's emotional state, neuroleptanalgesia has been suggested.

When the gas injected as contrast medium (henceforth referred to as contrast gas) does not have the same composition as the mixture of gases inhaled during general anesthesia (henceforth called anesthetic gas), some gas exchange occurs, affecting the behavior of CSF pressure. These phenomena would seem to account for certain untoward reactions observed during encephalographies performed under general anesthesia with air as contrast gas. For this reason they are discussed in this chapter, together with the techniques of general anesthesia and neuroleptanalgesia.

Preparation of the Patient before Encephalography without Anesthesia

Psychological preparation and local anesthesia in the lumbar region are often sufficient to ensure the patient's adequate cooperation for a correct encephalography. However, a few authors maintain that a pharmacological preparation is necessary. TAVERAS and WOOD [453] prescribe barbiturates and atropine before the examination; they claim that atropine eliminates the irritant effect of the air on neurovegetative centers which is what causes nausea, vomiting, and salivary and bronchial secretion. DELIGNÉ [110] and RUGGIERO [374] advise against the use of large doses of hypnotics or opiates whenever general anesthesia cannot be used. Unsatisfactory sedation halfway between wakefulness and sleeping would compromise the success of the examination.

In epileptic patients anticonvulsive drugs are discontinued the day before the examination.

"Classical" General Anesthesia

Premedication

Morphine and its derivatives must be avoided because of their depressant effects on respiration, with consequent hypercapnia and hypoxia, producing vascular congestion and edema of the brain. Chlorpromazine is also not advisable because of its vasoparalytic effects, producing instability of the arterial tension with pressure drops that are especially dangerous when the patient is in the sitting position.

Most authors believe that it is preferable to limit premedication to the administration of atropine (0.5 mg intramuscularly one hour before the induction of anesthesia). This allows the planning of a light general anesthesia followed by quick awakening. In children it is advisable to combine atropine and barbiturates (generally as suppositories at 5 mg/kg [196]). In apprehensive adults anxiolytic drugs of the benzodiazepine type, such as diazepam, may be helpful. A new analgesic drug, Pentazocine, has recently been introduced: it is not habitforming and can be advantageously used as a pre-anesthetic. It produces good analgesia without undesirable side effects, such as respiratory depression and vomiting.

Induction of General Anesthesia

In the adult 40 ctg pentobarbital and 10 ctg succinylcholine are generally injected intravenously. The patient is ventilated through a mask and then intubated.

In children narcosis is induced through a mask, usually in a non-rebreathing system, but sometimes with a by-pass system; the anesthetic gas consists of a 2:1 mixture of N_2O and oxygen with the addition of 0.5 to 1% fluothane.

When the corneal reflexes disappear, 3 mg/kg of succinylcholine is injected intramuscularly and the patient is ventilated artificially, and then intubated when curarization is complete. In pediatric radiology, Ketamine has recently been introduced as a substitute for fluothane; however, this drug is still undergoing evaluation [309, 460].

In newborns intubation may be made without previous induction. Contrary to what one might suppose, this method is neither difficult nor rough, and it avoids the drawbacks of mask induction, such as dropping of the epiglottis in front of the trachea, inhalation of saliva, and regurgitation.

In general anesthesia for encephalography the position and fixation of the tube are very important, as its distal extremity may penetrate a bronchus or slip out of the trachea during the various movements of head flexion and extension. Frequent thorax auscultation and careful observation of the anesthesia bag will warn of these accidents in good time. It is preferable to employ latex tubes with nylon spiral. Nasotracheal intubation has also been proposed because the movements of the tube in the larynx may produce cough reflexes during the examination, thus favoring cerebral edema. Surface anesthesia with a spray of 4% lidocaine should precede intubation; it is advisable to coat the tube with a layer of lidocaine jelly.

Maintenance of General Anesthesia

The main objective in the choice of equipment used for anesthesia is to avoid hypercapnia. For this reason, in children the open circuit system is the most appropriate; but nonrebreathing valves, such as Digby-Leigh's, can also be used. Ayre's T-tubes are also suitable, on account of their being easy to use and offering little resistance to the passage of gas. In the adult the systems most often used are the semi-closed and semi-open circuits, such as Magill's attachment. Spontaneous ventilation is preferable, so that possible signs of respiratory disturbances of central origin can be recognized. It is evident, however, that the ventilatory insufficiency, whatever its origin, must be immediately compensated for by manual assistance.

At present, fluothane is the volatile anesthetic most frequently used in neuroradiology because it is not explosive and allows rapid awakening; moreover, it is particularly suitable for pediatric anesthesia. However, there are also some disadvantages: a depressant effect on the respiratory centers that must be carefully controlled, especially in cases of overdosage and when the patient is prone; and the hypotensive effect on blood pressure, which is particularly to be feared when the patient is sitting. An increase in CSF pressure is observed in practically all cases in which fluothane is used.

The anesthetic gas must be compatible with the contrast gas. When this is air or oxygen, nitrous oxide should not be used as anesthetic because this gas dissolves in the blood and diffuses into the space occupied by the air, with a consequent increase in the intracranial pressure. The clinical importance of this phenomenon is considerable and is discussed in a special paragraph.

A technique developed especially for pneumoencephalography has been described by DELIGNÉ [110]: induction with pentobarbital and succinylcholine, intubation, ventilation with a mixture of nitrous oxide, oxygen and trichloroethylene. The patient is maintained in spontaneous respiration with an anti-rebreathing valve.

Post-Examination Care

Generally there are no considerable differences in the course of an encephalography with respect to anesthesia. Usually the examination is followed by a mild headache, the nature of which has been the subject of many hypotheses, which are beyond the scope of this paper. A preventive treatment with hydrocortisone (50 mg every 6 hours up to a total dose of 400 mg) has been proposed in view of its anti-inflammatory and anti-edematous effect.

To relieve the disturbances caused by encephalography, some authors [453] have proposed the administration of caffeine benzoate, first intramuscularly and then by the oral route in the form of a compound of caffeine, phenacetin, and aspirin. The tartrate of β-pyridylcarbinol has been used in encephalography [97] to reduce the duration of the headache. Perhaps it could also be used for fractional encephalography. When the patient suffers nausea and vomiting, we administer paranosine in suppositories, possibly adding 0.5 ml of haloperidol intravenously or intramuscularly. It can also be administered prophylactically. Another useful preventive measure may be the inhalation of oxygen for at least 6 hours under a tent, or of a mixture of 75% oxygen and 25% helium, thus facilitating the diffusion toward the lungs of the nitrogen contained in the air used as contrast gas (see Chap. I, p. 81).

In the course of an encephalography, more serious complications may occur as exceptions; they require prompt and up-to-date procedures of circulatory and respiratory resuscitation. For this reason every neuroradiological department should be equipped with all the necessary resuscitative facilities.

Anesthesia with γ-Hydroxybutyric Acid (g.h.b.a.)

Pharmacology

γ-Hydroxybutyric acid is a hypnotic agent of mild toxicity that is used intravenously at a dosage of 50–70 mg/kg. It has a rather slow action, producing in about 10 minutes a condition similar to physiological sleep, and lasting about 2 hours. Its analgesic action is weak. The chief advantage of the drug is the absence of any depressant effect on respiratory centers. However, it causes hypotonicity of the muscles of the face and pharynx; it is therefore necessary to use an oral airway. g.h.b.a. also causes bradycardia, arterial hypertension, and myoclonia. The cardiac rhythm is controlled by the atropine that for this reason is used as premedication. Because of these side effects, g.h.b.a. is not indicated in patients suffering from hypertension or epilepsy.

γ-Hydroxybutyric Acid in Encephalography

As early as 1961 LABORIT and KIND [243] suggested the advantages of g.h.b.a. in encephalography. In

Bologna it has been widely used (thus eliminating fluothane) for general anesthesia in encephalography [324]. The technique is the following: premedication with atropine and anxiolytic drugs; induction is associated in order to counteract the hypertensive effect of g.h.b.a. and to reduce the duration of the induction itself; ventilation through a mask, with a mixture of nitrous oxide and oxygen that the patient will inhale during the whole examination; intubation; a second injection of 2 g of g.h.b.a. Generally the anesthesia lasts from 60 to 90 minutes, and awakening is quiet. If necessary, it is possible to prolong the anesthesia by adding 1% fluothane; this is done routinely in children at the moment of the induction. The maximum dose of g.h.b.a. is 100 mg/kg.

With this technique, the CSF pressure measured at the beginning of the examination, before the injection of air, is equal to or even slightly below normal values. In this respect there is no difference from an encephalography performed without anesthesia [323].

Neuroleptonalgesia (NLA)

When neuroleptic and analgesic drugs are used in combination, the patient remains conscious, quiet, and indifferent, and all sensations of pain are abolished [109]. The most frequently used products are phenoperidine as analgesic and dehydrobenzperidol as neuroleptic drug. These drugs are generally injected intravenously, combined with muscle relaxants or local anesthetics.

Pharmacology

The cholinergic qualities of phenoperidine result in bradycardia that is suppressed with atropine [135]. The drug has a slight influence on the sympathetic nervous system: when given in the appropriate doses, it produces mild arterial hypotension and does not have any direct action on the heart. It acts on the bulbar centers, producing bradypnea, with reducction of the ventilatory volume. Generally, the depression of respiration acts directly on the heart. It acts on the bulbar centers, producing bradypnea, with reduction of the ventilatory volume. Generally, the depression of respiration is in direct proportion to the dose: with 2 mg of phenoperidine, analgesia is accompanied by drowsiness, while the administration of 6 mg may result in apnea. Nalorphine counteracts the action of phenoperidine in elderly patients and children, both of whom are particularly sensitive to it, whereas alcoholics and morphine addicts are resistant to it. Finally, it must be remembered that in asthmatic and emphysematous patients bronchial spasm may occur.

Dehydrobenzperidol increases the activity of the phenoperidine, causing a marked psychomotor sedation. Because of its action on the reticular system, dehydrobenzperidol "mineralizes" the patient, who becomes indifferent to pain. The drug does not exert any action on respiratory centers and its toxicity is very low.

Technique

Early experiments with NLA in encephalography were conducted on 53 patients in Bologna; those selected had a normal state of consciousness but were considered unsuitable for examination without anesthesia because of their apprehensiveness. In the first group of 35 patients conventional general anesthesia was combined with NLA; the anesthetics were then progressively reduced as experience with NLA increased. Thus, it was possible to determine the appropriate drug dosage in order to perform the examination with NLA alone.

NLA starts in the X-ray room, with trial doses of 0.1 mg (2 ml) of fentanyl and 20 mg (4 ml) of dehydrobenzperidol with continuous monitoring of pulse and respiratory rates. The effect of the drugs reaches its peak after 10 minutes then tends to remain constant. Generally, bradypnea appears and may reach 6 to 7 respirations per minute, but in a few cases polypnea appears and breathing becomes superficial. The heart frequency drops by about 20%. A mild clouding of consciousness is occasionally observed, but it never prevents the patient from cooperating. At this stage encephalography starts, after another administration of the two drugs, never exceeding half the initial dose. During the examination it is possible to continue the administration of dehydrobenzperidol, as it is quickly eliminated, and perhaps counteracts the depressant effects of fentanyl. NLA does not cause any rise in CSF pressure.

Up to the time of writing NLA had been used in Bologna in more than 200 cases, almost always with excellent results and without complications, except for one patient who showed a narcoleptic state with jaw-drop and airways obstruction, after which he had to be intubated. In Naples NLA has given equally favorable results (SMALTINO and MAZZARELLA [431]).

NLA has been used by us and by others [347] also during gas myelography. Today we tend to use NLA for all neuroradiological examinations.

NLA is a difficult technique. Good results are obtained by a perfect balance of the two drugs. This can be difficult to achieve because of the considerable variations in individual response; in a few cases, even with small doses, there can be respiratory depression to a degree rendering intubation necessary. It is therefore necessary to have the continuous assistance of an experienced anesthetist.

A few authors [209] use NLA to obtain a true anesthesia in the surgical sense of the word: considerable quantities of the drugs are used; the patient is intubated and sometimes ventilated mechanically, but with this method it is not always possible to obtain a rapid awakening [3].

Gas Exchange

Gases tend to diffuse. Therefore, we must expect exchanges to occur between the contrast gas present in the brain cavities and the anesthetic gas dissolved in the blood, as well as between the anesthetic gas dissolved in the blood and the gases present in the pulmonary alveoli. The rate of diffusion of an inert gas (nitrogen, nitrous oxide) through a membrane separating it from a fluid is proportional to the difference in the partial pressure of the given gas in the two media considered (the gas diffuses from the higher-pressure medium toward the lower-pressure one) and its solubility in the fluid. Diffusion also depends on the physical and anatomic characteristics of the membrane and on temperature. This relation explains why air reabsorption is slow after an encephalography (or a ventriculography) during which the patient is breathing air, as the partial pressures of nitrogen are almost equal in the lungs, blood, and tissues, and in the air injected as contrast medium. The situation is different if, for example, the examination is done under anesthesia, and the contrast gas is not the same as the anesthetic gas.

The Contrast Gas is Air and the Anesthetic Gas is Nitrous Oxide

When the patient, under anesthesia, is breathing a mixture consisting of 75% nitrous oxide and 25% oxygen, the nitrous oxide diffuses from the lungs toward the blood (where its partial pressure is lower) and takes the place of nitrogen which, in turn, diffuses in the pulmonary alveoli (where its partial pressure is lower than it was in the plasma) [345]. This phenomenon is called blood denitrogenation. In the case of pneumoencephalography, the air inside the skull is 80% nitrogen and 20% oxygen: the N_2O dissolved in the plasma consequently diffuses toward the air-filled ventricles and the subarachnoid space, where its partial pressure is zero [344]. Conversely the nitrogen contained in the air inside the skull diffuses toward the plasma. However, since in the plasma at 37° nitrogen is about 35 times less soluble than N_2O, only a few molecules of nitrogen leave the air contained in the skull, into which, on the contrary, a large number of nitrous oxide molecules penetrate. As a consequence of these exchanges, there is a considerable increase of gaseous particles in the space formerly occupied only by the air injected as a contrast medium, and hence an increase in CSF pressure that can be the cause of fatal accidents [481]. This increase occurs rapidly: 5 minutes after the injection of air, CSF pressure is 25% above the initial level [348]; it remains high for about 15 minutes, then returns to normal values after 30 minutes. The diffusion takes place also at the level of the ventricular system, but it is higher in the subarachnoid spaces, where after 10 minutes the quantity of nitrous oxide equals the volume of air injected [348]. Chromatographic analyses have confirmed these volumetric measures [343].

The above-mentioned phenomena can account for the accidents observed during encephalographies performed under these conditions, and would lead one to think that general anesthesia is contraindicated when the intracranial pressure is elevated. If general anesthesia is necessary in such cases, two procedures may be considered:

1. injection of air and inhalation of air
2. injection of nitrous oxide and inhalation of nitrous oxide.

The Contrast Gas is Nitrous Oxide and the Anesthetic Gas is Nitrous Oxide

As we have seen in Chap. I, p. 85, when the patient breathes air (as happens when the examination is performed with the patient awake), nitrous oxide is not suitable as a contrast because of its quick diffusion [344]. But it becomes an excellent contrast medium if the anesthesia is also performed with nitrous oxide [36, 345, 346]. In this case, on awakening, when the patient stops inhaling N_2O and breathes air again, there is very rapid reabsorption (practically complete 1 hour after the examination) of the nitrous oxide contained in the skull, and CSF pressure falls below the initial values. This phenomenon can be explained as follows: when the patient breathes air and no longer nitrous oxide, the partial pressure of the latter in the blood decreases; then the nitrous oxide contained in the skull diffuses into the blood.

Inhalation of Oxygen after Encephalography Performed with Air or Oxygen

As early as 1937 SCHWAB *et al.* [412], by having the patient inhale almost pure oxygen (95%) after a global encephalography performed with air, obtained a considerable alleviation of secondary symptoms. These results were confirmed by CLEVELAND and END [81] and by KORNREICH [229]; in 1957 ROBERTSON systematically used oxygen therapy after fractional encephalography performed with air or oxygen. Radiological monitoring shows that alleviation of the secondary symptoms coincides with an increase in the rate of reabsorption of the contrast gas. The attractiveness of the method has recently been pointed out by HAUKE *et al.* [203]. The principle consists in creating a physical medium devoid of nitrogen in order to obtain denitrogenation of blood and tissue; the injected nitrogen can thus diffuse more rapidly toward the blood and lungs. The patient is placed under a tent to breathe 70–80% oxygen for 24 hours and 50% oxygen for another 24 hours. With this technique, the time of air reabsorption is reduced to one-half.

General Anesthesia with Ketamine

MERCADER and CABORROCAS [299] in 1971 and ENGEL [139] in 1972 presented their experience with Ketamine (o-chlorophenyl-2-methylaminocyclohexanone) in neuroradiology. The use of this drug for general anesthesia was suggested by CORSSEN [89] in 1967. According to ENGEL [139], who used the method in a large number of encephalographies, Ketamine is very useful but it should be limited to the newborn and to children. This is in agreement with our own experience. In our department the anesthetists [325] use a dose of 10 mg/kg body weight in patients up to 12 years of age. If this dose is exceeded, muscular hypertonus may occur, so that whenever prolonged anesthesia is necessary (with 10 mg/kg body weight the anesthesia usually lasts about 1 hour) repeated administration is preferred to a higher dosage. According to the above authors, Ketamine offers two advantages: quick recovery from anesthesia without respiratory depression (for this reason the patient does not require endotracheal intubation); and the swallowing reflex is not impaired.

Ketamine is contraindicated in adult patients. All authors have observed cases with marked hypertonia of catatonic type. The presentation of ENGEL'S paper [139] at a meeting of neuroradiologists in Bologna was followed by a great deal of discussion. The consensus is that Ketamine is certainly very useful, but that it is too early to assess whether or not it should be the only drug for general anesthesia in children.

Conclusions

In most cases, psychological preparation and local anesthesia will obtain from the patient sufficient cooperation to enable a correct encephalography to be carried out without general anesthesia. However, this is not possible with children, with patients who are irrational and/or uncooperative, and with patients whose consciousness is impaired; in other words, in all those patients in whom neurological symptoms lead one to suspect a lesion capable of causing respiratory distress during encephalography. In these cases it is necessary to resort to general anesthesia with an anesthetic gas as similar as possible to the contrast gas, i.e. air and fluothane when atmospheric air is injected, N_2O when pure N_2O is injected. This will prevent the intracranial hypertension that often follows an encephalography performed under conventional general anesthesia (injection of air and inhalation of N_2O).

Another element that might contribute to an increase in CSF pressure during conventional general anesthesia is the cardiac-respiratory depression produced by fluothane. This can be avoided by performing anesthesia with g.h.b.a., but we must admit that the use of a volatile anesthetic is easier, and above all more useful, when sudden complications of an uncertain nature occur.

There are cases where the behavior of emotional or apprehensive patients makes the examination difficult and troublesome. It is here that NLA finds its main indication since, though producing considerable sedation, it does not deprive the body of its own defenses. A few of us (G. R., F. F.) are most favorably impressed by NLA and tend to use it with increasing frequency, thus reducing the use of both local and general anesthesia. However, NLA is a very delicate technique, requiring the continuous assistance of an experienced anesthetist. NLA is contraindicated in children, elderly patients, alcoholics and morphine addicts.

21. Complications

Introduction

A monograph on the subject of complications was published in English by RUGGIERO *et al.* [386] in 1969. Further experience has confirmed the conclusions stated in that work, so at first we were tempted to refer the reader directly to it. However, we have changed our minds and have decided to write the present chapter in order to give the complications of encephalography the same emphasis that we gave complications of ventriculography (both gaseous and with positive contrast). This chapter is in fact a résumé of the monograph by RUGGIERO *et al.* [386] and includes, without modifications, some of its most interesting passages.

A preliminary remark is necessary: the analysis of the literature *does not* give a true idea of the complications of encephalography for many reasons, the most important of which are:

1. It is impossible to discuss the publications on fractional and total encephalography separately. For instance, a paper classed as technically "good" does not usually hold the same value if it is viewed clinically, and vice-versa. This applies especially to earlier papers.
2. We have not been able to examine directly all the papers published, in spite of our request to medical documentation centers; some are thus quoted from other publications. This too applies chiefly to earlier papers.
3. Some papers fail to give important technical details, for example, whether the air was introduced by the lumbar or the suboccipital route; whether or not CSF was withdrawn and in what proportion; the kind of anesthesia performed, if any; etc.
4. The clinical material is not homogeneous because often the nature of the disease is not mentioned. Obviously, no comparison can be made between data relating to patients in poor condition, suffering from tumors and intracranial hypertension, and data gathered from examinations made of patients without tumors or in good general condition.

The above remarks, however, do not diminish the value of the analysis of literature made by RUGGIERO *et al.* [386]. This analysis shows that only 44 deaths were reported in 13065 encephalographies. Nevertheless, the authors have demonstrated, on the basis of the study of their personal cases, that a thorough, comparative study of the nature of the lesion and of the patient's condition is indispensable for the evaluation of the risks of an encephalography.

Results of Ruggiero, Cristi, and Trevisan [386]

There are two series: 523 patients examined between May 1964 and January 1966, and 500 cases examined more recently. The results of the second series are not reported since they confirm those of the first and demonstrate that in our department encephalography is tolerated better and better by the patients as a result of constant improvements in technique.

To evaluate the "clinical aspect" of encephalography, we considered two different periods: 1. the time spent by the patient in the X-ray room, 2. the interval between the end of the examination and the time when the patient is discharged from the department. The accidents observed during the first period are recorded on the forms shown in Chap. I, p. 12, Fig. 1.11 Complications arising during the second period are noted by the doctor in a special notebook. This is possible because the organization of our department allows the physician who performs the examination to take care of the patient personally afterward.

Syncope is the most frequent accident during encephalography. It is essential for the neuroradiologist to be able to recognize it and not to confuse it with acute cerebellar or temporal herniation, as has unfortunately occurred too often.

The pages of the monograph by RUGGIERO *et al.* [386] dealing with the physiopathogenesis of syncope are now reported almost in their entirety.

Syncope is a clinical entity which has been known for a long time, although it was only recently (1956–1960) that GASTAUT and coworkers (165–173) of Marseille described its etiology and the clinical and electroencephalographic features and presented a convincing physiopathogenic interpretation. This chapter derives mainly from their research.

Two types of syncope may be described, the cardio-inhibitory and the vasodepressor. The first involves cardiac arrest, while the second, which is much less frequent, involves a marked fall in blood pressure with no change in heart rate. In addition to these two forms, a mixed variety with prevalence of one of the other reaction is sometimes encountered. The outcome is always cerebral ischemia, the duration and extent of which determine the severity of the symptoms.

A cardiac arrest of less than 6 seconds produces no clinical signs. With one that lasts 6–8 seconds, pallor, respiration, impairment of consciousness, and slight diminution of muscular tone (head drop) will occur. Should the arrest last 8 to 10 seconds, the patient will lose consciousness, with extreme pallor, loss of upright posture, and upward deviation of gaze. With any arrest over 10 seconds convulsions appear, with one or more generalized clonic attacks preceding or following a tonic seizure in opisthotonus or emprosthotonus.

The duration of syncope rarely exceeds 15 seconds. On some occasions loss of consciousness and convulsions are accompanied by incontinence, together with excessive salivation and nausea, with or without vomiting. It is important to point out that at this stage the EEG will not disclose any epileptic patterns but only retardation of the cortical rhythm (which may go as far as electrical silence) and reticular overactivity. On cessation of syncope the rhythm is fast. Bradycardia may persist, with pallor and nausea of varying duration.

The physiopathogenic mechanism of syncope is that the bulbomesencephalic structures are released from the inhibiting action of the cortex and diencephalon, which are more sensitive to anoxia and consequently present early signs of disturbance.

A vagal discharge causes cardiac arrest and/or vasodepression. This discharge may be considered to be due primarily to congenital vagal hypertonus that undergoes spontaneous enhancement. However, because of the important afferent impulses, which are capable of activating the bulbar vagal centers and the surrounding reticular formation, it is more logical to consider the discharge as secondary to impulses coming from different sources (such as an intestinal contraction or a coughing spell) and directed to the vagal nuclei; the impulses might even arise from an emotional influence. GASTAUT (1956) [165, 169, 173] demonstrated in vagotonic subjects that syncope with anoxic-type seizures may be precipitated by intranasal or intra-auricular installations, by pharyngeal stimulation, or even simply by the anal introduction of a thermometer or suppository. It is therefore quite understandable that syncope may occur at the beginning of encephalography immediately after lumbar puncture, when the patient is tense and apprehensive, or even at the time of local anesthetic infiltration. The writers have observed four such cases; three other cases observed by CALABRÒ [70] are not included in the present material.

Therefore, although the precipitating factors may be many and difficult to classify, the writers think on the basis of the above considerations that the reason for which the patient receiving an encephalography probably influences the occurrence of syncope less than constitutional factors. Furthermore, it would appear that a peculiar vegetative reactivity plays an important role in this complication. A short report of a case observed recently, and not included in the present series, may be of interest.

The patient was a 31-year-old male with post-traumatic epilepsy. His normal blood pressure was 110/80 mm Hg at the time of encephalography, and it was 120/80 mm Hg prior to the lumbar puncture; the patient was quite apprehensive. After the lumbar puncture, performed with the Claude manometer connected to the needle by the technique described by RUGGIERO (1963) [378], the patient developed syncope. The CSF pressure was 54 ml and the systolic blood pressure 105. The syncope lasted 30 seconds, but the blood pressure did not rise in spite of the intramuscular administration of ephedrine. It was considered preferable to discontinue the examination; it was concluded successfully three days later with the patient under adequate sedation. No cause other than neurovegetative lability could explain the syncope: the patient had no intracranial tumor, was not hypertensive, and no spinal fluid had been withdrawn. The relationship between changes in blood pressure and syncope was proved, while there was no evidence of any variation in CSF pressure. The examiner did not record CSF pressure on the form before withdrawing the needle but he remembers that there was no significant variation. The occurrence of syncope need not therefore be considered serious (when encephalography is performed in ideal technical conditions); under no circumstances does it contraindicate the examination or call for its interruption. It is conceivable that, when the whole clinical picture is reconsidered in the light of this finding, premedication of patients will be undertaken.

The complications observed during the examination or persisting after it were divided by RUGGIERO *et al.* [386] into two groups: poorly tolerated and very poorly tolerated encephalographies. The authors analyzed the most serious cases very carefully, and demonstrated how difficult it is to make an objective evaluation of the causes of death. At any rate a positive relationship between death and encephalography was present in 0.76% of cases. Such a percentage is actually very low if we consider that the authors' data included many cerebral tumors.

Different factors in the complications were considered: age, sex, quantity of air introduced and CSF withdrawn, behavior of CSF pressure and blood pressure, state of the ventricular system, anesthesia, patient's condition at the time of the examination, duration of the examination, and neuroradiologist's experience.

The result of this study indicates that complications of encephalography depend essentially on four factors, which are in order of importance:

1. poor condition of patient
2. examination performed under general anesthesia
3. ventricular dilatation
4. presence of a tumor.

The depth of a tumor is more important than its supra- or infratentorial location. The dilatation of the ventricles has an effect independent of the increase of intracranial pressure. The fact that the patient is in poor condition at the moment of the examination and general anesthesia are the most negative factors in encephalography, while the presence and site of a tumor and ventricular dilatation must be regarded as only contributory factors. It is obvious, however, that patients with tumors are usually in poor condition.

Surprisingly, the amount of air injected and of CSF withdrawn did not seem to have much influence on tolerance of the examination. However, we are dealing here with "fractional" encephalography, i.e. an examination always performed with relatively small amounts of air and a moderate withdrawal of CSF, if any.

In conclusion, both the study by RUGGIERO *et al.* [386] and our subsequent experience prove that encephalography is a harmless procedure, and we absolutely deny that it is contraindicated in endocranial hypertension and tumors of the posterior fossa. A check of the vegetative and psychological condition of the patient is fundamental. The taboo of injecting a very small quantity of air or of rigorously conserving the proportion between air injected and CSF withdrawn then disappears.

Chapter II. Gas Ventriculography

Gas ventriculography is a radiological study of the ventricular system performed by replacing the CSF by air introduced into the lateral ventricles after they are punctured.

1. Historical Background

Ventriculography was proposed in 1918 by DANDY [100] who, on the basis of LUCKETT's accidental observation [265] of one case of post-traumatic spontaneous pneumoencephalon, understood the enormous diagnostic value of a study *in vivo* of the ventricular system. The method was quickly universally accepted but soon showed its limitations above all, the risk related to the noxious effect of air introduced into the ventricles under pressure. A number of papers were devoted to attempts at reducing these risks. First, it seemed sufficient to avoid hyperpressure (GARDNER and FRAZIER [162] and DEERY [108]), but later the opinion prevailed that the amount of contrast ought also to be reduced. This led to the advent via LYSHOLM [268–270] and TWINING [461, 462] of modern ventriculography, in which the "static" visualization of the ventricular system through total substitution of the CSF by air, is replaced by a "dynamic" fractionated study. This is usually carried out with a relatively small amount of contrast and necessitates special maneuvers and projections which must be performed by an experienced neuroradiologist.

More recently, the increasing use of encephalography and of neuroradiology in general has much restricted the indications for ventriculography. In supratentorial pathology the method is reserved almost exclusively for those cases where, owing to the extent of the lesion, communication between the supra- and intratentorial parts of the ventricular system is interrupted. However, in many departments ventriculography is still widely used for the pneumoencephalographic examination of the posterior fossa, since encephalography is considered dangerous, or because the indispensable conditions to perform it correctly cannot be obtained.

2. Technique

Introduction

Ventriculography consists of three stages: surgical, radiological, and mixed. The surgical stage is represented by skull trepanation and ventricular puncture; the mixed stage—radiological and surgical—is that of air injection, which should preferably be carried out with TV monitoring and in any case in the X-ray room; the pure radiological stage consists of the various projections and maneuvers which are necessary to visualize the different portions of the ventricular system.

The description of the surgical stage goes beyond the scope of this work. For this reason, together with TAVERAS and WOOD [453], we refer the reader to the neurosurgical textbooks, where the details of skull trepanation and ventricular puncture are described more precisely than we could do here.

From the radiological viewpoint, it is possible to distinguish two types of ventriculography: the conventional techniques (of which LYSHOLM'S [268–270] is the best in our opinion) and the "selective" technique, devoted to the study of special regions of the ventricular system. On the other hand, at the present time LYSHOLM'S technique may also be considered selective, since its main indication is the study of the posterior fossa, for which a special maneuver is necessary.

The principle of the conventional technique is as follows: the contrast medium is injected into the lateral ventricles, which are examined first; then the air is moved by appropriate maneuvers into the other portions (occipital and temporal horns, posterior portion of the third ventricle, aqueduct, and fourth ventricle), according to diagnostic needs.

The principle of the selective technique is to try to inject the air directly into the ventricles. A moderate amount of air should be sufficient and would reduce the risk of the examination.

There is in our opinion a preliminary reservation concerning these selective techniques, i.e. the difficulty of extending the examination, if necessary, to the whole ventricular system, since it is never possible to anticipate the site of the lesion with absolute certainty.

The radiographic technique for the ventriculographic study of the supratentorial portion of the ventricular system, including the temporal horns and the anterior portion of the third ventricle, is as described in Chap. I, to which we refer the reader. Here we deal only with the techniques suggested for studying the posterior portion of the third ventricle, the aqueduct, and the fourth ventricle. We shall only mention certain other techniques having merely historical value.

"Ventriculography without Air Injection" Gardner and Frazier [162] (1929)

The patient is supine, with shoulders raised and head flexed forward and elevated about 30 cm. A cannula is introduced into each occipital horn and CSF pressure is checked. One ml of indigo-carmine is injected into a single ventricle to verify whether the intraventricular communication is preserved.

The head is then lowered to the horizontal position and turned to one side. In this position the two cannulae lie in different planes, and the lower one acts as a siphon so that, as the fluid comes out, an equivalent amount of air is inspired through the upper cannula. CSF ejection is effected by jugular compression.

With this technique it would be possible to obtain the total replacement of the ventricular CSF by air without causing any severe pressure imbalance inside the brain.

Deery's Technique [108] (1931)

Deery's technique is also based on the principle of spontaneous air inspiration into the ventricles, after expression of the CSF. The filling of the ventricles is made easier by flexio-extension and rotation movements of the head.

Lysholm's Maneuver [268–270] (1935) for the Visualization of the Aqueduct and the Fourth Ventricle

After examination of the frontal horns in the supine position, the head is hyperextended to allow the contrast to accumulate in the third ventricle; the patient is then rapidly rotated while his head is kept lower than his body. At the end of the rotation the head is raised again, and with the patient in this prone position radiographs are taken in lateral, postero-anterior, postero-anterior half-axial, and oblique projections. The mechanism of the maneuver is that the contrast passes into the aqueduct and the fourth ventricle, and it is retained there when, after the rotation, the head returns to a horizontal position. In the absence of a block, the maneuver prevents the air from leaving the ventricular system through the foramina of Luschka and Magendie; this is also the reason why the maneuver must be rapid.

Twining's Maneuver [461, 462] (1939) for Filling the Third Ventricle, the Aqueduct, and the Fourth Ventricle

Soon after the publication of Lysholm's "Das Ventrikulogramm" [268–270], two important papers on ventriculography were published by Twining [461, 462], who suggested five maneuvers. The most important one was conceived essentially for studying the third ventricle and the aqueduct, but with slight modifications it serves also for the examination of the fourth ventricle. Ventricular puncture is performed with the patient in supine decubitus on a tilting table, which is later set in the Trendelenburg position. Then the head is hyperextended so that the air can fill the aqueduct. Radiographs are taken quickly, then the patient is returned to the horizontal position. Before carrying out the maneuver, it is necessary to establish exactly the height of the

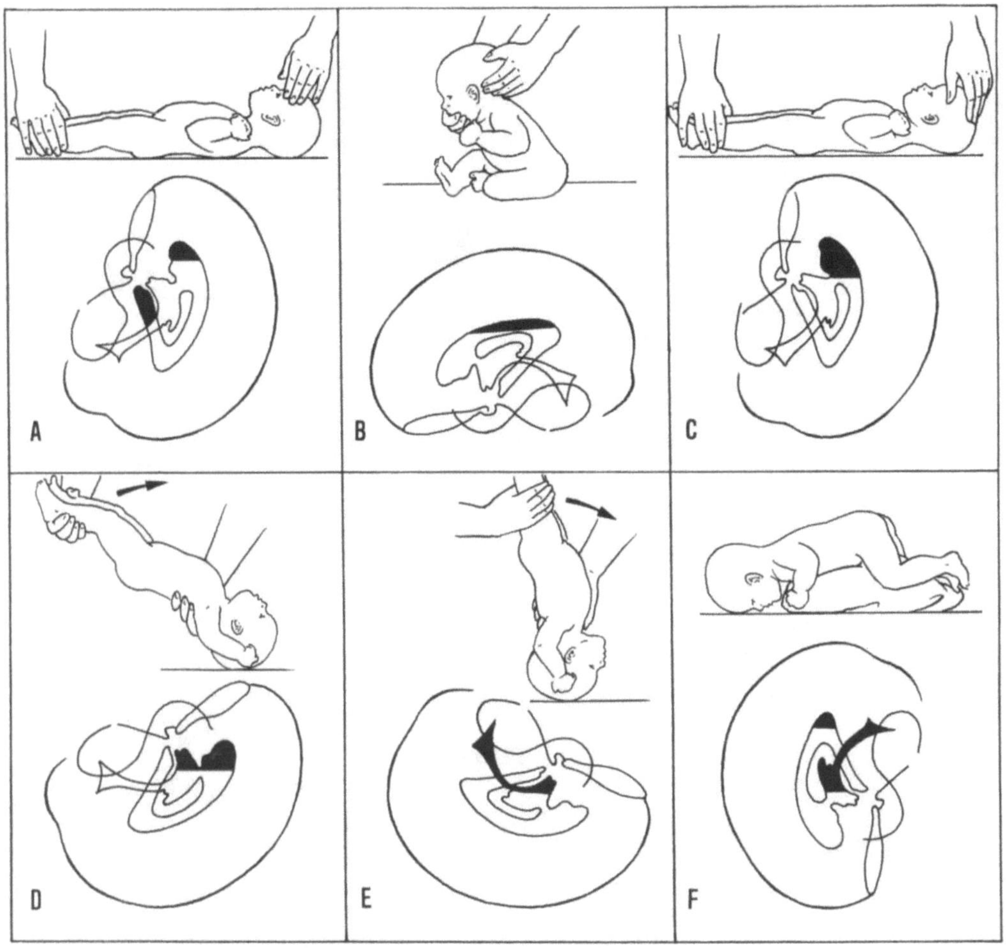

Fig. 2.1. Schematic drawing illustrating ZIEDSES DES PLANTES' technique for the examination of the third ventricle, the aqueduct, and the fourth ventricle

X-ray tube from the ground and the degree of inclination of the tilting table, so that the base of the skull is parallel to the floor; this is necessary to avoid the accumulation of the contrast in the temporal horns as a result of exaggerated hyperextension. The other four of TWINING's maneuvers [461, 462] were conceived for the study of the fourth ventricle. They are carried out with the patient in the prone position, and their principle is very similar to that of Lysholm's maneuver, of which they represent, in some way, separate stages.

Twining's maneuvers, especially his Number 1 and Number 4, seem to be the substratum of the technique suggested in 1957 by LAINE *et al.* [245, 246]; there is no reference in their text to TWINING's papers [461, 462], but they are mentioned in the bibliography.

Verbiest's Technique [468, 469] (1947)

After puncture of the two occipital horns, all the ventricular CSF is replaced by air. The usual projections are performed; then, with the patient prone, either a physiological solution or the previously drawn CSF (which has been preserved under sterile conditions) is introduced alternately into either ventricle, until it runs out on the opposite side. This outflow indicates that the two lateral ventricles and that part of the third ventricle anterior to the foramina of Monroe are filled with fluid, while the rest of the ventricular system is occupied by the air. This enables isolated images of the posterior portion of the third ventricle, of the aqueduct, and of the fourth ventricle to be obtained; their quality can be further improved by an additional intraven-

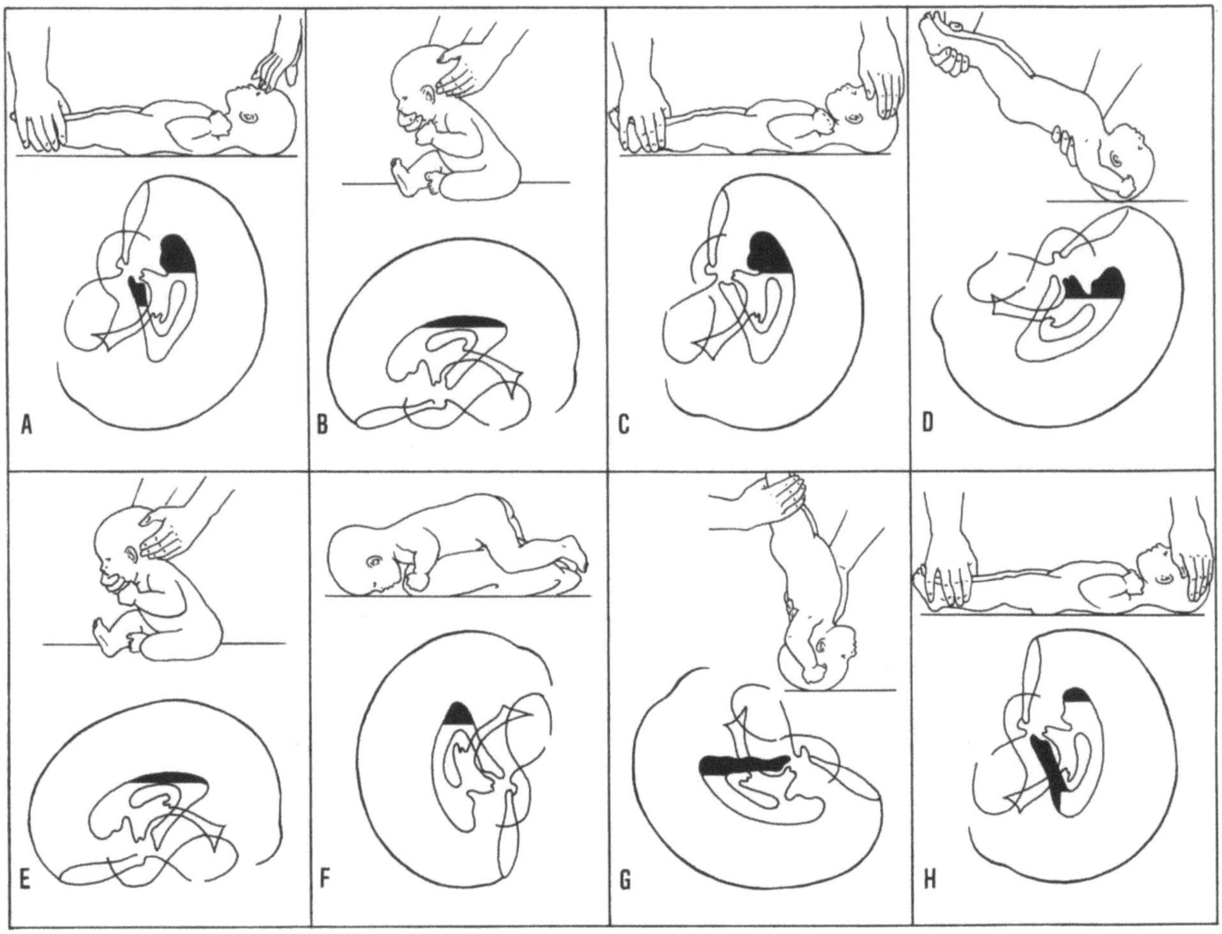

Fig. 2.2. Schematic drawing illustrating ZIEDSES DES PLANTES' technique for the examination of the temporal horns

tricular injection of fluid, causing a certain degree of intracranial hypertension.

In 1949 MALMROS [247] described an analogous technique, in apparent ignorance of VERBIEST'S paper [468].

Ziedses des Plantes' Maneuvers [487, 488] (1953) for the Study of the Third Ventricle, Aqueduct, and Fourth Ventricle, and for the Study of the Temporal Horns

This is the famous somersault that the author employs for pneumoencephalography in children, and which Figs. 2.1 and 2.2 demonstrate better than any verbal description. This maneuver is performed nowadays with motorized rotating chairs, of which ZIEDSES DES PLANTES' somersault can be considered a precursor.

For adults ZIEDSES DES PLANTES [487, 488] suggested a maneuver similar to LYSHOLM'S [268–270], the only difference being that the patient is placed in the Trendelenburg position.

Central Ventriculography of Azambuja, Arana-Iniguez, Sande, and Garcia-Guelfi [19] (1956)

The patient is supine on the operating table. One frontal horn is punctured about 2.5 cm from the midline and immediately before the coronary suture. The needle is inserted perpendicularly, then withdrawn, leaving a hole through which is intro-

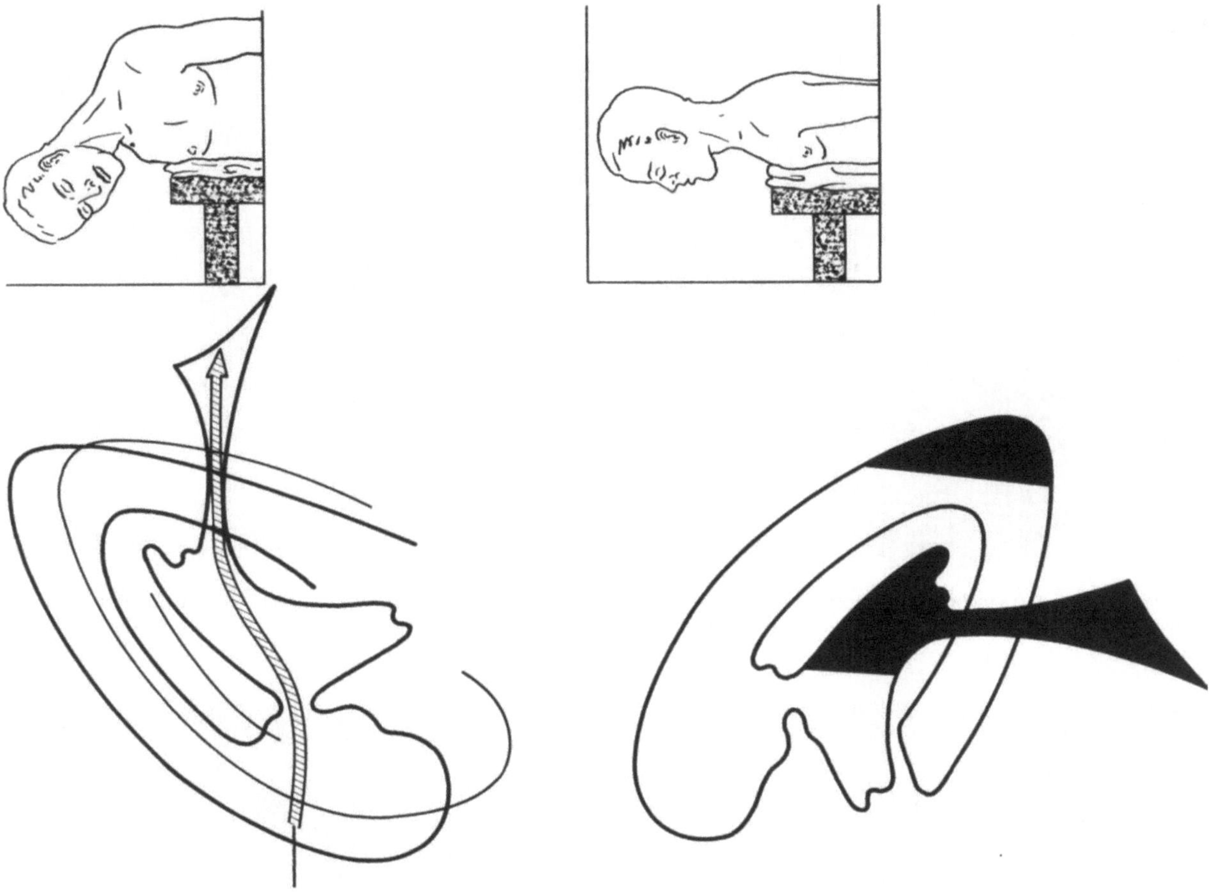

Fig. 2.3. Schematic drawing illustrating the mechanism of the first stage of CALABRÒ's techniques. Air collects in the posterior part of the third ventricle

duced a rubber catheter that crosses the frontal horn, then penetrates the foramen of Monroe to reach the third ventricle. This can be "felt", as its floor offers resistance to the penetration of the catheter. Once correctly placed in the third ventricle, the catheter is secured to the skin, but it still remains somewhat mobile. Now the patient is carried to the X-ray room, where the position of the catheter is checked radiologically in the prone position. If it is considered correct, 10 ml of air is injected in 10 seconds, and a lateral radiograph is taken with a horizontal central beam; 10 ml of CSF is withdrawn to balance the pressure, and further radiographs are taken in the usual postero-anterior projections. If the amount of air is not sufficient, further injections of air are performed, alternating with CSF subtraction. Once the study of the posterior fossa is finished, the patient is placed supine for examination of the anterior portion of the third ventricle.

Fractional Ventriculography by Laine, Riff, Delandtsheer, and Galibert [245, 246] (1957)

We have already mentioned this method when dealing with TWINING's technique [461, 462]. Usually the left frontal horn is punctured to facilitate a right frontal flap in case it should be necessary to open the supra-optical lamina before the tumor exeresis. In order to avoid pressure disequilibrium, not more than 10 ml of air is injected in small amounts, 2–3 ml at a time, alternating with the withdrawal of 2–3 ml of CSF.

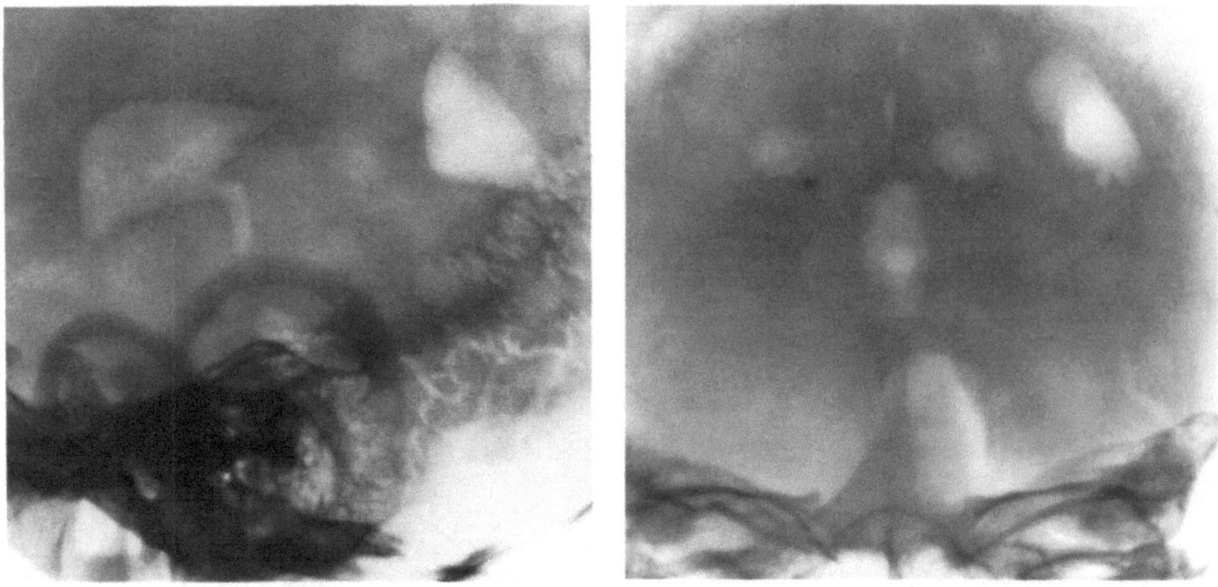

a b

Fig. 2.4a, b. CALABRÒ'S technique for posterior fossa ventriculography for right cerebellar astrocytoma. Almost the entire amount of air collects in the posterior part of the third ventricle, aqueduct, and fourth ventricle. Little air remains in the left lateral ventricle

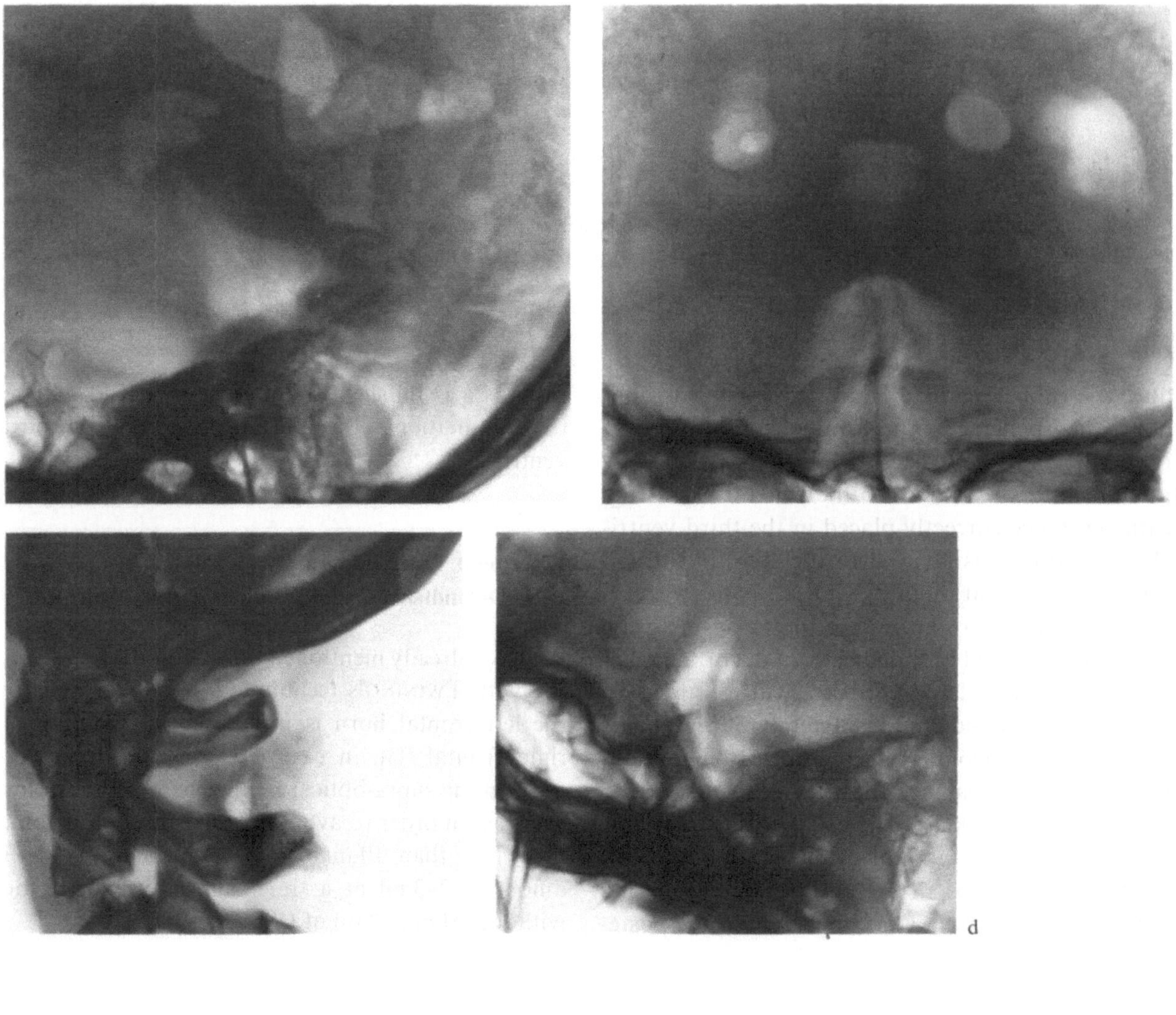

a b c d

Once the radiographic part of the examination is finished, the frontal horn is punctured again to let the contrast escape.

Rostotskaya's Technique [372] (1958)

In principle this technique is similar to the one suggested 40 years ago by GARDNER and FRAZIER [162], although the author seems unaware of this. The differences are that the frontal horn is punctured instead of the occipital horn, and the CSF is reinjected into the ventricles at the end of the examination.

Calabrò's Technique [70] (1967)

Frontal burr holes are made in the operating theater. The patient is moved to the X-ray room and positioned prone, with the head and breast (up to the level of the mammillary line) projecting from the radiological table. The head is flexed until the orbito-meatal line is parallel to the floor. The head is then turned through 50–60° toward the side opposite to the ventricle to be punctured, which will therefore lie posteriorly and at a lower level than the other one. Fifteen ml of CSF is withdrawn and 10 ml of air injected into the frontal horn in about 20 seconds.

This maneuver is performed twice. The second injection is made rapidly (7–9 seconds); and the head position, which had remained unchanged during the first 3–4 seconds, is modified during the following 4–5 seconds, reducing first the flexion, then the rotation, until the orbito-meatal line is perpendicular to the floor. At this moment the needle is withdrawn and the radiological stage begins. Lateral (with a horizontal beam) and postero-anterior radiographs are taken. If there is no block in the ventricular system, one can proceed to study the subarachnoid space: again, the head is strongly flexed; then, after a quick rotation, the patient is positioned supine while his head remains flexed. The usual radiographs are taken. The mechanism of the technique is as follows: when the head is stationary, the air moves from the frontal horn toward the posterior portion of the third ventricle; then it enters the aqueduct, the fourth ventricle, and the great cistern. In a second stage that could be called "dynamic" in opposition to the previous one, the progressive reduction of the head flexion and rotation prevents the contrast from leaving the ventricular system in the absence of a block (Figs. 2.3, 2.4). (Usually some contrast also enters one or both lateral ventricles, but this is not a drawback, as it may be useful later for the study of the anterior portion of the third ventricle.) In the final stage, when the head is again markedly flexed, the air collects, through the foramen of Magendie, in the great cistern, and in the cervical subarachnoid space. When the patient is rotated, the air moves in the opposite direction from these structures, toward the intracranial subarachnoid space (Fig. 2.5). This generally allows a good visualization of the interpeduncular, chiasmatic, and lamina terminalis cisterns (Fig. 2.6).

3. Complications

Introduction

The main difficulty in evaluating the risks of a ventriculography is that such an examination is in most cases immediately followed by a surgical operation. Consequently, only complications observed during the ventriculography or immediately after it can be noted; one cannot study the late complications, as is possible for encephalography. A thorough study of the subject is nevertheless fully justified, as will be demonstrated, we feel, by the following paragraphs.

Ventriculography is very seldom performed in the neuroradiological department of the Ospedale Maggiore. For this reason the material of this study is based chiefly on the cases treated in the neuroradiological department of the University Neurological Institute and the Ospedale Cardarelli in Naples. Paralleling what has been done for encephalography, the complications of ventriculography

◅ Fig. 2.5a–d. Second stage of CALABRÒ's technique: study of the subarachnoid space. After the examination of the infratentorial part of the ventricular system (a, b) the head is markedly flexed and the air enters the spinal subarachnoid space (c). Finally the head is rotated and the patient is set again in the supine position: the air fills the cisterns of the skull base (d)

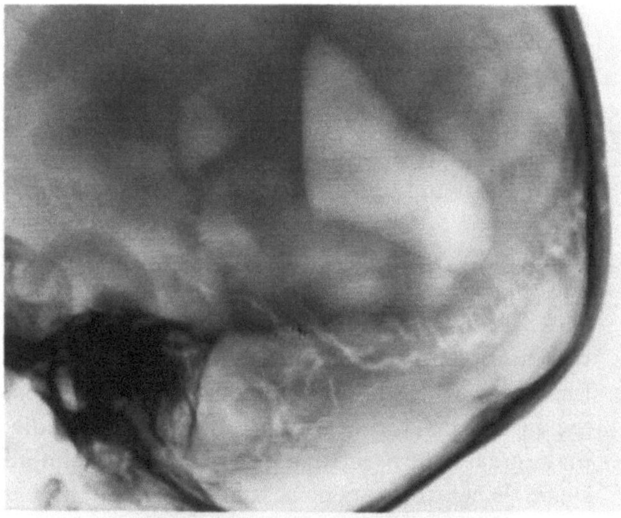
a

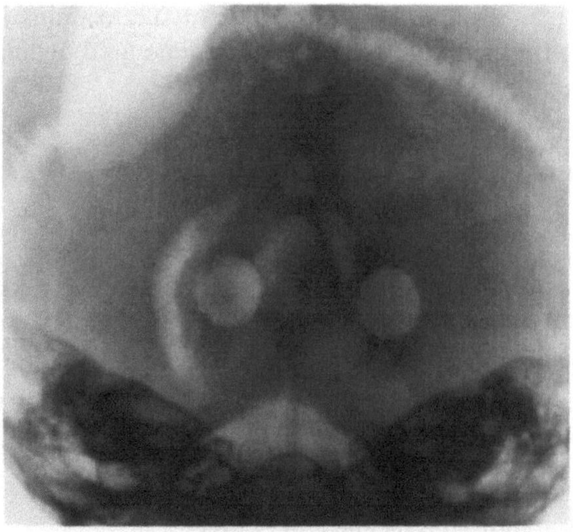
b

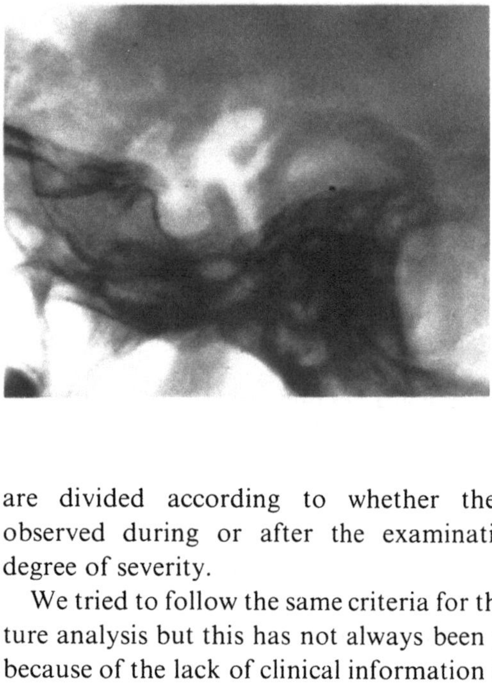
c

Fig. 2.6a–c. CALABRÒ's technique for posterior fossa ventriculography. Fourth ventricle papilloma. After the examination of the infratentorial part of the ventricular system (a, b) the air is directed toward the subarachnoid space. The pontine, interpeduncular, and chiasmatic cisterns are perfectly visualized, as well as the convexity subarachnoid sulci (c)

are divided according to whether they were observed during or after the examination and degree of severity.

We tried to follow the same criteria for the literature analysis but this has not always been possible because of the lack of clinical information in many papers. Another difficulty is that the number of examinations performed is seldom noted in the various publications.

Analysis of the Literature

Headache has been particularly studied by BREWER [56] on 86 ventriculographies performed in 77 patients (68 tumors). Both ventricles were punctured in 17 cases (14 times the occipital horns and 3 times the frontal horns) and only one ventricle in 69 cases (51 times the frontal horn). The air–CSF exchange was performed by fractions of 5–20 ml, and the total amount of the air injected, calculated on the basis of the presumed volume of ventricles, was less than the CSF removed. In most cases the introduction of air did not cause headaches. A frontal headache was frequent in cases of elevated intracranial pressure: it occurred when the CSF was being withdrawn and was attenuated with the air injection. This was observed whether a tumor was present or not.

According to most authors (RIGGS [368], TAVERAS and WOOD [453], VERBIEST [469]), vegetative troubles such as nausea, emesis, pallor, salivation, and cold sweat are constant. A slowing of the cardiac rate with hypothermia is also frequent, whereas an increase in cardiac and respiratory rhythms and in body temperature is seldom observed.

Bleeding has been observed by various authors: FALK [143] carried out in 203 cases a radiographic follow-up from 1 month to 15 years after ventriculography. Calcifications were present in 27 cases (13.3%); in 9 they had a ribbon-shaped aspect and were located between the burr hole and the lateral ventricle; in 18 cases the calcium deposit was of the "nodular" type and located immediately below the burr hole, probably in an extracerebral situation. FALK thinks these calcifications were the result of bleeding that occurred at the moment of the puncture, either along the path of the needle or around the dura mater.

LINDGREN [258] also pointed out dots indicative of bleeding along the needle's path.

DYKE, ELSBERG, and DAVIDOFF [134] discovered a filling defect near the choroid plexus in 6 out of 100 ventriculographies. Since there was no possible relationship with the symptoms, this feature was ascribed to an edema or bleeding caused by the puncture of the plexus or of the ventricular wall. In one case the hypothesis was confirmed at autopsy. No such feature was ever found in 1400 cases of encephalography.

TAVERAS and WOOD [453] described a case of "swelling" of the parietal region, presumably caused by an intracerebral hematoma following a difficult ventricular puncture. They warn that such a complication may lead to an incorrect diagnosis of a parietal tumor.

GROTJAHN and FRENCH [190] have observed 7 cases of akinesia after ventriculography in a series of 89 young people from 7 to 19 years of age.

When the occipital horn is punctured, it is not rare to observe impairment of visual acuity and/or visual field. As far as we know, these complications were first pointed out by MASSON [287], who among 100 patients observed 6 cases of temporary blindness. In two cases the blindness occurred during the examination and in 4 it was noticed respectively 2, 3, 4, and 16 hours later. The longest duration of the blindness was 3 days, but partial troubles were still observed for some weeks. Other cases of temporary cortical blindness were quoted by BAUDOUIN *et al.* [27], LOSSIUS [263], REDSLOB and DIEFFENBACH [364], and RINALDI *et al.* [369]. The mechanism of these troubles was attributed by MASSON [287] and BAUDOUIN *et al.* [27] to injury of the occipital cortex and/or the posterior portion of the occipital tracts caused by bleeding and/or edema. LOSSIUS [263] thinks it is a disorder reflex of the cerebral vasomotor control which causes vasoconstriction and consequent cerebral anemia and anoxia. According to RINALDI *et al.* [369], the pressure imbalance produced by ventriculography would cause temporal and cerebellar herniation with compression of the posterior cerebral arteries against the tentorium, with consequent anemia of the occipital cortex.

LINDGREN [258] and SCHWARZ and ROSNER [413] pointed out that a transtentorial herniation can arise or become worse as a consequence of a ventriculography.

SCHUPFER [409] has described a case of retinal hemorrhage.

Mortality

FALK [143] and LENZI [250], who made an extensive analysis of the literature, report that the mortality rate in ventriculography varies from 3 to 10%. According to FALK [143], however, such a finding is not very significant in itself, since fatalities were mostly connected with the nature of the disease for the diagnosis of which the patient underwent the ventriculography.

We have collected from the literature 81 cases in which death was clearly associated with ventriculography. We summarize them below.

MCCONNELL [292] (1923): 3 cases of posterior fossa tumor with compression of the brain stem; in one of them the fatal outcome occurred even before the air injection, after a single ventricular puncture which caused a fall in CSF pressure.

PENFIELD [336] (1925): 1 case where death occurred suddenly 36 hours after the ventriculography at the end of which the air had been allowed to escape through the ventricular puncture. The author neither describes the patient's condition nor gives any information on the nature of the disease.

GRANT [179, 180] analyzed both his personal cases (392 cases) and FREIZE's (160 cases); there were 32 deaths (8%) among his own patients and 10 (6.5%) among FREIZE's. Among his own cases, GRANT [179, 180] observed 19 gliomas, but apart from this fact we have no information about either the lesions or the patients' condition at the time of the examination. According to GRANT [179, 180], death is a result of intraventricular hemorrhage and/or sudden impairment of the endoventricular pressure followed by brain-stem edema. We were unable to read personally the two papers by GRANT [179, 180]; what we have reported here was quoted by RIGGS [368].

RIGGS [368] (1933): 12 cases (11 brain tumors and 1 syringobulbia) out of 148 ventriculographies. The cause of death was respiratory paralysis after more or less prolonged stupor and hyperthermia. In 31 cases the patient became worse after the examination. This was considered by RIGGS to be due to disequilibrium in the intracranial pressure.

CRAWFORD [92] (1933): 13 cases out of 169 examinations (7.7%). This paper too could not be examined personally by us, and what we report here comes from FALK's publication [143]. CRAWFORD [92] considered the presence of the tumour to be the direct cause of death in 6 cases, while in the others the fatal outcome was probably due to the effects of the "combination of pressure and cerebral anoxia" or, as happened in 2 patients, to a hemorrhage caused by the puncture. The author did not specify whether an autopsy had been done.

PEET [331] (1940): 1 case, a hydrocephalic child. Death was caused by bilateral epidural hematoma that occurred after the ventriculography.

In a case of corpus callosum astrocytoma described by FALK [143] in which there had probably been bleeding along the needle path a thalamic hemorrhage was demonstrated at autopsy.

In 1952 HEPPNER [208] observed a rather rare complication: in a case of septum pellucidum glioblastoma death occurred suddenly, 8 hours after the ventriculography. Autopsy demonstrated two findings: a torn ependymal vein, 2 mm in diameter along the needle path, and a cardiac gaseous embolism. The author did not hesitate to correlate them.

DAVID *et al.* [102] (1953) had 3 deaths among 23 ventriculographies performed in cases with brain tumors: an extracerebral tumor of the foramen magnum with marked herniation of the tonsils, a deep temporal glioma, and a pontine glioma. In a case of intraventricular extracerebral tumor, the ventriculography was followed by coma that, however, cleared up after the operation.

RUGGIERO [374] (1957) reported 2 deaths. In one case the autopsy showed an old softening of the left striated body and small, well limited, recent foci in both caudate nuclei; the diameter of these foci clearly corresponded to that of the ventriculographic parenchyma in the attempt to reach the ventricles. In the other case, not verified at autopsy, the fatal outcome was probably to be ascribed to subacute edema of the brain stem. In a third case a coma occurred in the night following the examination, but fortunately it regressed after a ventricular puncture.

TAVERAS and WOOD [453] (1964) had 1 death, a child suffering from a congenital anomaly. The patient died from a hemorrhage that occurred during the ventriculography, probably due to the opening of an abnormally located dural sinus.

Material and Methods

Our series consists of 300 examinations performed from 1960 to 1966. Two hundred and fifty patients were examined with Lysholm's technique [268–270] and 50 with the selective technique described by CALABRÒ [70]. The age of the patients ranged from 7 months to 72 years, with a higher percentage (42%) in the first 10 years of life. With the exception of a few cases, from 1960 to 1963 the examinations were performed under general anesthesia in children and under local anesthesia in adults. Later on, neuroleptanalgesia was employed for patients of any age, except babies. The type of lesion as well as the number and type of complications are summarized in Table 2.1.

As in the chapter on encephalography, the accidents that occurred during ventriculography are considered separately from those that appeared after it. The complications have been divided in three groups, according to their seriousness:

1. *Light:* rise in body temperature to 38° C; headache of variable intensity and duration; slight vegetative troubles.
2. *Serious:* high fever (over 38° C); severe headache; intense vegetative troubles; transitory psychological impairment of the sensorium; other neurological symptoms such as epileptic fits, transitory vision impairment, and/or aphasia.
3. *Very Serious:* progressive impairment of consciousness, associated with serious respiratory and circulatory disorders, up to the fatal outcome.

Table 2.1. Complications in ventriculography

Type of lesion	Classical technique					Calabrò's technique		
	Number of cases		Light	Severe	Very severe	Number of cases		
Infratentorial expansive processes	128					32		None
Anterior part of the posterior fossa		33		1	1		7	
Posterior part of the posterior fossa		95	6	5	—		25	
Supratentorial expansive processes	69					—		
Hemispherical		44	2	1			—	
Mid-line		25		1			—	
Non tumoral diseases	38					18		
Non communicating hydrocephalus		24	3				13	
Communicating hydrocephalus		11	1				5	
Pseudotumor		3	2				—	
Negative	15		2			—		
Total	250		16	8	1	50		

Comment

Six patients developed serious troubles during the examination. In 3 of them the symptoms were acute.

In a 27-year-old man with a third ventricle epidermoid cyst, generalized epileptic seizure occurred after the introduction of 20 ml of air. The crisis was accompanied by cyanosis and abundant transpiration and lasted about 30 seconds. The air injection was suspended and the patient improved but died suddenly 3 days later.

The second case was a 7-year-old child with a medulloblastoma of the vermis. A syncope occurred when the patient was positioned prone to fill the infratentorial portion of the ventricular system. He recovered from this crisis as well as from other serious vegetative disorders, and was successfully operated on the next day.

Cessation of breathing was observed also in a third case, a 12-year-old child with a right cystic cerebellar astrocytoma. He recovered spontaneously and was successfully operated on later.

Of the three patients who showed complications after ventriculography, one died. This was a man aged 22 who had been suffering for several months from symptoms of increased intracranial pressure with papilloedema. An encephalography was first performed showing nonfilling of the ventricular system with evident cisternal signs of an expansive posterior fossa process. A ventriculography was performed a few days later, affording the diagnosis of a large bulbo-pontine tumor; the ventricles were very much dilated. At the end of the examination body temperature rose to 39° and resisted medical treatment for 2 days. The third day after the examination Cheyne-Stokes respiration set in and the blood pressure dropped to 70 mm Hg. The patient died. The diagnosis was confirmed at autopsy, which showed a bulbo-pontine glioma; the cardio-circulatory system was undamaged.

In another case of pontine tumor—a 15-year-old girl in fair general condition—headache, high fever, twilight state, clouded consciousness, dyspnea, and cardiac arhythmia occurred immediately after the examination, during which 30 ml of air had been injected. A right hemiparesis appeared 2 hours later. All these symptoms became worse and the patient was discharged three days later at her family's request. Although the patient left the hospital alive, we fear this case must be included in the group of fatal outcomes.

The third case was a man aged 53 in good general condition. Immediately after the ventriculography—which showed a tumor in the right pulvinar region—severe headache, emesis, and tendency to dizziness occurred. These symptoms were followed 2 hours later by generalized seizures. The symptoms cleared up in 3 days with anti-edema therapy, and the patient was transferred to the radiotherapy department.

No complications were observed with Calabrò's [70] technique (Table 2.1). The results of the study of the ventriculographic material are less reliable than those obtained from the analysis of the encephalographic material. The ventriculographic case histories come from two different departments and the doctor who performs the examination is usually not able to follow the patient afterward.

Conclusions

1. The rapid evolution of radiological technology (tomography, TV monitoring, motorized rotating chairs) has increased the diagnostic value of all methods. Consequently, the differences among the various techniques of ventriculography have also been much reduced. For example, the distinction between Lysholm's and Ziedses des Plantes' techniques has practically disappeared with the use of the somersault technique. Ziedses des Plantes' maneuver, however, is still used with children who are difficult to manage in a motorized chair.
2. Ventriculography is an examination not without risks; it is certainly more dangerous than encephalography. The data that we could collect from our analysis of the literature and the study of our own material give only an approximate idea of the risks. Ventriculography is very often followed by a surgical operation; therefore it is not possible, if the patient's condition worsens, to distinguish the effects of the operation itself from what could be ascribed to the preceding ventriculographic examination.

Chapter III. Positive-Contrast Ventriculography

1. Introduction

Iodoventriculography, the radiological examination of the ventricular system by means of an opaque contrast medium, was introduced by BALADO [23–25] in 1928. In 1964 PORTERA [354–356] suggested employing iodate emulsions which diffuse through the CSF. With this technique (which the author named panventriculography) all parts of the ventricular system can be visualized simultaneously.

Iodoventriculography is one of the most controversial neuroradiological procedures: while many authors consider it of great diagnostic value, thanks to the fine outlining of the ventricles usually obtained with the positive contrast, others consider this examination dangerous. The opaque contrast media are liposoluble and not reabsorbable in CSF; their toxicity has been for many years the subject of heated controversies. While there are authors who consider these substances absolutely harmless, others judge them to be dangerous to the point of proscribing their use.

Before we can reach a definite conclusion on the usefulness of iodoventriculography, the problem of the toxicity of iodinated oil has to be solved. For this reason we decided to summarize the subject of these oils from the very beginning. The result is a rather heterogeneous chapter, since the papers on this subject are scattered in the literature of both ventriculography and myelography as well as that of experimental pharmacology.

2. Iodinated Oils

Analysis of the Literature

Iodinated oils were introduced in 1921 by SICARD and FORESTIER [422, 423]. The first compound was lipiodol, employed by SICARD *et al.* [424] to explore the spinal canal and by BALADO [23] to examine the ventricular system. After an initial success in South America (BALADO [23–25], CARILLO [73], and AMEZUA [11]), the usefulness of iodoventriculography was reviewed in many papers dealing with the risks of using lipiodol even in myelography. LYSHOLM [271] obtained successful diagnostic results with lipiodol but soon abandoned it because of its irritating effect on the arachnoid. As a contrast medium instead of lipiodol he suggested air, which was later adopted by his pupils in Sweden and in many other countries.

Opaque contrast media were again brought to the attention of radiologists in 1942 when STEINHAUSEN *et al.* [435] suggested using Pantopaque in myelography. Pantopaque is more fluid than lipiodol and therefore easier to withdraw after the examination. The great popularity of Pantopaque led to its use for ventriculography as well. In 1952 BULL [66] reported satisfactory results obtained in 80 cases in which ventriculography had been performed with Myodil, which is the British equivalent of Pantopaque.

The problem, however, remained unsolved; soon many authors expressed the same reservations as regards Pantopaque and similar products as had been made for lipiodol. Meanwhile in France lipiodol was replaced by Etiodol (ultrafluid lipiodol) and later by Discolipiodol. These compounds were manufactured by the producers of lipiodol; they are quite different from lipiodol, but for a long time they were confused with it and so considered dangerous.

In 1964, after the introduction of PORTERA'S [354–356] panventriculography, the toxicity of the emulsions came under discussion and was the subject of a great deal of experimental research.

In 1966 GUERBET *et al.* [191, 192] introduced a new contrast medium, Duroliopaque. To our knowledge there are no publications on this product in iodoventriculography, but in view of the experience with myelography of BORIES *et al.* [49] and HELLER [207] and of the results of PENNING and KERCKHOFF's experimental work [339] it is easy to foresee that Duroliopaque will replace all the positive contrast media used to the present day.

We conclude this paragraph with a brief mention of attempts to use triiodate water-soluble contrast media. Their use in iodoventriculography must be proscribed because of the severe secondary reactions (CAMPBELL *et al.* [72, 204]). Among these compounds, however, methylglucamine salts seem to be less toxic than sodium salts. Thorotrast was abandoned a long time ago. The papers of ALEXANDER *et al.* [7], VILLACA [470], SCHOENFELD and FREEMAN [408], and TWINING and ROWBOTHAM [463] are therefore mentioned here only because of their historical significance.

Chemistry and Physics

The characteristics of the various compounds are summarized in Table 3.1. Opacity is expressed by the number of grams of iodine present in 1 ml of the substance, and viscosity is expressed in poises.

Iodinated oils are divided into three groups:

Table 3.1. Characteristics of the various compounds for positive contrast ventriculography

Compound	Density at 15°	Opacity	Viscosity at 15° (in poises)
Lipiodol LAFAY	1.36	0.54	20
Lipiodol F.	1.32	0.52	2
Lipiodol U. F.	1.28	0.48	0.65
Pantopaque	1.25	0.38	0.60
Discolipiodol	1.15	0.32	0.25
Duroliopaque	1.14	0.32	0.28

Lipiodol and its Derivatives

Lipiodol

Lipiodol is also called Lipiodol Lafay and is iodinated clove oil. Its formula is not very well defined: it is a mixture of fatty acids, including about 76% diiodostearic and approximately 12% monoiodostearic. Lipiodol is the oldest and most toxic iodinated oil. It is very viscous (20 poises at 15° C) and does not compare favorably with other compounds, from any point of view. Therefore it must definitely be abandoned.

The derivatives of lipiodol are its ethyl esters which are listed below:

Fluid Lipiodol

Fluid lipiodol has practically the same opacity as lipiodol but it is ten times more fluid. Nevertheless its viscosity is still too high and it cannot be withdrawn with ease from the subarachnoid space. Fluid lipiodol is better than lipiodol; but since its properties are inferior to those of more recent compounds, it is hard to understand why it is still used in some departments.

Ultrafluid Lipiodol, or Etiodol

Ultrafluid lipiodol has the same viscosity as Pantopaque and can rather easily be withdrawn after the examination.

Discolipiodol

Discolipiodol has more or less the same opacity as Pantopaque but is three times more fluid. It has not yet been employed in iodoventriculography.

Ethyl Iodophenylundecylate

Ethyl iodophenylundecylate is manufactured under the names of Pantopaque, Myodil, and Etiodan. These products are used chiefly in the Anglo-Saxon countries and in South America. They are considerably less opaque than lipiodol and fluid lipiodol but provide satisfactory contrast for clinical use. Pantopaque is three times more fluid than fluid lipiodol and can be more easily withdrawn after the examination. This is one of the main reasons for its popularity and that of its derivatives.

Ethyl Monoiodostearate

Ethyl monoiodostearate is sold under the name Duroliopaque. It is the most recent and the least toxic liposoluble contrast medium. It has practically the same viscosity and opacity as Discolipiodol.

Pharmacology

GUERBET *et al.* [191, 192] made a comparative study on the toxicity of lipiodol derivatives (which is the same for all compounds) and of Pantopaque.

Oral Administration

Pantopaque is much more toxic than lipiodol derivatives. In the rat LD_{50}* is 1.2 g/kg body weight, whereas with the compounds of the lipiodol series it is 20 g/kg body weight; 5 g/kg has only a laxative effect.

Intraperitoneal Administration

Even by this route, Pantopaque reveals itself as much more toxic: LD_{50} is 4.6 g/kg body weight in the mouse, and 19 g/kg body weight in the rat. LD_{50} of lipiodol and Duroliopaque is 60 g/kg body weight in both mouse and rat.

Intraspinal Administration

Intraspinal administration is dealt with in the section below on clinical and experimental research with the various compounds. Here we only mention that in the experiments made by GUERBET *et al.* [191, 192], dogs injected with Pantopaque showed much more severe meningeal reactions than those receiving Duroliopaque.

Local Complications

In man the subcutaneous injection of 2 ml of Duroliopaque does not produce any local inflammatory reaction. However, pain is experienced for 24 to 48 hours at the site of the injection.

Reabsorption

The rate of reabsorption varies according to the route of administration. Pantopaque and Duroliopaque are very slowly reabsorbed when injected subcutaneously: in rats 1 ml of such compounds takes a year to disappear. With intraperitoneal injections reabsorption is faster and the same for both compounds.

According to GUERBET *et al.* [191, 192], more than half of the Duroliopaque injected into dogs is reabsorbed within one month; later reabsorption is much slower. Pantopaque reabsorption is faster but the difference is apparent only if a considerable amount of compound is employed. According to PEACHER and ROBERTSON [330], the reabsorption rate of Pantopaque is only 0.5–1 ml a year.

Metabolism

Duroliopaque is ethyl monoiodostearate. It is derived from the ethyl ester of stearic acid and is obtained by the substitution (in position 9 or 10) of one atom of hydrogen by one atom of iodine. The structure and the metabolism of Duroliopaque are thus analogous to those of the natural fatty acids and this substance is probably destroyed in the organism by β or ω oxidation without liberation of toxic compounds, while iodine is eliminated in the urine as sodium iodide. Pantopaque has a completely different structure. It is ethyl iodophenylundecylate; its degradation involves the liberation of a derivative of monoiodobenzene which is much more toxic than the degradation products of Duroliopaque.

Complications

The papers devoted to iodoventriculography are rather few, but all authors agree that the method is risk-free. As early as 1952 BULL [66] published 80 cases of Myodil ventriculographies without complications; JEFFERSON and OCCLESHAW [239] had an analogous experience with 67 cases; MORETTE and PARDAL [308] said they observed no accidents in a total of 1280 lipiodol iodoventriculographies performed between 1928 and 1937. According to CORNELIS and DEREYMAEKER [85], iodoventriculography gives the best diagnostic results and presents fewer drawbacks for the patient. DILENGE *et al.* [130, 131], on the basis of 300 stereotaxic procedures, conclude that the intraventricular injection of lipiodol is not dangerous. For MARTIN *et al.* [282, 283] extrafluid lipiodol should be employed to explore the posterior fossa, in particular the cerebello-pontine angle.

*LD_{50} is the "lethal dose" causing the death of 50% of the animals.

These arguments are surprising in view of the pessimistic literature in myelography where complications from iodinated oils appear to be frequent. At first we thought lipiodol was responsible for these accidents, as it was the first compound of this series to be prepared and the most frequently used. The main papers written on this subject are by BENEDEK and JOBA [35], BOLDREY and AIRD [46], BROWN and CARR [64], CROUET *et al.* [98], GAUTHIER [174], LINDBLOM [253], MACLAIRE [272], MARCOVITCH *et al.* [279], SIEBNER [425], and PINEAS [350]. But even after the appearance of Pantopaque, negative reports on lipiodol continued (BERING [37], DAVIES [105], ERICKSON and VAN BAAREN [142], GARLAND [163], GROSJEAN [188], HURTEAU *et al.* [217], LUCE *et al.* [264], MASON and RAAF [286], PEACHER and ROBERTSON [330], and TARLOV [450]).

Complications can be observed immediately (within hours of the examination) or later (months or years after it). DAVIES [105], who analyzed 125 Myodil ventriculographies, observed 56 cases of early complications. These are usually slight: elevation of body temperature (observed in 40 cases by DAVIES), headache, stiffness of the neck, nausea, vomiting, back pain; but there were also severe complications like meningism, paralysis of the cranial nerves, nystagmus, sphincter impairment. Later complications are represented by the so-called arachnoiditis, observed 14 times by DAVIES [105]. DAVIES thinks it is generally difficult to establish whether the arachnoiditis is due to the long residence time of the contrast medium in the subarachnoid space, the natural progression of the disease, or the sequelae of the surgical operation.

The relationship between arachnoiditis and iodinated oils is a proven one. In 5 patients of DAVIES' [105] series operated one year or more after a myelography and in 3 cases on whom autopsy was performed 1 to 4 years after operation, the findings were similar: a thick, white membrane adhering to the nerve sheaths (in one case enveloping the cauda equina). In one of these cases there was a thickening of the arachnoid at the level of the basal cisterns where some Myodil had accumulated. We recently observed [95] in our department a case of chiasmatic arachnoiditis after a myelography performed with ultrafluid lipiodol. Lesions of the same type were described by TARLOV [450], who was using Pantopaque. According to CROUET *et al.* [98], it is impossible to assess how often arachnoiditis is due to iodinated oil. BERING [37] never observed any cases in 106 myelograms.

MASON and RAAF [286] reported a fatal outcome due to aseptic meningitis from Pantopaque, but this was the only complication observed among 1500 myelograms performed over a period of 15 years. Two similar cases were described by LUCE *et al.* [264]. ERICKSON and VAN BAAREN [142] also reported one death. MARCOVITCH *et al.* [279] and PEACHER and ROBERTSON [330] observed three cases of arachnoiditis out of 150 and 60 myelograms, respectively.

GAUTHIER [174], in a recent paper, collected from the literature 29 observations of spinal arachnoiditis (20 from lipiodol and 9 from Pantopaque) and 4 cases of cisternal arachnoiditis.

Experimental Research

In 1925, in the early days of myelography, PEIPER and KLOSE [332] injected iodinated sesame oil into the rabbit by the cisternal route. They observed serious damage to spinal cord and brain but noticed that the same lesions were produced by non-iodinated oil. The lesions depend on the amount of compound injected: all rabbits that received 2 to 3 ml showed severe medullary lesions; the lesions were slight with smaller doses, and even absent with minimal doses of 0.05–0.1 ml.

Thus, this early work, the value of which is perhaps underestimated, proved that the toxicity of the iodinated oils is due to the oil and not to the iodine; moreover it demonstrates the importance of the *type* of compound used as well as of the amount remaining in the subarachnoid space after the examination.

DAVIES *et al.* [106], in 1930, injected into dogs 1.5 ml of lipiodol by the cisternal route. The animals were sacrificed at intervals ranging from 3 to 252 days. In all cases the histological examination revealed an aseptic meningitis and the presence of encysted fat corpuscles and degenerated gray matter. BRUSKIN and PROPPER [65] reported similar findings one year later following the injection of sesame oil. The discrepancy existing between the results of experimental work and the rarity of the complications observed in clinical practice encouraged CRAIG [91] to take up the subject again in

1942. Having in mind PEIPER and KLOSE's conclusions [332], he wanted to verify the importance of the amount of compound injected. For this reason he used a dose in proportion to the animal's weight: 0.073 ml/kg. In no dog were histological changes of the medulla and/or of the nerve roots found. The only pathological finding was some meningeal inflammation, which was more evident in dogs that had been sacrificed earlier. These experiments confirmed the importance of the quantitative factor in determining the toxicity of an oily contrast medium; they also demonstrated that a liposoluble myelography is contraindicated in the presence of any existing inflammation of the meninges.

MEACHAM and TOLCHIN [296] studied the effects of the intraventricular injection of Pantopaque. They filled with this substance the lateral ventricles of dogs in which an artificial obstructive hydrocephalus had been produced. There were no symptoms. More than six months later the animals were sacrificed: no ependymal, choroidal plexus, or parenchymal lesions could be demonstrated. Conversely, with lumbar injection acute inflammation of the arachnoid was observed, with a tendency to form chronic granulomas containing oily droplets. According to the authors, the ependymal epithelium and the pia mater always act as a protective barrier. SCHOBER [405–407] injected Pantopaque (0.1 ml/kg body weight) in the frontal subarachnoid space of the rabbit. Autopsy disclosed contrast deposits in nearby adhesions, and histological examination showed in all animals the presence of meningeal lesions, the extent of which was proportional to the duration of the experiment. According to the author, the irritation of the meninges is due to the action of the fatty acids resulting from the slow degradation of the iodinated esters—in this particular case undecylic acid, which does not saponify with the fluid. It is interesting to note, in this respect, that Etiodol and Duroliopaque are metabolized quite differently; their metabolism is more similar to the metabolism of the natural fatty acids, whose degradation products are less toxic.

The conclusions of the above experimental work can be summarized as follows:

1. Pantopaque irritates the meninges, and it appears that small doses of Pantopaque (not exceeding 0.1 ml/kg body weight) produce more serious changes than equal doses of iodinated oil.
2. There is no injury in either case to the cerebral parenchyma or medulla.
3. Both substances are much less toxic when injected (into the ventricles).

Recent attempts to use iodinated emulsions for both ventriculography and myelography gave rise to a series of very interesting experiments. We shall deal with them in detail in the chapter on panventriculography. Here we shall take into consideration only the additional information afforded by these works on the toxicity of iodinated oils, in particular of the most recent products: Pantopaque, Etiodol, and Duroliopaque.

FISHER [148], working on cats, noticed that the nonemulsified Pantopaque always produces either acute or chronic meningeal irritation. Such effects were not observed with emulsified Etiodol, which was completely reabsorbed in three months.

PENNING *et al.* [337–341] injected 3–4 ml of emulsified and nonemulsified lipiodol, Pantopaque, and Etiodol into the cerebral subarachnoid space of different rabbits. Only the nonemulsified contrast media produced toxic reactions. Pantopaque turned out to be by far the most toxic compound (even more toxic than lipiodol), whereas the toxicity of Etiodol seemed to be very low. Pantopaque proved to be more irritating than Etiodol, also when the two compounds—either pure or emulsified—were injected subcutaneously. Duroliopaque and Etiodol injected by the lumbar route proved to be much less toxic than Pantopaque and lipiodol. When injected subcutaneously, Duroliopaque and Etiodol did not produce reactions, and they also seemed to be nontoxic when the intraperitoneal route was used.

Presence of Blood in the Subarachnoid Space

HOWLAND *et al.* [215, 216] tried to explain why arachnoiditis from iodinated oil develops only occasionally. They thought that in some patients the arachnoid might be injured by the needle, with the consequent hemorrhage acting in turn as an irritant. In order to verify their hypothesis, the authors investigated the effect of both blood and Pantopaque on dogs. The results were very interesting; the animals that were injected with blood alone showed no histological modification of the arachnoid; those injected only with Pantopaque did not develop any clinical symptoms, but the autopsy showed a chronic meningeal inflammation; finally, dogs in which a mixture of blood and Pantopaque was injected had serious clinical reactions as well as considerable inflammation of the arachnoid, especially in the lower cervical region. Therefore, the presence of blood in the CSF has to be regarded as being more toxic than Pantopaque. This fact might account for the severe arachnoiditis that is sometimes observed in clinical practice. The lumbar puncture must therefore be performed with great care and, if bleeding occurs, the examination should be postponed. The same caution must be observed when the lumbar puncture is performed to withdraw the contrast medium after the examination.

HOWLAND *et al.* [215, 216], observed that, when corticosteroids are associated with Pantopaque, arachnoiditis is less frequent, even in the presence of hemorrhage.

Emulsions

The usefulness of emulsified Pantopaque in myelography has been pointed out by PIRKEY *et al.* [351] in 1950; by NOSIK [316] in 1951; and by BLEASEL [45] in 1961. The technique of intraventricular injection of iodinated emulsions is attributed to PORTERA [354–356] (1964), but before him (1960) MATSUBARA and NOMURA [289] pointed out that lipiodol emulsified with sodium lauryl sulfate gave good visualization of the ventricular system, without apparent complications. Such an emulsion, however, cannot be reabsorbed like the emulsion of Pantopaque and CSF used by PORTERA.

PORTERA in an 18-month follow-up of his patients did not observe any complications other than temporary febrile reaction and headache. Therefore panventriculography seems to be quite a promising technique. However, there are still many reservations regarding it, as reported in the next paragraph.

Toxicity

As early as 1950 JAEGER [230] demonstrated beyond all doubt by experiments in the dog that all emulsions are toxic. He tested several types of iodinated oil by emulsifying them with an equal amount of isotonic saline. He also added some gum arabic in order to facilitate molecular dispersion. By this method the author obtained a stable emulsion of similar pH to CSF and with particles small enough (less than 12 µm in diameter) to pass through the subarachnoid pathways. The results were disastrous: all the dogs died within 24 hours, whether the oil had been injected into the spinal subarachnoid space, the great cistern, or the cerebral ventricles. Such a harmful effect could not be attributed to the gum arabic, since this substance proved to be innocuous when injected alone in the course of other experiments. It seemed therefore justified to consider that the toxicity of iodinated oils increases considerably when these substances are emulsified. With Pantopaque the results were even worse, and all the animals died within 10 minutes of the injections.

MAUPIN *et al.* [290] in 1966 emulsified Pantopaque with five different agents: CSF, dextran (molecular weight 40000); dextran (molecular weight 75000); Ficoll (a dextran polymer, molecular weight 400000); and 25% human serum albumin.

The two dogs that had received the human serum albumin died rapidly owing to the anaphylactic phenomena; the other animals, unlike JAEGER's [230], survived, but many of them developed spastic paralysis of the hind limbs.

These experiments seem to condemn the emulsions of iodinated oils and Pantopaque without appeal. However, they contradict the previously quoted favorable clinical results. Why is this? Apart from gum arabic (which is harmless), the main difference between the emulsions used by JAEGER and PORTERA is that the first is stabilized and contains very small particles, whereas the second is coarse, as it is manually prepared without a stabilizer. Clearly, the problem is how to prepare the emulsion.

TEPLICK *et al.* [454], in 1964 injected into the subarachnoid space of the dog by the cisternal route Etiodol emulsified with different agents. There were no clinical complications and the autopsy showed only slight inflammation of the meninges, of the same type as that which could be observed with nonemulsified Pantopaque.

In 1965 FISHER [148] demonstrated in turn the harmlessness of Etiodol emulsified with lecithin, injected into the lumbar subarachnoid space of the cat.

PENNING *et al.* [337–341] injected into the subarachnoid space of the right cerebral hemisphere of the rabbit emulsions having a different degree of dispersion. Such dispersion is expressed by a coefficient K that is equal to the billions of particles contained in every gram of oil.

A first series of experiments was carried out, using emulsions of Pantopaque, lipiodol, and Etiodol with coefficients $K=2.5$ (average diameter of particles 28.8 µm), $K=5$ (average diameter 11.2 µm), and $K=20$ (average diameter particles 6.8 µm). There were no complications with $K=2.5$ and $K=5$ emulsions, regardless of the type of contrast medium used. On the contrary, with the $K=20$ emulsion, all the animals treated with Pantopaque died, whereas those receiving Etiodol showed no reaction. With lipiodol, the results were better than with Pantopaque, but much worse than with Etiodol. Finally, 8 animals received $K=40$ Etiodol emulsion: 7 showed no reaction; 1 had generalized seizures one hour after the injection and died two days later.

In a second group of animals PENNING *et al.* used two emulsions: Mulsopaque, which is a premanufactured emulsion of Pantopaque in which the average diameter of the particles is less than 1.6 µm, and GUERBET's "experimental emulsion 14" in which the average diameter of the particles is less than 0.8 µm. Of the 3 animals injected with Mulsopaque one died within 24 hours; two had generalized seizures, with one of them dying the following day. The GUERBET experimental emulsion 14 was tested in 5 animals; immediately after the injection, they appeared apathetic; later on, 3 had convulsions and 2 paralysis of the hind limbs. However, all of them improved. A third series of experiments was carried out with Duroliopaque. This compound showed the same toxicity as Etiodol; it is therefore less toxic than Pantopaque. In conclusion, the important work by PENNING *et al.* [337–341] proves that:

1. Emulsifying liposoluble contrast media considerably increases their toxicity.
2. Pantopaque is more toxic than Etiodol and Duroliopaque.
3. The toxicity of an emulsion depends on its degree of dispersion: coarse emulsions of $K=2$ or $K=5$ produce no reaction, even when prepared with Pantopaque, whereas emulsions having a higher coefficient give rise to serious complications as was demonstrated by JAEGER [230]. According to PENNING *et al.* [337–341], high coefficient emulsions contain a very large number of particles, and this would lead to an increase in their "total surface area" so favoring a more active meningeal response.
4. The emulsions, as well as the nonemulsified compounds, are better tolerated when they are injected into the ventricles. This is also the opinion of MARKESBERY and WILSON [281].

Conclusions

In the complex dispute on liposoluble contrast media a few important points can be singled out:

1. Liposoluble compounds are toxic and can produce chronic inflammatory changes in the arachnoid.
2. Toxicity is not the same for all compounds. Lipiodol is only of historical interest and must no longer be used. Pantopaque, Myodil, and Etiodan are more toxic than Etiodol and Duroliopaque.
3. The amount of substance remaining in the subarachnoid space has a considerable influence on the onset of secondary effects. After the examination it is therefore necessary to withdraw as much contrast as possible.
4. Emulsions should consist of rather large particles. The higher the degree of dispersion of the emulsion, the more toxic it is.

3. Techniques of Positive-Contrast Ventriculography

Balado's [25] and Amezua's [11] Technique

The ventricular puncture is performed in the operating room, with the patient prone. Two or 3 ml of contrast medium is injected, leaving a cannula in the ventricle (in order to inject air when it is also necessary to study the supratentorial portion of the ventricular system). The patient (still prone) is then moved to the X-ray room and placed on a tilting table. The examination includes three stages:

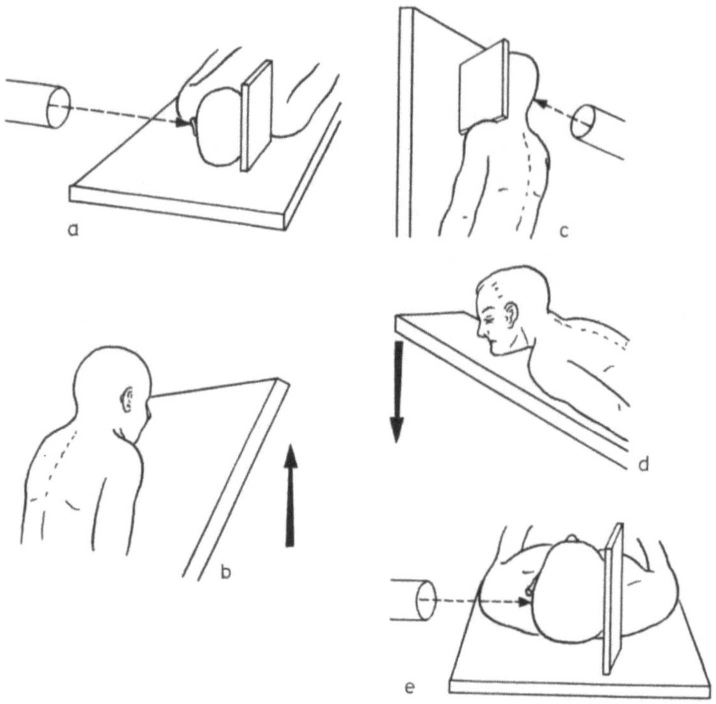

Fig. 3.1 a–e. Schematic drawings illustrating BALADO and AMEZUA's technique. See text, p. 114

1. Table horizontal. Radiographs in lateral projection to check the location of the contrast, which normally must lie in the frontal horn (Fig. 3.1 a).
2. Table almost vertical. Patient's head slightly turned, so that the side of the injection is higher (Fig. 3.1 b). The iodinated oil enters the anterior portion of the third ventricle which is then explored in lateral and postero-anterior projections (Fig. 3.1 c).
3. Table tilted down. The contrast remain in the anterior portion of the third ventricle (Fig. 3.1 d).

The patient is rapidly turned and placed in the supine position (Fig. 3.1 e), so that the posterior portion of the third ventricle, the aqueduct, and the fourth ventricle can be examined. If an obstruction exists, the patient is left supine for 10 minutes.

Bull's Technique [66]

BULL's technique has four main stages:

1. Supine position, head flexed and turned in such a way that the nose is slightly lower than the occiput. The contrast is introduced into the uppermost ventricle; it slides along the wall of the ventricle and settles on the floor of the frontal horn. If the third ventricle is normal, 0.5 ml of contrast is sufficient, but in cases of hydrocephalus it is necessary to increase the dose to 2–3 ml.
2. Sitting position, head flexed, then slowly deflected under radioscopic control so that the contrast moves through the foramen of Monroe into the anterior portion of the third ventricle (Fig. 3.2 a). A lateral rotation and also gentle shaking of the head is sometimes necessary to facilitate this passage.
3. Supine position. The contrast passes into the posterior portion of the third ventricle, the aqueduct, and the fourth ventricle (Fig. 3.2 b),
4. Sitting position again. The contrast goes into the spinal subarachnoid space from where it can be withdrawn.

Ruggiero's Technique [375]

The place where the contrast medium is injected is not important; it can be the surgical or radiological department. The position of the contrast medium in the ventricular system is radiologically checked; then the appropriate maneuvers are per-

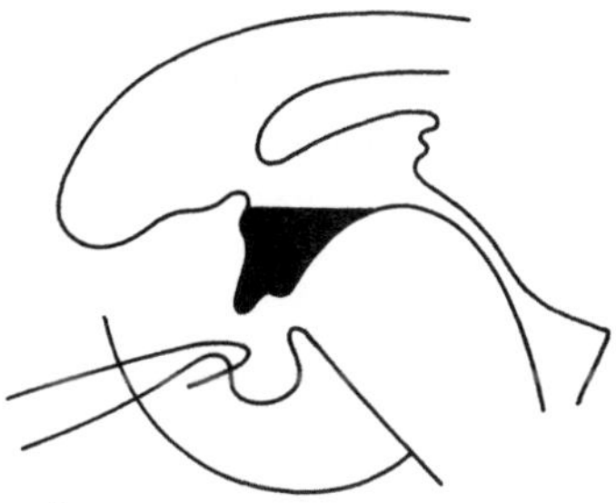
a

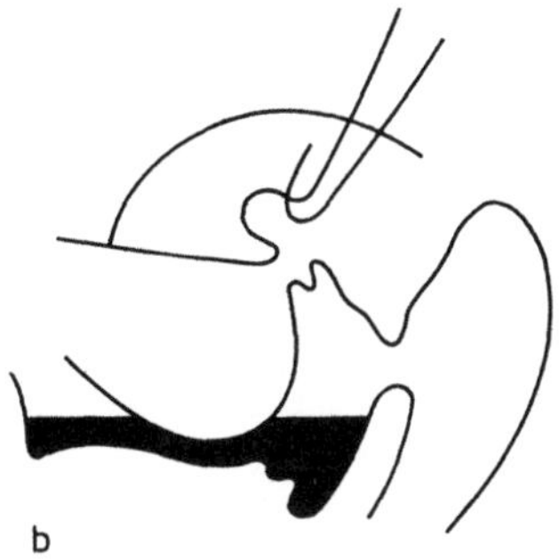
b

Fig. 3.2a, b. Schematic drawings illustrating BULL's technique. See text, p. 114

formed to visualize the desired structures. These maneuvers are the exact opposite of those used for air studies. With a TV-amplifier system, the whole procedure is controlled radioscopically and pictures are taken only when necessary.

Ralston, Gross, and Newman's Technique [362]

The patient is prone: 3 ml of contrast is injected into the frontal horn, either directly or via the occipital horn (Fig. 3.3a). Generally, 30–40 ml of air is injected, in addition to the iodinated oil. Then the head is deflected so that the orbito-meatal line is parallel to the table (Fig. 3.3b); thus the contrast passes through the foramen of Monroe into the third ventricle. For the visualization of the posterior portion of the third ventricle, aqueduct, and fourth ventricle, the supine position is resumed (Fig. 3.3c). With the head straight the posterior portion of the third ventricle and the aqueduct are visualized; with the head slightly flexed (Fig. 3.3d) the contrast passes into the fourth ventricle. The authors consider fluoroscopy useless. One of the advantages of the technique would be the simultaneous visualization of the posterior portion of the ventricular system with opaque contrast and of the frontal horns with air.

Dilenge, David, and Talairach's Technique [130]

The patient is sitting, head slightly flexed: 1–1.5 ml of lipiodol is injected into the frontal horn (Fig. 3.4a) and a lateral radiograph is made. The head is then slightly extended to allow the contrast to reach the foramen of Monroe. Generally 5 to 6 minutes are necessary for a good visualization of the third ventricle (Fig. 3.4b). A further extension of the head will bring the contrast into the initial portion of the aqueduct to demonstrate any existing stenosis. If the aqueduct is patent, part of the contrast will flow through the aqueduct (Fig. 3.4c) and a lateral radiograph must be taken immediately after the head extension to catch the contrast during its passage. For a good visualization of the fourth ventricle it is necessary to place the patient supine (Fig. 3.4d). When the fourth ventricle is grossly enlarged, only its posterior portion can be visualized (Fig. 3.4e). In this case it is necessary to complete the examination with a film taken in the prone position (Fig. 3.4f).

Some reservations should be made regarding this technique, as the aqueduct seems to be studied only in the lateral view.

Portera's Panventriculography [354–356]

From a frontal burr hole 8–15 ml of CSF is withdrawn from the right lateral ventricle in a sterile syringe to which are added Pantopaque to the amount of one-quarter of the volume of CSF extracted and 5 ml of air. The contents of the syringe are then shaken for 50 seconds. The air is expelled from the syringe and the emulsion is injected into the ventricle. Films are taken in lateral and antero-posterior projections. Taking a series of two radiographs per second the authors showed that the emulsion enters the ventricle with some turbulence, causing the contrast to spread quickly throughout the ventricular system, which is completely visualized within 3 seconds. After 5 minutes the emulsion breaks and the Pantopaque settles in different parts of the ventricles.

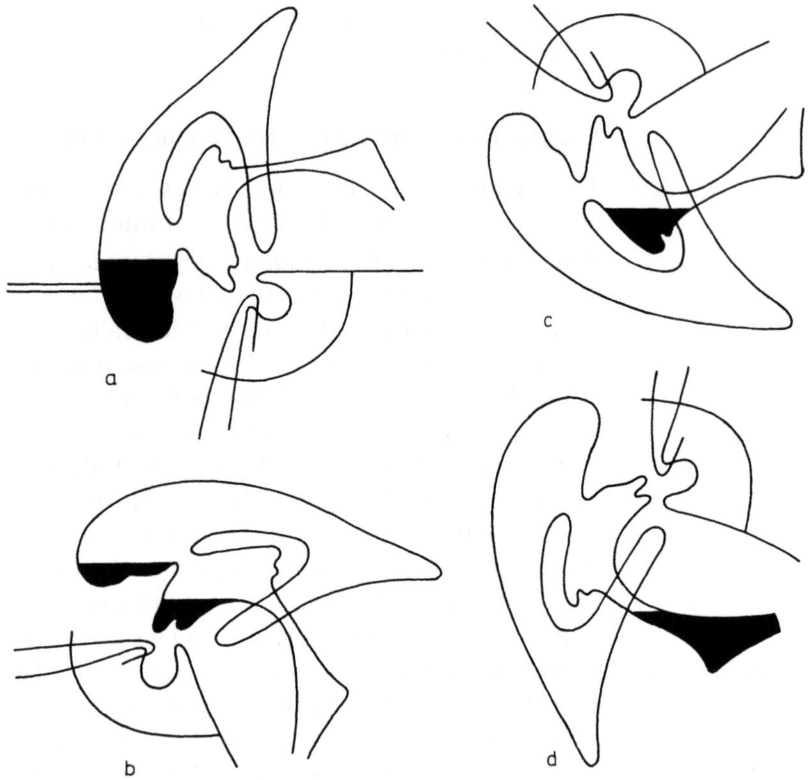

Fig. 3.3a–d. Schematic drawings illustrating RALSTON, GROSS, and NEWMAN'S technique. See text, p. 115

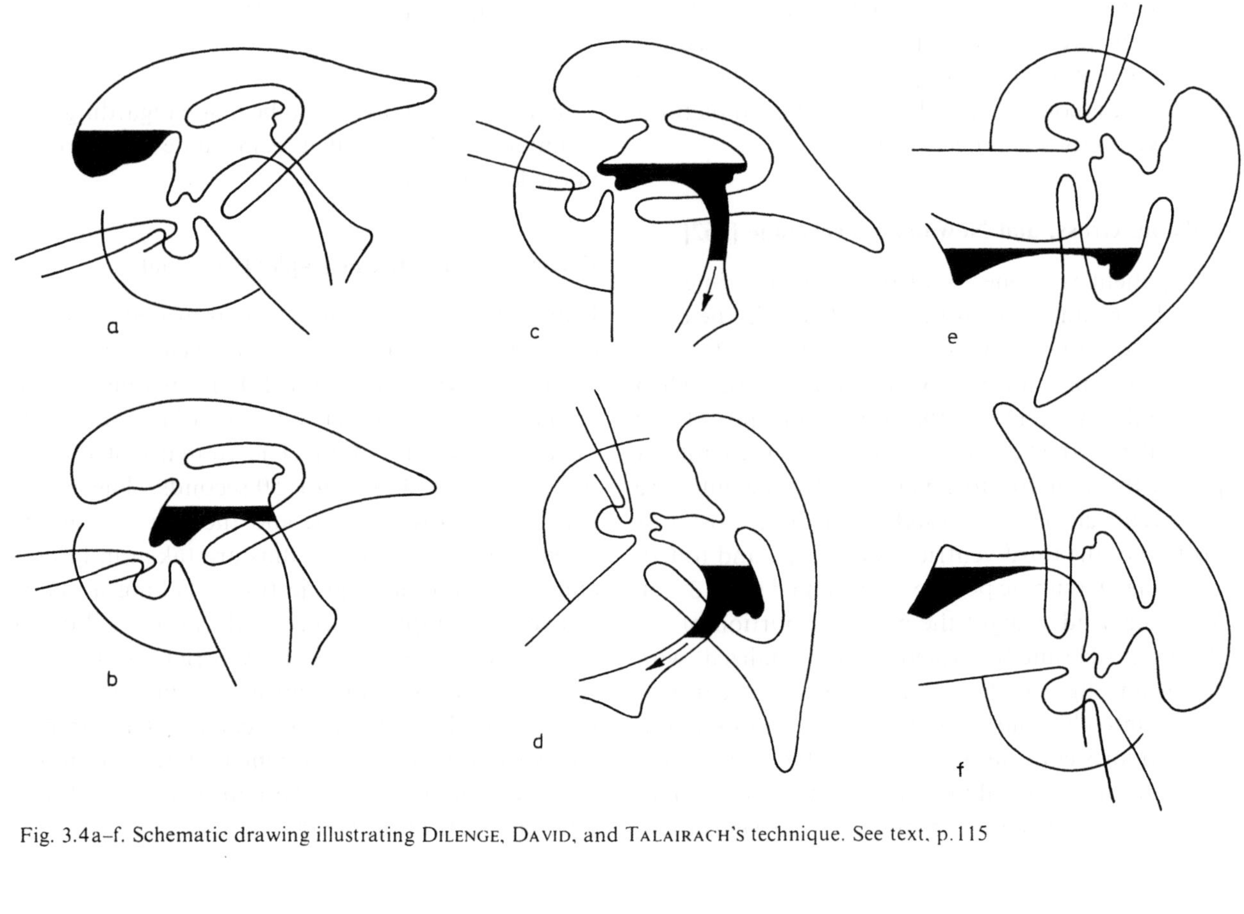

Fig. 3.4a–f. Schematic drawing illustrating DILENGE, DAVID, and TALAIRACH'S technique. See text, p.115

4. Positive-Contrast Ventriculography with Water-Soluble Contrast Media

Papers by CAMPBELL *et al.* [72] and HEIMBURGER *et al.* [204] seem to indicate that small amounts (2 to 3 ml) of 60% methylglucamine iotalamate diluted 2 to 6 times, are not toxic, whereas serious complications (chiefly convulsive seizures) occur with larger amounts. However, this technique is still undergoing experimentation so that at present its use in clinical practice is still unwarranted.

Recently IIZUKA and WAPPENSCHMIDT [218] proposed stereoencephaloscopic ventriculography. This examination entails endoscopy of the ventricular system by means of a special instrument followed by direct injection into the third and fourth ventricles of 1–2 ml of Conray, previously diluted in CSF or saline and then warmed. In the authors' opinion this method does not cause injury to the nervous tissue; consequently, the complications of water-soluble positive-contrast ventriculography can be avoided.

Chapter IV. Positive Contrast Cisternography of the Posterior Fossa

1. Literature

As far as we know, the first attempt to study the posterior fossa radiologically was made by BROWN and AYE [63] in 1955. However, these authors only succeeded in showing the "negative" image of the vertebral artery but did not obtain any further information on the anatomy and pathology of the cerebello-pontine angle.

In 1958 MALIS [273] suggested a technique for exploring the region of the occipital foramen and clivus based on the indirect visualization of vessels of vertebro-basilar circulation after the injection of 30 ml of Pantopaque by the lumbar route. MALIS did not try to let the contrast collect in the cerebello-pontine angle cistern because he was afraid it might prove impossible to withdraw it after the examination.

"Myeloencephalography" was proposed by MONES and WERMANN [307]. After a lumbar injection of 9–12 ml of Pantopaque, the patient is set in 45–55° Trendelenburg position. The third and fourth ventricles, the great cistern, and indirectly, the posterior border of the occipital foramen are visualized. Diagnostic results were good in tumors of the foramen magnum and the brain stem, as well as in cases of Arnold-Chiari malformation and aqueduct stenosis. No complications were observed in 40 cases. According to the authors, the main limitation of air encephalography is the superimposition in postero-anterior view of the cisterns upon the aqueduct and the fourth ventricle, while in a lateral view the fourth ventricle can be masked by air present in the mastoid cells.

From his experience with 204 cases, BAKER [22] states that positive-contrast cisternography is useful for the diagnosis of pontine and cerebello-pontine angle tumors, lesions of the jugular foramen, and vertebro-basilar aneurysms. His technique is as follows: the patient is prone in the Trendelenburg position with the head hyperextended. Six to 12 ml of Pantopaque is injected by the lumbar route and directed toward the skull under radioscopic control. When the contrast is collected over the clivus, the head is rotated so that the oil can enter the cerebello-pontine angle cistern and the internal auditory meatus. Pictures in both lateral and frontal views are taken; then the maneuver is repeated on the opposite side. After that, the patient is placed in a supine position, with his head hyperflexed, while the table is set first in moderately (6–7°) inverted Trendelenburg position and then again in the Trendelenburg position so that the contrast can collect in the great cistern, outlining the cerebellar tonsils. It is also possible to fill the fourth ventricle by means of flexion-extension movement of the head. In the stages of the examination performed in the Trendelenburg position, one must take care not to have the table tilted more than 45°; otherwise, there is the risk of seeing the contrast penetrating the middle or even the anterior cerebral fossa.

GASS [164] described a technique practically identical to that of BAKER. He was able to diagnose a nasopharyngeal carcinoma invading the clivus, an acoustic neurinoma, and a meningioma of the cerebello-pontine angle. GASS [164] called the technique "Pantopaque anterior basal cisternography of the posterior fossa."

SCANLAN [398] examined 100 patients (among whom 45 cases had tumors of the cerebello-pontine angle cistern) with the following technique: the patient is prone, head extended; after injection of 10 ml of Pantopaque, the head is rotated 45°, the side to be examined downward; then the table is tilted to a 45° Trendelenburg position. The tilting maneuver should be gentle to prevent the contrast from passing over the tentorium. Once the cerebello-pontine angle cistern is filled with oil, the head is placed perpendicular to the table in order to radiograph the internal auditory meatus in lateral projection. According to the author, in the case of intracanalicular tumors it is necessary to fill the cistern up to the vestibule; for this the Valsalva maneuver may be useful. SCANLAN's conclusions [398] are as follows: examination by positive-contrast medium of the cerebello-pontine angle cistern and the internal auditory meatus has definitely improved the diagnosis of acoustic neurinoma by supplying the surgeon with useful information about the relationship between the tumor and the large adjacent vessels. With this technique it is also possible to exclude the presence of an intracanalicular tumor when the internal auditory meatus is enlarged due to a congenital anomaly. However, SCANLAN [298] thinks only the diagnosis of extracanalicular tumors is certain; the diagnosis of intracanalicular tumors can be very difficult, since arachnoiditis or some anatomical anomaly can also cause nonfilling of the cistern and/or the meatus. Fortunately, such cases are rare.

SHARRON and WIENER [419] have suggested a technique slightly different from SCANLAN's [398]: after tilting the table, the head of the patient is positioned almost as for a Stenvers projection. The tumor is shown by a filling defect or a bulging of the oil column. With this technique SHARRON and WIENER [419] were able to diagnose 1 meningioma and 3 neurinomas of the cerebello-pontine angle. They do not say in how many cases their technique had been employed.

Using a technique similar to that described by BAKER [22], REESE and BULL [365] have examined the internal auditory meatus, the cavum Meckelii, the jugular foramen, and the cerebello-pontine angle cistern. These authors give an accurate description of the anatomic-radiologic appearance of these structures, which are better demonstrated in oblique views. The cerebello-pontine angle cistern looks like a triangle, the base of which is formed by the impression of both the basilar and the vertebral arteries and with the apex directed to the side. At its center the internal auditory meatus appears as a rounded-tip cavity about 10 mm deep and 4 mm wide, in which one can distinguish both the facial and the acoustic nerves. The cavum Meckelii also appears as a cavity, smaller than the internal auditory meatus. Such a cavity is situated laterally to the internal auditory meatus and is directed forward and downward, while the similarly shaped jugular foramen is directed downward and slightly backward, and is situated immediately behind the internal auditory meatus.

BURROWS [68] performed 74 positive contrast cisternographies and demonstrated 12 acoustic neurinomas. The amount of contrast medium is 6–9 ml of Pantopaque, and the radiological technique is not very different from those already mentioned. BURROWS' description of the procedure can be simplified as follows: the cerebello-pontine angle cistern is examined with the head hyperextended, the head is then placed in a normal position; all the contrast with the exception of that located in the internal auditory meatus reaches the clivus and the cervical region, which can now be examined in their turn. At this moment, if one desires a full visualization of the internal auditory meatus in lateral view, it will be sufficient to hyperextend the head, as at the beginning of the examination. Tomography can also be performed in all these projections. The diagnosis is made on the appearance of a "filling defect" in the contrast spot due to a bulging of the medial border of the lesion: sometimes its appearance is polylobate, and sometimes it has the shape of a half-circle, which would indicate that the tumor is extracerebral. In the latter case the size of the lesion is calculated by measuring the distance between the two extremities of the half-circle, as seen on the frontal projection. Its relationship to the brain stem could be a function of the distance between the basilar artery and the half-circle itself: the smaller the distance, the closer the tumor should be to the midline.

According to BURROWS [68], in cerebello-pontine angle tumors opaque cisternography gives more accurate information than any other method, since encephalography seldom indicates the size of the tumor and ventriculography shows it only indirectly, through the displacement of the fourth ventricle. Another advantage of this method is its reliability: when this technique is used correctly, there is always a good filling of the cerebello-pontine angle cistern and the internal acoustic meatus; consequently the nonfilling of these structures must be regarded as pathological. There are only two exceptions: severe cervical spondylo-arthrosis and intracranial hypertension, both of which cause obliteration of the cisterns. These occurrences should therefore be considered a contraindication of opaque cisternography.

BURROWS' technique [68], on the other hand, is not very satisfactory in small, purely intracanalicular tumors. Here diagnosis may be difficult, since the nonfilling of the internal acoustic meatus does not necessarily indicate a neurinoma but can also be due to arachnoiditis.

VALVASSORI [466] suggested injecting 2–3 ml of Pantopaque by the lumbar route, the patient being in lateral decubitus in the Trendelenburg position. The oil is directed toward the posterior fossa under fluoroscopy and collects in the cerebello-pontine angle cistern; at this moment the patient's head is rotated to assume at first a Stenvers, then a classical postero-anterior projection. This last view is a very important one, since the whole internal acoustic meatus is visualized on it. Spot radiographs and, if necessary, also tomograms, are taken during the maneuver. VALVASSORI [466] advises that when a tumor is present, no contrast should be withdrawn, since it could be useful later for a postoperative radiological check-up. VALVASSORI'S cases [466] include 85 expansive processes of the cerebello-pontine angle: 78 neurinomas, among which are 7 intracanalicular, 3 meningiomas, 2 epidermoids, 1 cyst, and 1 case of aneurysm of the internal auditory artery.

BRITTON *et al.* [58] suggested a particular technique for examining intracanalicular neurinomas. After an intrathecal injection of 1 ml of Pantopaque, together with 40 mg of methyl prednisolone acetate, the patient is kept for 2 minutes in a lateral position, with the side to be examined downward and the table tilted in a 45° Trendelenburg position. During this time the contrast collects in the cerebello-pontine angle cistern and the internal acoustic meatus. Then the table is set horizontal, the head is rotated through 45° as in a Stenvers projection, and the X-ray tube is tilted 15° caudally. Stereographic pictures are taken. Again the head is put in lateral position and the Potter and X-ray tubes are positioned for a postero-anterior trans-orbital projection. New stereoradiographs are taken in which the internal acoustic meatus appears in the center of the orbit. Finally, an axial projection is performed. These authors do not make use of fluoroscopy; they consider the Polytome the most suitable apparatus for the demonstration of the borders of the internal acoustic meatus. In 1969 at the World Congress of Radiology, LING LEE [261] presented 35 cases of acoustic neurinomas examined with positive-contrast cisternography. LING LEE considers this method more useful than encephalography and ventriculography in the case of small tumors.

This is also the opinion of VALVASSORI [466], who feels that in encephalography the amount of air present in the cerebello-pontine angle cistern and inside the internal acoustic meatus is insufficient to outline small lesions. WENDE and LÜDECKE [475] also consider positive-contrast cisternography especially indicated for small tumors.

2. Discussion

The above analysis of the literature needs a brief comment.

There is no doubt that opaque cisternography can give very clear pictures of the internal acoustic meatus.

However, we do not endorse the reasons put forward by the authors of these articles who prefer this method to encephalography. For example, MONES and WERMANN'S statement [307] that in encephalography the images are confused due to the superimposition of cisterns and ventricular system should be ignored because it is practically impossible to confuse them. A precise demonstration of how to interpret the encephalographic pictures of posterior fossa structures was given by RUGGIERO [374] in 1957, not to mention the work of LINDGREN [257], LYSHOLM [268–270], TWINING [461, 462], and ROBERTSON [371].

Many authors stress that with positive contrast it is possible to visualize the vertebro-basilar vessels indirectly, and consider this an advantage of the method. But this visualization is much more easily and clearly obtained by vertebral angiography.

SCANLAN [398] states that only with positive-contrast medium can one exclude the presence of a tumor in the cerebello-pontine angle cistern, the visualization of which is essential for the diagnosis of tumors in that region. But BURROWS [68] has shown that failure to visualize the cerebello-pontine angle cistern can also occur in cases of intracranial hypertension. This seems to us to be an important deficiency of this method; as a matter of fact, a more or less marked increase in endocranial pressure exists in almost every case of cerebello-pontine angle tumor.

For Reese and Bull [365], nonfilling of an internal acoustic meatus, even if it must always be considered pathological, does not necessarily indicate the presence of a tumor since it can also happen in cases of adhesive arachnoiditis. This statement, too, seems to us to throw doubt on the diagnostic utility of opaque cisternography. On the other hand, with encephalography the differential diagnosis between the arachnoiditis and the tumors is usually easy: in the former the cistern is not visualized; in the latter it is occupied by the tumor.

Burrows [68] thinks that one of the merits of positive-contrast media is that they show the size of the tumor, which is revealed by the dimensions of the filling defect. This does not seem correct to us: the most one could speak of is the size of the implantation of the tumor. The size of the tumor itself is a question of volume. Thus it cannot be given by a method in which the contrast medium tends to stratify, whereas it can be given by air because it occupies the whole cistern.

The authors of the present book have not had significant experience with positive-contrast cisternography. The excellent results that they obtained with air did not encourage them to change their technique. However, this method might be useful in the case of small tumors, especially intracanalicular neurinomas.

Chapter V. Radioisotope Examination of the CSF Pathways

1. Literature

As far as we are aware, the first attempt to study the spinal subarachnoid space by radioactive isotopes was made in 1953 by BAUER and YUHL [28], who injected by the lumbar route ^{131}I to verify whether the spinal arachnoid spaces were pervious or not.

The physiology of the CSF was investigated by means of various radioisotopes (radioiodine human serum albumin = RIHSA, ^{38}Cl, ^{42}K) by SWEET and LOCKSLEY [447] in 1953, SWEET *et al.* [446], in 1954, and CHOU and FRENCH [79] in 1955. The first two groups of authors injected the radioactive compound by the ventricular route, the last group by the subarachnoid route. In 1960 VAN WART *et al.* [467] injected RIHSA in the cisterna magna of narcotized dogs and recorded its presence in blood samples.

The modalities of CSF reabsorption were studied by MIGLIORE *et al.* [305] (1961), who injected RIHSA and ^{24}Na by the lumbar route, and by ATKINSON and FOLTZ [16] (1962), who injected RIHSA by the ventricular route. These investigations were made on both normal and hydrocephalic subjects. DI CHIRO [120, 122] (1964, 1966) and BROCKLEHURST [59, 61] (1967, 1968) also studied by means of external scanning both the diffusion and the reabsorption of RIHSA injected by either the ventricular or the lumbar route.

Isotopes were associated with coloring substances to study hydrocephalus and to verify the efficiency of surgical shunts. In 1957 BELL [30] measured the radioactivity of RIHSA injected into the ventricular system along the cerebrospinal axis. Other publications appeared later by BELL [31], MIGLIORE *et al.* [306], KAGEN *et al.* [222], and SCHLESINGER *et al.* [403].

In 1962 MEALEY [297] performed external scanning of the cerebral convexity in cases of subdural hematoma. He injected RIHSA through the bregma in children, and through a burr hole in adults. The same technique was employed later by GROS *et al.* [185] for diagnosis of subdural hematoma in children. In 1966 MEALEY and CAMBELL [298] reported "isotope subdurography" using transferrin labeled with ^{113m}In or ^{99m}Tc-HSA.

In a series of papers [117, 119–122, 124–128, 321, 367] from 1962 onward, DI CHIRO with several coworkers described "RIHSA cisternography" and "RIHSA ventriculography." According to the author, these techniques make it possible to study the physiology of the CSF and the appearance of both the subarachnoid space and the ventricular system. The radiocompound can be introduced by the ventricular, the lumbar, or the suboccipital cisternal route.

2. Choice of the Radiocompound

The radiocompound which has always attracted the attention of most authors is human serum albumin labeled with ^{131}I (RIHSA) [references are 8, 26, 119, 120, 125, 127–129, 157, 185, 187, 205, 228, 232, 275, 284, 317, 322, 342, 451]. RIHSA is a large protein molecule (molecular wt. 70000) bound to ^{131}I ion, has a half-life of 8.3 days, and emits beta and gamma radiations. The great majority of the beta radiations consist of 608 keV radiations, while most of the gamma radiations are of 364 keV. Both the physico-chemical and biological characteristics of RIHSA are ideal for the study of the subarachnoid spaces and cerebral ventricles. In fact, because of the considerable size of the albumin molecule to which the radioactive ion is bound, the latter diffuses spontaneously, and when injected by the lumbar route, is carried by the ascending currents present in the CSF [119, 122, 124, 231]. The protein content of RIHSA is similar to that of CSF; therefore RIHSA is absorbed along CSF pathways and can be followed up to the granulations of PACCHIONI [1, 205, 231]. However, the ease of RIHSA reabsorption along the CSF pathways may also represent a contraindication of the method. HARBERT *et al.* [202] measured radioactivity absorbed by the lumbar medulla following the injection of 100 μCi* of RIHSA: the result was 7.4 rads** in normal subjects, 12.3 rads in hydrocephalic subjects, and 58.7 rads in cases of cervical block. These last doses are high. Another complication of RIHSA can be the presence of symptoms in relation to the albumin injected [references are 32, 119, 124, 228, 231, 320, 328] To avoid them, DI CHIRO [121, 126] and later other authors [228, 232, 320, 451] utilized RIHSA with high specific activity, i.e. a compound with considerable radioactivity and a small amount of albumin.

RIESELBACH *et al.* [367] tried (first in monkeys and then in man) colloidal gold (^{198}Au) and Rose Bengal labeled with ^{131}I (in man only gold) injected by the lumbar route; but these drugs were soon abandoned because they did not diffuse well in the most cranial segments of the subarachnoid space and also because they were responsible for a chronic inflammatory reaction in the surrounding tissues.

DI CHIRO [120, 122, 128] (1964, 1966) employed the patient's own CSF labeled with ^{131}I. This compound is, however, difficult to prepare and is less convenient than RIHSA as a routine clinical procedure [128].

DI CHIRO and GROVE [120, 125] also tried technetium. The radioisotope employed was ^{99m}Tc-pertechnetate (Na-^{99m}TcO$_4$), which has a low molecular weight (163) and a physical half-life of 6 hours. It is devoid of beta emission, and emits only gamma radiations (140 keV [124, 125]). Na-^{99m}TcO$_4$ is especially indicated when there is a need for a quick answer (isotopic ventriculography, verification of the patency of a surgical shunt [120, 124, 125, 231]). On the other hand, Na-^{99m}TcO$_4$ is not suitable for cisternography since it diffuses quickly in the blood, but does not move easily in CSF because its molecule is small [120, 122, 127, 231]. Technetium has been employed by STERN *et al.* [436] to label human serum albumin (^{99m}Tc-HSA). However, when injected by he lumbar route, this radiocompound showed little specific activity [211].

^{99m}Tc-HSA is not commercially available but must be prepared ad hoc; the procedure takes time, and there is risk of infection [212]. DI CHIRO *et al.* [127] (1968) and OMMAYA *et al.* [321] (1968) used some technetium compounds of high specific activity, modifying the technique RICHARDS and ATKINS' technique [366], as it already been done with iodine. These radiocompounds can be used in very high doses, thus retaining the advantage of low risk with technetium [124, 211] (short physical half-life) yet excluding the disadvantage of too rapid reabsorption. This technique allows very accurate examinations to be made in a very short time [231] and is particularly useful in children [199]. According to HARBERT [199], the amount of radiation absorbed at the level of the lumbar spine after the injection of 100μCi of ^{99m}Tc-HSA is: 0.27 rad in normal subjects, 0.46 rad in cases of hydrocephalus, and 0.54 rad in cases of cervical block. These doses are far lower than those absorbed in the same conditions when RIHSA is used. However, the short physical half-life of technetium precludes scanning 24–48 hours after the radiocompound injection. DI CHIRO *et al.* [124, 127] (1968) tried to solve this problem by means of a "double-tracing" technique, i.e. by injecting ^{99m}Tc-HSA and RIHSA together at a high specific activity; with the former radiocompound one investigates the early phenomena, while the latter can be used to study the late phenomena.

BELL *et al.* [32] (1969), in experimental work on *Macacus rhesus*, suggested binding ^{99m}Tc with inulin which, being of low molecular weight and quick diffusibility, would allow a rapid cisternography. HARBERT [199] does not trust this method because in his opinion it fails to reveal a block at the level of the base of the skull, owing to too rapid reabsorption of the compound at the level of the spine.

Mercury (Neohydrin ^{203}Hg) has physico-chemical and biological characteristics that are intermediate between RIHSA and ^{99m}Tc-HSA. It has been used by SENIN *et al.* [416] (1966) to study the spinal subarachnoid spaces, and later by SIGNORINI *et al.* [426] (1968) and BRICOLO *et al.* [57] (1969). Neohyd-

* A Curie (Ci) is a unit quantity of any radionuclide in which exactly 3.7×10^{10} disintegrations occur per second.

** A rad is a unit of absorbed dose of ionizing radiation equal to 100 erg/g of irradiated material.

rin ^{203}Hg is a mercurial diuretic radiocompound; it emits beta and gamma radiations and has a physical half-life of 46 days. However, it remains in the subarachnoid space for only a short time because of its high diffusibility through the meningeal barrier [427]. CABASSA *et al.* [69] (1967) observed that only 30% of the radiocompound is still present in the human body 48 hours after its subarachnoidal injection; the remaining part being eliminated by the renal route. The molecular weight of Neohydrin ^{203}Hg is low; therefore this radiocompound does not easily reach the convexity of the brain, but stops at the level of the base of the skull [427]. Another disadvantage of Neohydrin is the high dose of radiation delivered to the kidney, for which the patient must be prepared with mercurial diuretics for several days beforehand.

MCQUEEN and ABBASSIOUN [295] (1968) used positive-emitting isotopes such as radioarsenic (^{74}As) and radiogallium (^{68}Ga). These radioisotopes have very low radiation doses (15–50 mrad with 500 μCi of radiogallium in children and 2 mCi in adults), but their indication is limited because of their very short physical half-life and their high diffusibility in the blood.

TAUYA [452] (1969) has recently proposed the use of colloidal indium (^{113m}In). This radiocompound emits monochromatic radiations of 390 keV [210]; it is easy to prepare but has a very short physical half-life (1.66 hours) so that it cannot be used in prolonged examinations of the CSF circulation.

WAGNER *et al.* [472] and JAMES *et al.* [231, 232] (1970, 1971) experimented with ytterbium-169 bound with diethylenetriamine-pentaacetic acid (^{169}Yb-DTPA), which had previously been used by HOSAIN *et al.* [176] (1969) for cerebral scanning. The characteristics of ^{169}Yb-DTPA are as follows:

1. high specific activity (400 μCi/mg)
2. long physical half-life (32 days)
3. short biological half-life (10 hours)
4. gamma radiations of 177 and 198 keV
5. rather low molecular weight (600).

Consequently, ytterbium can be injected in high doses because it is rapidly eliminated through the kidneys [214, 472]. The radiation dose to nervous structures is five times higher than with ^{99m}Tc but is still well below danger level. Ytterbium-169-DTPA is well stabilized from both the chemical and physiological viewpoints, and therefore does not require preliminary checking, like technetium and indium.

BELL *et al.* [32] (1969) summarized the characteristics of the ideal radiocompound for isotope cisternography as follows:

1. nonantigen
2. short physical life
3. rapid clearance from blood
4. insoluble in the lipids, i.e. no infiltration of the nervous tissues or pial vessels
5. rapid diffusion toward the convexity subarachnoid spaces
6. nonirritant
7. not metabolized in CSF
8. easily labeled with suitable gamma emitter
9. easily sterilized
10. nonpyrogenic
11. nontoxic.*

3. Diffusion of the Radiocompound

After the first papers by DI CHIRO and coworkers [120, 128], the modality of diffusion of the radiocompound in the ventricular system and subarachnoid space has been the object of much research [8, 231, 317, 426, 451]. All authors seem to be in agreement on the following fundamental points:

1. A radiocompound injected by the lumbar route does not penetrate the ventricular system. When injected directly into the ventricular system, however, it tends to escape through the aqueduct and the fourth ventricle, collecting in the basal cisterns and then in the subarachnoid space.
2. To diffuse from the spine to the skull, the radiocompound follows the anterior route of the basal cisterns [122, 231].
3. The reabsorption of the radiocompound takes place chiefly in the proximity of the superior longitudinal sinus.

GROS *et al.* [187] think that the radiocompound may sometimes diffuse toward the great cistern; TATOR *et al.* [451] exclude this eventuality. According to JAMES *et al.* [231] there are two main pathways: one central and one lateral. The central path-

* Recently, technetium chelated with DTPA or EDTA has been used at the dosage 30 μCi for Kilogram of bodyweight. This compound has the physical advantages of technetium and the chemical and biological advantages of DTPA and EDTA. (SOM, P., HOSAIN, F., WAGNER, H. M., and SCHEFFEL, V.: Cisternography with chelated complex of ^{99m}Tc. J. Nucl. Med. 13, 551 (1972).)

way can also be divided into two directions: an upper direction (from the suprasellar cisterns to the parasagittal region through the lamina terminalis, and the corpus callosum and interhemispherical cisterns); and a lower direction (from the basal cisterns to the parasagittal region through the circumpeduncular and posterior part of the corpus callosum cisterns). The lateral pathway goes to the parasagittal region along the Sylvian cisterns and the sulci of the convexity. Some radioactivity around the cerebellum has been recorded in a few cases.

What is the mechanism regulating the diffusion of the radiocompound in the subarachnoid space? According to DI CHIRO [122], who carried out research with the patient's own CSF, there are some ascending currents in CSF which are probably responsible for carrying the isotope from the lumbar region to the skull base and convexity, whatever the patient's position [119, 120, 231].

In the opinion of ALKER and LESLIE [8] the mechanism of the diffusion of a radiocompound is still unknown.

4. Technique

Preparation of the Patient

In order to avoid an accumulation of iodine in the thyroid it is necessary to halt the activity of this gland. Lugol's solution or iodine is therefore administered to the patient in the days preceding the examination [61, 125, 127, 186, 228, 373]. HOLMES [213] suggests blocking the salivary gland with atropine when technetium is used. Mercurial diuretics are indicated when mercurial radiocompounds are used [432].

Lumbar puncture must be performed with caution. TATOR *et al.* [451] advise having the patient lie in lateral decubitus and using a thin needle to avoid lacerating the meninges [8, 127, 212, 228]. Such a laceration might cause extravasation of the tracing [433] from the subarachnoid space, reducing the amount of radiocompound which is able to reach the skull, and produce false images of block [125, 187, 228, 231] or interfere with CSF circulation. When the radiocompound penetrates the epidural veins [124, 127], one can observe a partial picture of cerebral isotope scanning. It has been suggested that either 5 ml of air or 2 ml of Pantopaque be injected before the radiocompound in order to check that the needle is correctly positioned [212, 228].

Some authors dilute the radioactive compound injected by the lumbar route with 5 [228] or 10–20 ml [124, 127, 128, 228, 342, 451] of CSF withdrawn from the patient. In this connection, it seems that the speed of endocranial diffusion of the radiocompound depends on the amount of solvent injected [122, 128, 231]. A cortisone compound may be injected through the same needle immediately following the radioactive compound to prevent allergic symptoms or aseptic meningeal reactions (BAGGIO and MORGANDO [21], SIGNORINI *et al.* [426], and SCIALFA [415]).

Doses of Radiocompound and Injection Route

These two problems have to be discussed together since the dose varies according to the characteristics of the radiocompound itself (specific activity, reactions of the patient, etc.) and the route of its introduction [426].

The physical half-life and molecular size of the isotope are very important. The larger its molecules, the longer it takes for the isotope to leave the subarachnoid space; on the other hand, when using radiocompounds with a long physical half-life (low elimination rate), one should inject only moderate doses [231, 472].

The injection route is also important. If the radiocompound is injected by the lumbar route, the dose must be high because of the dispersion during the ascension. According to DI CHIRO [120, 122] and MCQUEEN and ABBASSIOUN [295], only 20–35% of the radiocompound injected reaches the endocranial subarachnoid spaces. The amounts required are smaller when the radiocompound is injected by the suboccipital or ventricular routes [119, 120, 124].

The doses suggested for each radiocompound are:

RIHSA. By the lumbar route (which is the one used by the majority of authors [26, 119, 128, 284, 342, 373, 433]) 100 μCi is usually injected in adult patients; some authors [187, 288], however, go up to 200–500 μCi. In children the average dose is 50 to 75 μCi [284]. By the suboccipital route the dose is the same as by the lumbar route [451]. By the ventricular route the dose usually is 50 μCi in adult patients [8, 61, 119, 128]. By the bregmatic route doses vary between 50 and 75 μCi [185, 187].

^{99m}Tc-*HSA*. By the lumbar route 2 [124] to 3 [227] mCi are usually injected in adult patients, and 1 mCi [227] in children. By the suboccipital route the average dose is 500 μCi in adult patients [284]. By the ventricular route 1 mCi is injected in adult patients.

Na-$^{99m}TcO_4$. The radioisotope is injected by the ventricular route or directly through a shunt tube. The amount is between 100 and 500 μCi [125].

Radioarsenic (^{74}As). 750 μCi is usually injected by the lumbar route in adult patients, and 75 μCi in children [295].

Radiogallium (^{68}Ga). The average dose is 2 mCi by the lumbar route in adult patients and 750 μCi in children [295].

Neohydrin (^{203}Hg). 200 μCi is injected in adult patients by the lumbar route; only 100 μCi is injected by the suboccipital route [426, 427].

^{169}Yb-*DTPA*. In adult patients 1 mCi of compound is injected by the lumbar route and 0.5 mCi by the suboccipital or ventricular routes [231].

The choice of injection route depends mainly on the clinical problem [119, 128]. When the CSF dynamics has to be investigated, the lumbar route can be considered the most physiological [119, 120, 122, 124, 231]. The suboccipital route must be chosen to obtain a detailed visualization of the basal cisterns [231, 426], while both suboccipital [321] and lumbar routes [127, 228] are appropriate to demonstrate small fistulae.

Some authors [284] prefer to use the suboccipital route in all cases because it shortens the length of the examination—an advantage in the case of emotional patients and children. A ventricular injection is indispensable in studying the appearance of the ventricular system and to check the efficiency of a surgical shunt [119, 128]. An injection via the bregma or through a burr hole is indicated to study the convexity sulci in patients suffering from subdural hematoma [185, 187, 212, 297].

The choice of introduction route also depends on the speed with which the radiocompound diffuses into the endocranial cisterns; a radiocompound with a short physical and biological half-life can be utilized for a complete exploration of the intracranial subarachnoid space only if it is injected by the suboccipital or the ventricular route [124, 231].

Scanning Apparatus

Linear Scanner

The linear scanning device consists of a small lens (5 in. × 5 in.) fixed to a moving support which explores a limited zone of the radioactive surface. A semiconical collimator "focalizes" a certain level according to a sort of tomographic mechanism. Recording is effected by measuring the difference in intensity of a monochromatic hatch and/or by means of color or a photographic device.

The linear scanner was the first apparatus employed for isotope cisternography.

According to Di Chiro *et al.* [124] and also Signorini *et al.* [426], linear scanning offers the advantage of greater resolving power than the gamma camera; moreover, there is only a slight deformation of the image.

James *et al.* [231] pointed out that with a linear scanner it is possible to record both low-energy (for example, ^{99m}Tc: 140 keV) and high-energy (for example, RIHSA: 364 keV) radiation. A drawback of the linear scanner is the time required [124] (several minutes), especially when the scan must be repeated for four projections. The tetrascanner and the biscanner were suggested by Di Chiro [117, 122] (1963, 1966), Di Chiro and Matthews [126] (1969), and Martini and Oberson [284] (1969). Di Chiro and Matthews [126] used the tetrascanner, while Martini and Oberson [284] used the biscanner. These apparatuses shorten the examination considerably, since more than one scan can be performed simultaneously.

Gamma Camera

The use of a gamma camera for isotope cisternography was suggested and then employed by Di Chiro and coworkers [122, 124] (1966, 1968); by Signorini *et al.* [426] (1968); and by others. It consists of a 11.5 in. diameter lens which covers the whole surface to be scanned. The collimator "does not focalize;" thus it does not explore a plane but a volume. the image is obtained on a cathodic screen and can be photographed or filmed.

One drawback of the gamma camera is the wide area of the lens which consequently must be very thin (0.5 in.). Therefore only isotopes of energy less than 522 keV [327] can be recorded. According to JAMES *et al.* [231], even RIHSA (364 keV) is not an ideal radiocompound for gamma-camera scanning.

With a gamma camera the scanning is very quick (sometimes a few seconds) [124]. This means greater accuracy in the examination, since it is easier to keep the patient still for a short time; moreover, it is possible to follow almost second by second the progression of the radiocompound in the subarachnoid space. In addition, it is possible to do multiple projections which are very useful for some particular cases (CSF oto- and/or rhinorrhea) which need to be examined rapidly (DI CHIRO *et al.* [124]).

Finally, when positron-emitting radiocompounds such as ^{68}Ga or ^{74}As are used, the radioactivity can be recorded only by positron cameras [295].

In conclusion, linear scanning is particularly useful for the study of the anatomic appearance of the CSF pathways, while for the dynamic study of CSF a gamma camera is preferable.

Scanning Procedures

Patient's Position

Many authors think the patient's position does not influence the diffusion of the radiocompound [8, 119, 120, 231], KILGORE *et al.* [228], however, prefer the prone position.

Scanning Schedule

The intervals at which the various scans are performed depend on many factors: injection site, the physico-biological characteristics of the radiocompound, and the type of disease. The reabsorption time of a radiocompound in the endocranial subarachnoid space varies between 1 to 48 hours and seems to be shorter in children [119, 231]. Most authors agree with DI CHIRO that scanning should be done 1, 6, 24, and 48 hours after a lumbar injection. Usually the posterior fossa and brain stem cisterns are demonstrated 1 hour after injection, the suprasellar, Sylvian, and corpus callosum cisterns 6 hours later, and the subarachnoid spaces of cerebral convexity 24 hours later. Only slight radioactivity is recorded 48 hours after injection, mainly at the level of the parasagittal regions [26, 119, 122, 451]. In the lumbar region, at the level of the injection, some radioactivity is still present over 48 hours later [61, 122].

Immediate scanning is necessary when the radiocompound is injected into the ventricles. A few minutes after the injection, some radioactivity is recorded at the level of the cerebral ventricles and basal cisterns; 12–24 hours later, it is recorded at the level of the parasagittal regions [120]. When the suboccipital route is employed, controls are made in roughly the same way; the great cistern remains active for a few days due to the escape of the radiocompound through the puncture hole [451].

Where the diffusion or reabsorption of the radiocompound is delayed by a pathological condition, scanning might be necessary as long as 72 or 96 hours after injection [8, 26, 124, 231]. Obviously, in such cases the radiocompound used must have low reabsorption time, considerable molecular weight, and a long physical half-life, like RIHSA and ^{99m}Tc-HSA [231].

Examination of CSF Fistulae

The examination is performed with the patient in the position in which the liquorrhea occurs [127].

The elective scanning time usually varies according to the site of the fistula [127]: 30–60 minutes after the injection for the posterior cranial fossa, 60–120 minutes for the middle fossa, 3–5 hours for the anterior fossa. In the case of a subarachnoid cyst communicating with the nasal cavities, scanning should be done 24 and 48 hours later.

Verification of the Efficiency of Surgical Shunts

DI CHIRO and GROVE [125] suggested injecting the radiocompound directly into the tube and scanning immediately afterward. In ventriculo-atrial shunts scanning must include the cervical spine. HOLMAN and DAVIS [212] inject the radiocompound directly into the shunted ventricle and make scans 1 and 2 hours after the injection.

Projections

Many authors [142, 127, 284] use for isotope cisternography the four projections considered classical for the radiographic examinations of the skull: antero-posterior, postero-anterior, right lateral, and left lateral. These projections allow a three-dimensional study of subarachnoid spaces and cerebral ventricles. Other authors [26, 187, 228, 415, 451], however, perform only the antero-posterior and one lateral projection; the latter has to be performed with the patient prone and the head turned on one side. Where both antero-posterior and postero-anterior projections are used, on the former it looks like a heart; on the latter the temporal horns are also visible. James *et al.* [231], Bricolo *et al.* [57] and Holmes [312] suggested "vertex" and half-axial projections. "Vertex" projection is in effect an axial projection performed in the opposite way to that usually employed in radiology: the patient is prone and his neck is hyperextended. On this projection one can observe one central area of radioactivity and two lateral areas corresponding to the Sylvian cisterns. Half-axial projection is employed less often and is easier with the gamma camera. It allows differentiation between the quadrigeminal cistern and the basal and Sylvian cisterns [231].

Lateral projection is most useful in the case of anterior fistula [228], while frontal projections are preferred if the fistula is located in the posterior fossa [127]. For better localization of the fistula, marking points are set at the level of the nasion, external acoustic meatus, and inion. To check surgical shunts, the most useful projections are lateral (omolateral to the shunt) and postero-anterior.

Our Technique

In our department isotope cisternography has been routinely carried out since 1968 [99, 415, 416]. When this chapter was written our statistics covered 230 cases. Our technique is substantially the same as that described by Di Chiro. The patient is sitting. We use particular care in performing the lumbar puncture with a two-way, small-caliber needle. Immediately after the injection of RIHSA some cortisone preparation (usually 25 mg of sodium prednisolone succinate diluted in 1 ml of double-distilled water) is introduced into the subarachnoid space to prevent allergic phenomena. In our department RIHSA is injected only exceptionally into the ventricles and into the great cistern. We use linear scanning and make records 1, 4, 24, and 48 hours after injection of the radiocompound (Fig. 5.1). In the great majority of our cases radioisotope cisternography is performed in the course of an encephalography immediately after the air injection. This does not seem to influence the result in either of the two types of examination.

5. Anatomy

Some preliminary considerations must be kept in mind.

1. The ventricular system and the cisterns are demonstrated directly by the radiocompound they contain [231].
2. Linear scanners have a resolution limit of 2 cm. Consequently, the small cisterns cannot be identified as separate structures [231].
3. Scanning of the different structures should be done at the time when the radiocompound reaches its maximum concentration. The aspect of the ventricular system and the subarachnoid space in the various projections is outlined below.

Lateral Projections

The upper part of the cervical subarachnoid space, and the pontine, interpeduncular, and suprasellar cisterns appear as a radioactive band directed upward and onward. About the center of the base of the skull the radioactivity appears particularly intense because of the superimposition of the horizontal segments of the Sylvian cisterns on the suprasellar cisterns. With suboccipital injection, the great cistern is visible a few minutes later; it looks like a triangle. The superior longitudinal sinus appears on the vertex as a semicircular radioactive band.

Fig. 5.1 a–h. *Radioisotope Cisternography*. Lateral (a, c, e, g) and antero-posterior (b, d, f, h) scans recorded 1, 4, 24, and 48 hours after injection of 100 μCi of RIHSA ▻

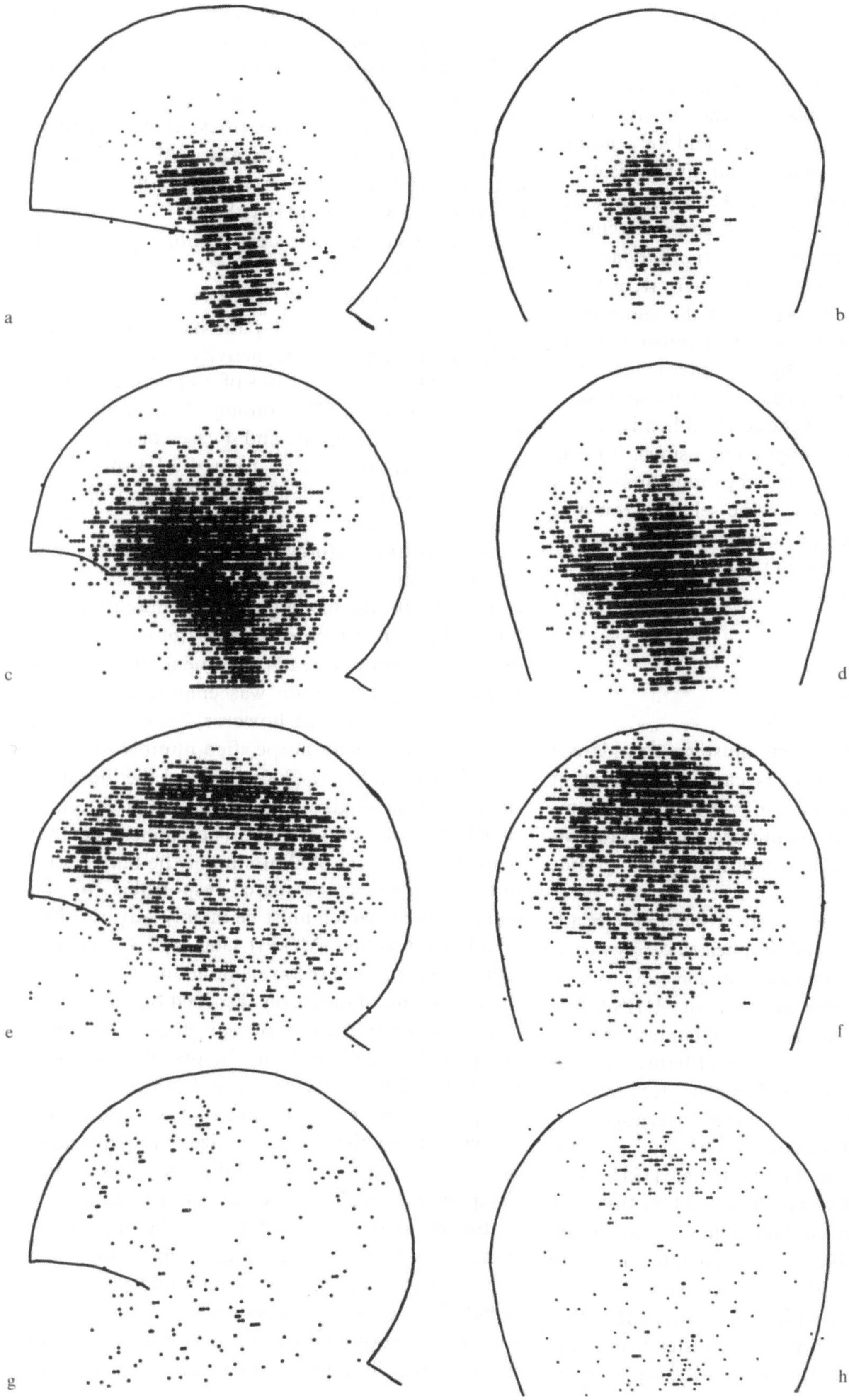
a
b
c
d
e
f
g
h

Antero-Posterior and Postero-Anterior Projections

There is a highly radioactive area at the center of the picture which is caused by the superposition of the cervical subarachnoid space, and the pontine, interpeduncular, suprasellar, and great cisterns. Above this area, about 6 hours later, three radioactive bands are visible, two lateral and one central. The lateral bands correspond to the Sylvian cisterns. The lower portion of the central band is formed by the superimposition of the suprasellar and brain stem cisterns; the upper portion of the central band is formed by the interhemispheric spaces (cistern of the corpus callosum and sulci of the internal surface of the cerebral hemispheres) and by the superior longitudinal sinus. In the antero-posterior projection the radioactivity is more evident at the level of the sellar region and Sylvian cisterns; in the postero-anterior projection, more radioactivity is seen at the level of the posterior fossa cisterns [231, 426].

6. Complications

Two types of complications must be considered: the "clinical" complications caused by injection into the subarachnoid space of particular radiocompounds, as previously mentioned; and complications resulting from irradiation of the nervous tissue.

Clinical complications range from simple headache, vomiting, fever, and dyspnea to cardiovascular failure. They were demonstrated in 1957 following the intraventricular injection of RIHSA [30, 222] and in 1965 also in cases of lumbar cisternography [368]. DETMER and BLACKER [113] (in an unspecified number of cases) and NICOL [315] (among 4 patients) observed after a lumbar cisternography, one case of aseptic meningitis thought to be caused by the buffer solution. For DI CHIRO [121], however, and for PATTEN and BENSON [328] the large amount of albumin contained in the radiocompound was responsible for such complication, and they considered it could be avoided by using radiocompounds of high specific activity where the albumin concentration is low. Thus, instead of 27 mg (DETMER and BLACKER) and 100–130 mg (NICOL) of albumin, DI CHIRO injects only 2–4 mg of albumin with high specific activity (250–500 μCi per mm^3). MCQUEEN and ABBASSIOUN [295] using ^{74}As observed 28 cases of aseptic meningitis which they attributed to colloidal impurities; they suggested the use of filtered material to prevent this complication. MARTINI and OBERSON [284] (1969) in a series of 20 patients examined with RIHSA observed headache, nausea, and fever of short duration in an unspecified number of cases.

ALKER and LESLIE [8] observed only one case of hyperthermia among 50 patients examined with RIHSA of high specific activity; OLDHAM and STAAB [320] observed 2 cases of aseptic meningitis; and KILGORE *et al.* [228] among 54 cases observed 5 cases of fever in adults and 4 cases of meningitis in children. KILGORE *et al.* injected RIHSA of high specific activity with 5 ml of CSF. In their opinion a feverish reaction can be observed even after a simple lumbar puncture and they consider the albumin (even in very low doses of 1–1.6 mg) to be responsible for the meningeal symptoms; they propose a further reduction of the albumin and the use of technetium instead of iodine as the radioactive isotope. Technetium was employed by BELL *et al.* [32], who observed, however, 2 cases of aseptic meningitis among an unspecified number of cases.

OLDHAM and STAAB [320] reviewed the literature on aseptic meningitis following lumbar injection of RIHSA and ^{99m}Tc-HSA. They concluded that neither the amount of albumin nor the buffer solution alone can be considered responsible for the complications, which must be mainly attributed to an allergic reaction. MERRIT [300] and ALKER and LESLIE [8] expressed the same opinion.

The amount of radiation absorbed by the patient following administration of a given dose of radiocompound depends on many factors: the bio-physico-chemical characteristics of the radiocompound [231], the type of impairment of CSF circulation shown by the patient [199], the size of the subarachnoid space, and the rate of diffusion of the radiocompound through the subarachnoid space and its reabsorption in the blood [212]. The site of the highest absorption, however, depends on the route of introduction of the radiocompound and on its metabolism. Radioisotopes such as ^{131}I and ^{203}Hg, which emit both gamma and beta radiations and have a rather long physical half-life, must be considered more dangerous than ^{99m}Tc, which emits only gamma radiations and has a physical half-life of 6 hours [211]. Obviously the irradiation of the medulla is poor when the radiocompound is introduced by the suboccipital or the intraventricular route. When iodine is used, there is also a considerable irradiation of the thyroid gland; with technetium the salivary glands (particularly the parotid) are irradiated as well as the nasopharyngeal and gastric mucous membranes [125]; with mercury and ytterbium the kidney is the most affected organ, besides the nervous system [69, 472]. At any rate, BANNISTER *et al.* [26] believe that, when normal radioisotopes are used, the irradiation of both the nervous system and the other organs is within the limits of safety even when pathological conditions mean that the radiocompound stays for a long while in the CSF [199, 202]. DI CHIRO *et al.* [126, 128] and TATOR *et al.* [451] stated that, following the lumbar introduction of 100 μCi of RIHSA, the radiation dose absorbed by the entire body is 100 mrad while that absorbed by the central nervous system is about 1 rad. These results were confirmed by BANNISTER *et al.* [26]. For BROCKLEHURST [60] the dose absorbed by the central nervous system after the injection of 100 μCi of RIHSA by the lumbar route is 3–4 rads when the CSF circulation is normal and 5 rads when it is impaired. For MCALISTER [291] this dose can reach 8 rads. GROS *et al.* [185] observed that cerebral cortex absorbs 3924 rads following the administration of 75 μCi of RIHSA injected through the bregma. GROS *et al.* [186] calculated that after injection through the lumbar route of 100–200 μCi of RIHSA, the dose absorbed by the medulla is about 15–20 rads. HODAK *et al.* [211], without giving any figures affirm that the radiation dose absorbed after the injection (either lumbar or intraventricular) of 2 mCi of ^{99m}Tc-HSA was inferior to that occurring with 100 μCi of RIHSA. According to ANCRI [15] and HOLMAN and DAVIS [212], the doses absorbed when using 1 mCi ^{99m}Tc are 0.3 rad at the level of the central nervous system and 0.01 rad at the level of the body. MCQUEEN and ABBASSIOUN [295] calculated the radiation dose absorbed after the injection of 500 μCi of radiogallium (^{68}Ga) in children and 2 mCi of same compound in adults. The result was 14, and 15–20 mrad, respectively. STAAB *et al.* [433] calculated that the radiation dose absorbed by monkeys following RIHSA cisternography varied between 15 and 60 rads. HARBERT [199] has recently made a comparative study of the absorbed radiation at the lumbar level following the injection of 100 μCi of RIHSA, ^{99m}Tc-HSA, ^{133}indium, and ^{169}ytterbium. He concluded that the absorption dose varies according to the radioisotope employed and that, when the same radioisotopes are used, doses are higher in patients with impaired CSF circulation (hydrocephalus, cervical block, etc.).

7. Indications and Results

In this paragraph we will make an exception by not confirming this work in the technical field. Radioisotope cisternography is still a rather unfamiliar technique and we deem it justifield to state its main indications on the basis of the results obtained.

CSF Fistulae

For DI CHIRO *et al.* [127, 128] radioisotope cisternography is the only technique allowing the direct demonstration of the path of a CSF fistula, especially in cases of spontaneous traumatic rhinorrhea. We agree that this technique is very important but we also feel on the basis of much personal experience that the results are difficult to evaluate. It is difficult to identify with certainty the course of the fistula, which is only indirectly revealed by radioactivity in the facial region. This opinion is shared by GROS *et al.* [187]. Three cases of CSF fistulae were diagnosed by MARTINI and OBERSON [284]. In 3 more cases observed by FRONT and PENNING [158] the diagnosis could be made only by radioisotope cisternography.

Atrophy, Hydrocephalus, and Malformations

Differential diagnosis between hydrocephalus and atrophy has become urgent since neurological pathology has recognized the so-called normal-pressure or occult hydrocephalus. Such a diagnosis is facilitated by isotope cisternography. In normal conditions a radiocompound injected by the lumbar or the suboccipital route does not enter the ventricular system; it does do so, however, in cases where there is an anomaly of the CSF circulation. According to many authors, such an anomaly would exclude the diagnosis of atrophy, unless it was coexistent [26, 206, 430, 451]. OBERSON *et al.* [319] have studied the "normal" appearance of CSF circulation in 150 cases, including elderly and adult patients, and children. They think that, though the "normal" appearance is variable, the passage of the radiocompound into the ventricular system (and of course into a fistula) must always be considered pathological.

There have, however, been some puzzling cases. Recently, MICHELSEN [304] observed that there are three possibilities in cases of normal-pressure hydrocephalus:

1. The radiocompound passes into the ventricular system.
2. It is stopped at the level of the base of the skull.
3. It passes into both the ventricular system and the subarachnoid space.

HEINZ *et al.* [206] affirmed that in cerebral atrophy the cisternographic picture is characterized by accumulation of radiocompound in the subarachnoid space of the atrophic zone. JAMES *et al.* [201, 232] confirmed their opinion, stating that a radiocompound accumulation is always observed when the subarachnoid space is dilated. This occurs not only in cases of cortical cyst—either cerebral or cerebellar—but also in meningo- or myelocele (in which it is possible to demonstrate the communication between lesion and subarachnoid space) and/or in Dandy-Walker malformations [200]. In this last case the same authors, in collaboration with CONWAY *et al.* [84] observed two different aspects: halting of the radiocompound at the level of the foramen magnum, or accumulation of radioactivity in the cystic cavity. In the latter case, however, the diagnosis is uncertain since a similar aspect can also be observed in normal cases if the great cistern is very wide. CASTELLINO *et al.* [75] employed radioisotope cisternography in children affected by Arnold-Chiari malformation.

Differential diagnosis as between normal-pressure hydrocephalus and atrophy is important from a practical viewpoint, too, since in the former a surgical shunt may be useful. The indication for this operation is based by many authors on the results of isotope cisternography, especially in cases of post-traumatic hydrocephalus and/or dementia with ventricular dilatation.

ALLEN *et al.* [10] were able to diagnose 58 cases of normal-pressure hydrocephalus by means of radioisotope cisternography, and in 20 of them the radiocompound entered the ventricular system. These 20 patients were operated on: 13 improved, but in 7 cases the symptoms remained unchanged. According to RUDD *et al.* [373], radioisotope cisternography is inadequate to differentiate a well-compensated hydrocephalus from a hydrocephalus out of balance, but the majority of authors [9, 228, 284, 373] agree in stating that it is the only method that permits a correct indication for a surgical operation. In our opinion, definite progress could only be achieved by a comparative study between pictures obtained by radioisotope cisternography and encephalography—of course, both performed at a similar technical level. To our knowledge, no such study exists in the literature. We are trying to make such a study in our department, but have encountered considerable difficulties, which will be described in another paper.

Expansive Processes

GROS *et al.* [185] performed RIHSA cisternography by the bregmatic route on 5 children with subdural hematoma. The results were good and the method is considered by these authors to be preferable, in such cases, to encephalography and even to cerebral angiography.

SIGNORINI *et al.* [427] injected Neohydrin ^{203}Hg by the lumbar route in cases of suspected tumor. The results were good in extracerebral, hemispheric, and parasellar tumors, but these authors consider radioisotope cisternography of no use in cases of posterior fossa tumors. MAMO *et al.* [275] observed a "silent" zone in the region of the pontine and cerebello-pontine angle cisterns in 7 cases of neurinoma of the cerebello-pontine angle. In 2 cases radioisotope cisternography proved to be fundamental for a correct diagnosis.

Addendum

The EMI-Scanner apparatus has now definitely entered—in a rather triumphal way—in Neuroradiological routine. This apparatus, a computerized analyzer of the absorbed radiations, actually opens new prospects in Neuroradiology. We have no personal experience on it, since it is not yet operating in our Department; however its utility for the study of the ventricular system appears quite evident from the papers already published. It seems therefore fair to us to pay a dutyful homage to the inventor of EMI-Scanner, Ing. G. HOUNSFIELD and to Drs. J. AMBROSE and J. BULL, the neuroradiologists who have introduced and emphasized respectively the clinical utility of this valuable machine.

AMBROSE, J., and HOUNSFIELD, G.: Computerized transvers axial tomography. Brith. Journal of Radiology. **46**, 148, (1973).
BULL, J.: Lectures on EMI-Scanner all over the world.

References

1. ABBOTT, M., ALKSNE, J. F.: Transport of intrathecal ^{125}I RIHSA to circulating plasma: a test for communicating hydrocephalus. Neurology **18**, 870 (1968).
2. ADSON, A. W.: The evaluation of pneumoventriculography and encephalography. Amer. J. Roentgenol. **27**, 657 (1932).
3. AGUADO MATORRAS, A., NALDA FELIPE, M. A., PERAITA, P.: Neuroleptoanalgesia asociada a la hiperventilaçion o a l'urea. Estudio comparativo de algunas costantes en pacientes neuroquirurgicos. Rev. esp. Oto-neuro-oftal. **23**, 155 (1964).
4. AIRD, R. B.: Experimental encephalography with anesthetic gases. Proc. Soc. exp. Biol. (N. Y.) **31**, 715 (1934).
5. AIRD, R. B.: Encephalography with anesthetic gases. Arch. Surg. **34**, 853 (1937).
6. ALBERTI, J., ANDREWS, I., WILSON, G.: Posterior fossa tomography during encephalography. Acta radiol. (Stockh.) **9**, 128 (1969).
7. ALEXANDER, L., JUNG, T. S., LYMAN, R. S.: Colloidal thorium dioxide. Its use in intracranial diagnosis and its fate on direct injection into the brain and the ventricles. Arch. Neurol. Psychiat. (Chic.) **32**, 1143 (1934).
8. ALKER, G. J., JR., LESLIE, E. V.: Isotope cisternography and ventriculography. Acta radiol. (Stockh.) **9**, 589 (1969).
9. ALKER, G. J. JR., LESLIE, E. V., GLASSAUER, F.: Five years' experience with isotope cisternography and ventriculography. Communication, IX Symposium Neuroradiologicum, Göteborg 1970.
10. ALLEN, J. H., STAAB, E. V., YOUNG, B., MEACHAM, W.: Correlation of isotope cisternography, pneumoencephalography and clinical data in selection of normal pressure hydrocephalus patients for shunt surgery. Communication, IX Symposium Neuroradiologicum, Göteborg 1970.
11. AMEZUA, L.: Yodoventriculografia de fosa posterior y de tercer ventriculo. Nueva tecnica de manejo rapida de la sustancia opaca. An. Neurocirugia **31**, 75 (1957).
12. AMPLATZ, K.: An improved chair for pneumoencephalography and autotomography. Amer. J. Roentgenol. **90**, 184 (1963).
13. AMUNDSEN, P.: Gas encephalography on the polytome. Communication, Annual Meeting of the European Society of Neuroradiology, Bologna 1972.
14. AMUNDSEN, P., DUGSTAD, P., GRIMSRUD, O. K.: Gas encephalography with hypocycloidal tomography. Correlation with anatomic cast. Acta radiol. (Stockh.) **9**, 134 (1969).
15. ANCRI, D.: Exploration du liquide céphalo-rachidien dans son segment médullaire par les radio-isotopes. Traité de Radiodiagnostic. Neuroradiologie **15**, Paris: Masson et Cie. 1971.
16. ATKINSON, J. R., FOLTZ, E. L.: Intraventricular RIHSA as a diagnostic aid in pre- and postoperative hydrocephalus. J. Neurosurg. **19**, 159 (1962).
17. Autotomography. Editorial. Brit. J. Radiol. **35**, 415 (1962).
18. AZAMBUJA, N.: Round table on the technique of encephalography. Annual Meeting of the European Society of Neuroradiology, Bologna 1972.
19. AZAMBUJA, N., ARAÑA-INIGUEZ, R., SANDE, M. T., GARCIA-GUELFI, A.: Central ventriculography. Acta neurol. lat.-amer. **2**, 58 (1956).
20. BACIOCCO, A., CHIAPPETTA, F.: L'impiego dell'urea come elemento facilitante nella esecuzione della pneumoencefalografia. Radiol. med. **50** 765 (1964).
21. BAGGIO, G. F., MORGANDO, E.: La mieloscintigrafia nello studio delle affezioni vertebro-midollari. Riv. Pat. nerv. ment. Speçial issue for XV Congress of the Italian Society of Neurology; Symposium on "L'applicazione dei radioisotopi per lo studio delle malattie del sistema nervoso" 1965.
22. BAKER, H. L.: Myelographic examination of posterior fossa with positive contrast medium. Radiology **81**, 791 (1963).
23. BALADO, M.: Radiografia del tercer ventriculo por medio de inyeccion intraventricular de lipiodol. Arch. argent. Neurol. **4**, 69 (1928).
24. BALADO, M.: Diagnostico de las obstruciones ventriculares por inyeccion intraventricular de lipiodol. Arch. argent. Neurol. **5**, 85 (1929).
25. BALADO, M.: Tecnica de la ventriculografia con lipiodol. Arch. argent. Neurol. **6**, 34 (1930).
26. BANNISTER, R., GILFORD, E., KOCEN, R.: Isotope encephalography in the diagnosis of dementia due to communicating hydrocephalus. Lancet ii, 1014 (1967).
27. BAUDOUIN, A., HARTMANN, E., PUECH, P.: Cécité temporaire et troubles du champ visuel après ventriculographie. Rev. neurol. **65**, 167 (1936).
28. BAUER, K., YUHL, T.: Myelography by means of ^{131}I. The myeloscintigram. Neurology (Minneap.) **3**, 341 (1953).
29. BEGHÉ, R., TUGNOLI, F.: Trattamento dell'ipertensione endocranica mediante urea endovenosa. Minerva neurochir. **6**, 27 (1962).
30. BELL, R. L.: Isotope transfer test in the diagnosis of ventriculo-subarachnoidal block. J. Neurosurg. **14**, 674 (1957).
31. BELL, R. L.: Isotope transfer test in the diagnosis and treatment of hydrocephalus. Int. J. appl. Radiat. **5**, 89 (1959).
32. BELL, E. G., SUBRAMANIAN, G., ROSS, G. S., MCAFEE, J. G.: Gamma-cisternography—an evaluation of short-lived radioactive agents. J. nucl. Med. **10**, 321 (1969).
33. BELLONI, G.: Pneumographische Passageprüfung der Arachnoidalräume. Zbl. Neurochir. **6**, 43 (1941).
34. BELLONI, G.: Pneumographie des espaces arachnoidiens encéphaliques. Bull. schweiz. Akad. med. Wiss. **5**, 147 (1949).
35. BENEDEK, L., JOBA, A.: Blocages tardifs au cours de la lipiodographie. Dtsch. Z. Nervenheilk. **151**, 55 (1940).

36. Bergström, K., Hogström, S., Lödin, H.: Experiences with nitrous oxide-oxygen as contrast medium in encephalography and ventriculography performed under general anesthesia. Ann. Radiol. **10**, 189 (1967).
37. Bering, E.A., Jr.: Notes on retention of Pantopaque in subarachnoid space. Amer. J. Surg. **80**, 455 (1950).
38. Berney, J., Werner, A.: Value of tomography in gasmyelography and pneumoencephalography. J. Indian med. Ass. **47**, 162 (1966).
39. Bernini, F.P., Calabrò, A., Mazzarella, B., Smaltino, F.: L'iperventilazione polmonare controllata in encefalografia frazionata. Communication, Annual Meeting of the European Society of Neuroradiology, Bologna 1972.
40. Bétoulières, P., Lafon, R., Temple, J., Labauge, R., Pelissier, M., Paleirac, R.: L'apport de la pneumostratigraphie simultanée dans l'exploration des structures du tronc cérébral. J. Radiol. Électrol. **37**, 956 (1956).
41. Bétoulières, P., Latour, H.: La pneumostratigraphie. Paris: Masson et Cie. 1955.
42. Bétoulières, P., Paleirac, R., Labauge, R., Bassède, J.: La pneumostratigraphie encéphalique. J. Radiol. Électrol. **35**, 27 (1954).
43. Betz, H.: Pneumotomographie der hinteren Schädelgrube. Fortschr. Röntgenstr. **109**, 319 (1968).
44. Betz, H.: Correlations of clinical symptoms with radiographic finding in pneumotomography of the posterior cranial fossa. Radiologe **9**, 488 (1969).
45. Bleasel, K.: Nerve root radiography. Brit. J. Radiol. **34**, 596 (1961).
46. Boldrey, E., Aird, R.B.: The effects of iodized poppy seed oil and iodine clorine in peanut oil in the subarachnoid space of animals. J. nerv. ment. Dis. **99**, 521 (1944).
47. Bonkalo, A.: The filling of subarachnoid spaces over the convexity in encephalograms of normal and tumour cases. Acta psychiat. scand. **25**, 323 (1950).
48. Bories, J.: La technique de l'encéphalographie avec le Neurocentrix. Communication, Annual Meeting of the European Society of Neuroradiology, Bologna 1972.
49. Bories, J., Bamberger-Bozo, C., Rosier, J.: Mono-iodostéarate d'éthyle et myélographie. Acta radiol. (Stockh.) **9**, 686 (1969).
50. Bories, J., Fredy, D., Rosier, J.: Tomo-encephalography. Technique and normal images. Neuroradiology **1**, 200 (1970).
51. Bories, J., Fredy, D., Rosier, J.: Étude tomoencéphalographique des atrophies cerebelleuses. Communication, IX Symposium Neuroradiologicum, Göteborg 1970.
52. Bories, J., Zecques: Le Neurocentrix. Personal communication.
53. Bourdon, R., Fischgold, H., Gilles, E., Herdner, R., Lenzi, M., Lombardi, G., Mascherpa, F., Oliva, L., Piazza, A., Porcher, P., Vallebona, A.: Cranial tomography in neuroradiology. Acta radiol. (Stockh.) **40**, 272 (1953).
54. Bozza, M., Rossanda, M., Visca, A.: I diuretici osmotici in Neurochirurgia. Minerva neurochir. **6**, 80 (1962).
55. Bradac, G.B., Wackenheim, A.: The normal and pathologic pneumostratigraphic radioanatomy of the presellar and the inferomedial frontal regions. Ann. Radiol. **11**, 217 (1968).
56. Brewer, E.D.: Etiology of headache; occurrence and significance of headache during ventriculography. Bull. neurol. Inst. N.Y. **6**, 12 (1937).
57. Bricolo, A., Marabini, A., Bazzan, A., Dalle Ore, G.: Isotope subarachnoidography with ^{197}Hg and ^{203}Hg chlormerodrin. Minerva neurochir. **13**, 237 (1969).
58. Britton, B.H., Hitselberger, W.E., Hurley, B.J.: Iophendylate examination of posterior fossa in diagnosis of cerebello-pontine angle tumours. Arch. Otolaryng. **88**, 608 (1969).
59. Brocklehurst, G.: Observations on C.S.F. flow using isotope ventriculography. J. Neurol. Neurosurg. Psychiat. **30**, 587 (1967).
60. Brocklehurst, G.: Radiation dose in isotope encephalography. Lancet ai, 358 (1968).
61. Brocklehurst, G.: Use of radio-iodinated serum albumin in the study of cerebrospinal flow. J. Neurol. Neurosurg. Psychiat. **31**, 162 (1968).
62. Bronisch, F.W.: The 24-hour encephalogram. J. nerv. ment. Dis. **116**, 892 (1952).
63. Brown, F.M., Aye, R.C.: Myelographic demonstration of basilar artery. Amer. J. Roentgenol. **73**, 32 (1955).
64. Brown, H.A., Carr, J.L.: The effect of lipiodol in the subarachnoid space. Surg. Gynec. Obstet. **68**, 945 (1939).
65. Bruskin, J., Propper, N.: Experimentelle Myelo-Encephalographie an Hunden und über den Einfluß von Iodopin und Lipiodol auf das Rückenmark, Gehirn und dessen Häute. Z. ges. exp. Med. **75**, 34 (1931).
66. Bull, J.W.: Positive-contrast ventriculography. Acta radiol. (Stockh.) **34**, 253 (1950).
67. Burrows, E.H.: An autotomographic appliance. Amer. J. Roentgenol. **87**, 366 (1962).
68. Burrows, E.H.: Positive-contrast examination (cerebellopontine cisternography) of extrameatal acoustic neurofibromas. Brit. J. Radiol. **42**, 902 (1969).
69. Cabassa, N., Donati, E., Bazzan, A., Marabini, A.: Studio sulla distribuzione e diffusione nell'uomo del ^{203}Hg Chloromerodrin somministrato nello spazio subaracnoideo del midollo spinale. Radiol. med. **53**, 501 (1967).
70. Calabrò, A.: Ventriculographie gazeuse du III ventricule, de l'aqueduc et du IV ventricule. Acta radiol. (Stockh.) **9**, 154 (1969).
71. Campbell, C.B.: The value of autotomography in the demonstration of the mid-line ventricular system of the brain. Radiol. Techn. **41**, 65 (1969).
72. Campbell, R.L., Campbell, J.A., Heimburger, R.F., Kalsbeck, J.E., Mealy, J.: Ventriculography and myelography with absorbable radiopaque medium. Radiology **82**, 286 (1964).
73. Carrillo, R.: Ventriculografia de fosa posterior. Buenos Aires: El Ateneo 1938.
74. Carrillo, R., Oribe, M., Malenchini, M.: Tomo-encephalografia. Sem. méd. (Paris) **2**, 472 (1937).
75. Castellino, R.A., Zatz, L.M., DeNardo, G.L.: Radioisotope ventriculography in the Arnold-Chiari malformation. Radiology **93**, 817 (1969).
76. Catalano, S., Sassaroli, S.: Comportamento della pressione endoventricolare durante l'encefalografia frazionata. Rass. Neuropsichiatria **9**, 99 (1955).
77. Cestan, R., Riser, M.: La ventriculographie par la pneumorachie. Sem. Hôp. Paris **48**, 953 (1924).
78. Chechan, C.: Quoted by 112.
79. Chou, S.N., French, L.A.: Systemic absorption and urinary excretion of RIHSA from subarachnoid space. Neurology (Minneap.) **5**, 555 (1955).
80. Chrzanowski, R., Wackenheim, A.: Pneumostratigraphie frontale du tronc cérébral. Ann. Radiol. **9**, 872 (1966).
81. Cleveland, D., End, E.: Helium in encephalography. Surg. Gynec. Obstet. **74**, 760 (1942).

82. COLLAN, R.: Cardiac arrest caused by rapid elimination of nitrous oxide from cerebral ventricles after encephalography. Canad. Anaesth. Soc. J. **16**, 519 (1969).
83. CONTE, M., D'ELIA, E., SIMONETTI, N.: L'impiego dell'urea nell'edema cerebrale traumatico. Acta chir. ital. **17**, 489 (1961).
84. CONWAY, J.J., YARZAGARAY, L., WELCH, D.: Radionuclide evalution of the Dandy-Walker malformation and congenital arachnoid cyst of the posterior fossa. Amer. J. Roentgenol. **112**, 306 (1971).
85. CORNELIS, C., DEREYMAEKER, A.: L'iodoventriculographie dans les affections de la fosse postérieure. Acta radiol. Diagn. **1**, 828 (1963).
86. CORRALES, M.: A radiologic investigation of the fourth ventricle. Thesis. Stockholm 1972.
87. CORRALES, M., GREITZ, T.: The fourth ventricle. Normal appearance and changes in expanding lesions of the posterior fossa. Communication, IX Symposium Neuroradiologicum, Göteborg 1970.
88. CORRALES, M., GREITZ, T.: El cuarto ventriculo. Aspecto normal y cambios en procesos expansivos de la fosa posterior. II Congresso Latino-Americano de Neuroradiologia, Punta del Este 1971.
89. CORSSEN: Quoted by 139.
90. COVA, P.L., POMPILI, G.: Tomografia a strato spesso. Radiol. med. (Torino) **43**, 1057 (1957).
91. CRAIG, W.M.: Effect of iodized poppy seed oil in spinal cord and meninges. Arch. Neurol. Psychiat. (Chic.) **48**, 799 (1942).
92. CRAWFORD, A.S.: Method of ventricular puncture and studies in cerebral pneumography. Yale J. Biol. Med. **11**, 473 (1939).
93. CREZEE: Quoted by 17.
94. CRISTI, G.: Anatomia encefalografica del IV ventricolo. Radiol. med. (Torino) **57**, 676 (1971).
95. CRISTI, G., SCIALFA, G., DI PIERRO, G., TASSONI, A.: Su un caso di rara complicazione da mielografia liposolubile. Communication, LXXX Raduno Emiliano-Marchigiano della S.I.R.M.N., Pesaro 1971.
96. CRONQVIST, S., LUNDBERG, N., PONTÉN, U.: Cerebral pneumography with continuous control of ventricular fluid pressure. Acta radiol. (Stockh.) **1**, 558 (1963).
97. CROSBY, R.M.: Treatment of post-pneumoencephalographic headache with pyridil carbinol tartrate. Amer. J. med. Sci. **61**, 225 (1953).
98. CROUET, P.L., FAIVRE, G., LAMY, P., LARCAU, A.: Séquelles neurologiques graves du lipiodol-diagnostic. Sem. Hôp. Paris **32**, 4 (1956).
99. DALBUONO, S., BRADAC, G.B., RUGGIERO, G.: Cisternografia con radioisotopi. Boll. Soc. Med. Chir. Bologna **1**, 78 (1969).
100. DANDY, W.E.: Ventriculography following the injection of air into the cerebral ventricles. Amer. Surg. **68**, 5 (1918).
101. DANDY, W.E.: Roentgenography of the brain after the injection of air into the spinal canal. Amer. Surg. **70**, 397 (1919).
102. DAVID, M., RUGGIERO, G., TALAIRACH, J.: L'encéphalographie en neurochirurgie. Rev. neurol. **88**, 287 (1953).
103. DAVIDOFF, L.M., DYKE, C.G.: The normal encephalogram. Philadelphia: Lea & Febiger 1946.
104. DAVIDSON, KC., CLARK, L.: An autotomographic device for pneumoencephalography and ventriculography. Radiology **87**, 950 (1966).
105. DAVIES, F.L.: Effect of unabsorbed radiographic contrast media on the central nervous system. Lancet ii, 747 (1956).
106. DAVIES, H., HAVEN, H.A., STONE, T.T.: The effect of injections of iodized oil in the spinal subarachnoid space. J. Amer. med. Ass. **94**, 772 (1930).
107. DAVINI, V., GHIRARDI, L.: Studio radiografico stratigrafico e ventricolografico in un caso di asimmetria craniocerebrale. Sist. nerv. **1**, 37 (1949).
108. DEERY, E.M.: A method of ventriculography. Bull. neurol. Inst. N.Y. **1**, 193 (1931).
109. DELIGNÉ, P.: Nouveaux neuroleptiques dans différents types d'anesthésie; indications en anesthésiologie neurochirurgicale. Agressologie **2**, 363 (1961).
110. DELIGNÉ, P.: Anesthésie au cours des examens électroradiologiques en neurologie. Cah. Anesth. **11**, 36 (1962).
111. DENK, W.: Über Encephalographie und ihre Ergebnisse. Z. ärztl. Fortbild. **20**, 426 (1923).
112. DESCUNS, P., VIALLET, P., CHEVROT, L., AUBRY, P.: L'encéphalographie gazeuse à l'ozone. J. Radiol. Électrol. **38**, 1045 (1957).
113. DETMER, D.E., BLACKER, H.M.: A case of aseptic meningitis secondary of intrathecal injection of ^{131}I human serum albumin. Neurology (Minneap.) **15**, 642 (1965).
114. DETTORI, P., FINIZIO, F.S., BERNARDI, L.: Further experience with urea in encephalography. Communication, Annual Meeting of the European Society of Neuroradiology, Bologna 1972.
115. DI BIAGIO, F., SASSAROLI, S.: Quadro pneumografico di ipereplezione cervicale come segno di preincuneamento delle amigdale. Ann. Radiol. diagn. (Bologna) **32**, 264 (1959).
116. DI CHIRO, G.: An atlas of detailed normal pneumoencephalographic anatomy. Springfield: Charles C. Thomas 1961.
117. DI CHIRO, G.: Anatomical, tridimensional brain scanning. In: Radioisotopes et affections du système nerveux central. Paris: Masson et Cie. 1963.
118. DI CHIRO, G.: Axial transverse encephalography. Amer. J. Roentgenol. **92**, 441 (1964).
119. DI CHIRO, G.: New radiographic and isotopic procedures in neurological diagnosis. J. Amer. med. Ass. **188**, 524 (1964).
120. DI CHIRO, G.: Movement of the cerebrospinal fluid in human beings. Nature (Lond.) **204**, 290 (1964).
121. DI CHIRO, G.: Specific activity of radio-iodinated serum albumin for intrathecal injection. A correction. Neurology (Minneap.) **15**, 950 (1965).
122. DI CHIRO, G.: Observations on the circulation of the cerebrospinal fluid. Acta radiol. Diagn. **5**, 988 (1966).
123. DI CHIRO, G.: An atlas of pathologic pneumoencephalographic anatomy. Springfield: Charles C. Thomas 1967.
124. DI CHIRO, G., ASHBURN, W.L., BRINER, W.H.: Technetium Tc99^{m} serum albumin for cisternography. Arch. Neurol. (Chic.) **19**, 218 (1968).
125. DI CHIRO, G., GROVE, A.S.: Evaluation of surgical and spontaneous cerebrospinal fluid shunts by isotope scanning. J. Neurosurg. **24**, 743 (1966).
126. DI CHIRO, G., MATTHEWS, W.H.: The tetrascanner: a device for rapid three-dimensional brain scanning. J. nucl. Med. **7**, 330 (1966).
127. DI CHIRO, G., OMMAYA, A.K., ASHBURN, W.L., BRINER, W.H.: Isotope cisternography in the diagnosis and follow-up of cerebrospinal fluid rhinorrhea. J. Neurosurg. **28**, 522 (1968).
128. DI CHIRO, G., REAMES, P.M., MATTHEWS, W.H.: RIHSA-ventriculography and RIHSA-cisternography. Neurology (Minneap.) **14**, 185 (1964).

129. Dietz, H. E., Zeitler, E., Wolf, R.: Die szintigraphische Darstellung der Liquorräume mit 131-J-markiertem menschlichen Serumalbumin (RIHSA). Fortschr. Röntgenstr. **105**, 537 (1966).
130. Dilenge, D., David, M., Talairach, J.: A propos des indications de la technique de l'iodoventriculographie. Neurocirugia **6**, 347 (1960).
131. Dilenge, D., David, M., Talairach, J.: Technique de la iodoventriculographie par lipiodol. Ann. Radiol. **4**, 912 (1961).
132. Dilenge, D., Deligné, P., David, M., Calabrò, A., Metzger, J.: Intérêt de l'urée-mannitol en neuro-radiologie. In: La radiographie des formations intrarachidiennes. Paris: Masson et Cie 1965.
133. Dulac, C. L.: Études sur la précision en radiodiagnostic. Techniques d'un nouveau craniographe. Paris: Masson et Cie. 1956.
134. Dyke, C.G., Elsberg, C.A., Davidoff, L.M.: Enlargement of the defect in the air shadow normally produced by the choroid plexus; its occurrence after ventricular puncture. Amer. J. Roentgenol. **33**, 736 (1935).
135. Eagle, C.L., Froman, C.: Neuroleptanalgesia for neuroradiological procedure. S. Afr. med. J. **43**, 654 (1969).
136. Edholm, P., Quiding, L.: Elimination of blur in linear tomography. Acta radiol. (Diagn.) **10**, 441 (1970).
137. Eley, R.C., Vogt, E.C.: Encephalography in children: further observations in children with fixed lesions of the brain. Amer. J. Roentgenol. **27**, 686 (1932).
138. Elsberg, C.A., Southerland, R.W.: Etiology of headache: I. Headache produced by injection of air for encephalography. Bull. neurol. Inst. N.Y. **3**, 519 (1934).
139. Engel, Ph.: Encéphalographie gazeuse du nouveau-né et du petit enfant. Anesthésie à la Ketamine. Communication, Annual Meeting of the European Society of Neuroradiology, Bologna 1972.
140. Engeset, A., Hauge, T.: Urea as an aid in encephalography. Acta radiol. Diagn. **1**, 565 (1963).
141. Epstein, B., Davidoff, L.: Use of laminography with encephalography in the diagnosis of mid-line and subtentorial brain's tumours. Amer. J. Roentgenol. **55**, 675 (1946).
142. Erickson, T.C., Van Baaren, H.J.: Late meningeal reaction to ethyl-iodophenylundecylate used in myelography; report of case that terminated fatally. J. Amer. med. Ass. **153**, 636 (1953).
143. Falk, B.: Calcifications in track of needle following ventricular puncture. Acta radiol. (Stockh.) **35**, 304, (1951).
144. Fauré, C., Gruson, B.: L'exploration radiologique des craniopharyngiomes de l'enfant (à propos de 17 observations). Ann. Radiol. **3**, 197 (1959).
145. Figaard, A.: Changes in ventricular size during pneumoencephalography. Neuroradiology **3**, 8 (1971).
146. Fischgold, H.: Visibility of the cranial nerves in pneumography. Bibl. psychiat. neurol. Supp. 10, **40**, 143 (1970).
147. Fischgold, H., Bonnemazou, A., Fredy, D., Metzger, J.: The opto-chiasmatic cistern and its contents. I. Normal aspects. II. Pathologic aspects. J. Radiol. Électrol. **50**, 12 (1969).
148. Fisher, R.L.: An experimental evaluation of Pantopaque and other recently developed myelographic contrast media. Radiology **85**, 537 (1965).
149. Foerster, O.: Encephalographische Erfahrungen. Z. ges. Neurol. Psychiat. **94**, 512 (1924/1925).
150. Fournier, A.M.: L'hélium comme moyen de contrast clair. J. Radiol. Électrol. **40**, 77 (1959).
151. Fredy, D.: Étude tomographique de la citerne opto-chiasmatique pathologique. Thèse de Paris. 1968.
152. Fredy, D., Bories, J.: A tomographic study of the temporal horn. Neuroradiology **4**, 96 (1972).
153. Fredzell, G., Greitz, T., Grepe, A., Holmström, L.: Mimer III and rotating chair. Acta radiol. Diagn. **7**, 543 (1968).
154. Fredzell, G., Lindgren, E.: Mimer. Acta radiol. (Stockh.) **53**, 209 (1960).
155. Fremont-Smith, F., Putman, J.J.: Quoted by 311.
156. Friedman, E.O.: Further experiences with encephalography and its evaluation in clinical neurology. Int. Clin. **1**, 54 (1930).
157. Front, D., Beks, J.W.F., Georganas, Ch.L., Beekhuis, H., Penning, L.: Abnormal patterns of cerebrospinal fluid flow and absorption after head injuries; diagnosis by isotope cisternography. Neuroradiology **4**, 6 (1972).
158. Front, D., Penning, L.: Occult spontaneous cerebrospinal fluid rhinorrhea diagnosed by isotope cisternography. Neuroradiology **2**, 167 (1971).
159. Gaist, G., Martelli, A.: Il valore della indagine cisternografica nelle sindromi ottico-chiasmatiche. Riv. oto-neuro-oftal. **3**, 187 (1956).
160. Ganglberger, J.: Zur Frage der Pneumoenzephalographie mit einem Kombinationspräparat von Theophyllin-Ephedrin und Oxyäthylthiophyllin. Wien. med. Wschr. **119**, 646 (1969).
161. Garcia, O.: Quoted by 195.
162. Gardner, W.J., Frazier, C.H.: Ventriculography without air injection. J. Amer. med. Ass. **93**, 193 (1929).
163. Garland, L.H.: Effect of iodized oil on meninges of spinal cord and brain. Radiology **35**, 467 (1940).
164. Gass, H.: Pantopaque anterior basal cisternography of posterior fossa. Amer. J. Roentgenol. **90**, 1197 (1963).
165. Gastaut, H.: La syncope nocturne des hypervagotoniques, sa différenciation avec l'épilepsie morphéique. Rev. neurol. **95**, 420 (1956).
166. Gastaut, H.: Polygraphische Differentialdiagnostik der fokalen und generalisierten ischämischen und epileptischen Anfälle. Zbl. Neurol. Psychiat. Neurochir. **13**, 161 (1961).
167. Gastaut, H., Bostem, F., Fernandez-Guardiola, A., Naquet, R., Gibson, W.C.: L'activation hypoxique de l'EEG par inhalation d'azote. Premiers résultats obtenus dans les épilepsies partielles. Rev. neurol. **102**, 356 (1960).
168. Gastaut, H., Bostem, F., Naquet, R., Fernandez-Guardiola, A.: L'activation hypoxique de l'EEG par inhalation d'azote. I. Premiers résultats obtenus dans les épilepsies généralisées. Rev. neurol. **100**, 501 (1959).
169. Gastaut, H., Fischer-Williams, M., Lugaresi, E.: Étude électroencéphalographique des syncopes. II. Corrélations électrocliniques chez 25 sujets enregistrées pendant leur syncope. Rev. neurol. **95**, 542 (1956).
170. Gastaut, H., Gastaut, Y.: Syncopes et convulsions. A propos de la nature syncopale de certains spasmes du sanglot et de certaines convulsions essentielles hyperthermiques ou à froid. Rev. neurol. **96**, 158 (1957).
171. Gastaut, H., Gastaut, Y.: Étude électroclinique des syncopes posttraumatiques. Rev. neurol. **96**, 423 (1957).
172. Gastaut, H., Gastaut, Y.: Étude électroencéphalographique et clinique des convulsions anoxiques de l'enfant. Leur situation dans le cadre des convulsions infantiles. Rev. neurol. **99**, 100 (1958).

173. Gastaut, H., Navarranne, P., Pitot, N., Salamon, G.: Étude électroencéphalographique des syncopes. I. Corrélations électrocliniques chez 150 sujets présentant des syncopes vasovagales. Rev. neurol. **95**, 541 (1956).
174. Gauthier, G.: Les accidents de la myélographie avec produits de contraste non résorbables. In: La radiographie des formations intra-rachidiennes. Paris: Masson et Cie. 1965.
175. Geilfuss, C.J., Shargest, T.: A modification of the Amplatz pneumographic chair for better head stabilization. Radiology **97**, 685 (1970).
176. Gilday, D.L., Reba, R.C., Hosain, F., Longo, R., Wagner, H.: Evaluation of Ytterbium-169 Diethylenetriaminepentacetic acid as a brain-scanning agent. Radiology **93**, 1129 (1969).
177. Giovine, G.P., Riva, M.: L'air sous-dural du «deuxième jour» après l'encéphalographie dans les séquelles de traumatisme cranien. Neuro-chirurgie **3**, 47 (1957).
178. Gozzano, A., Moselli, M.: L'urea ipertonica per il controllo dell'edema cerebrale acuto traumatico. Minerva chir. **16**, 152 (1961).
179. Grant, F.C.: Ventriculography: a review based on the analysis of 392 cases. Arch. Neurol. Psychiat. (Chic.) **14**, 513 (1925).
180. Grant, F.C.: Ventriculography and encephalography; their value in the localization and treatment of intracranial lesions. Arch. Neurol. Psychiat. (Chic.) **27**, 1310 (1932).
181. Greitz, T.: Some technical aspects of the pneumoencephalographic and ventriculographic examination of the posterior fossa. Communication, Annual Meeting of the European Society of Neuroradiology, Bologna 1972.
182. Greitz, T., Grepe, A.: Mimer II and rotating chair. Stockholm: Elema-Schönander 1967.
183. Gros, C.M.: Discussion on the "Tomography in neuroradiology". Acta radiol. (Stockh.) **40**, 280 (1953).
184. Gros, C.M.: Aspects angiographiques dans l'oedème cérébral. In: L'oedème cérébral, by G. Lazorthes and L. Campan. Paris: Masson et Cie. 1963.
185. Gros, C.M., Schneegans, E., Wackenheim, A., Oberson, R., Haarscher, A.M.: Examen scintigraphique des espaces péri-cérébraux et péri-médullaires. I. Scintigraphie de l'hematome sous-dural du nourrisson. J. Radiol. Électrol. **46**, 453 (1965).
186. Gros, C.M., Wackenheim, A., Vrousos, C.: La scintigraphie des espaces sous arachnoidiens du canal rachidien. J. Radiol. Électrol. **46**, 457 (1965).
187. Gros, C.M., Wackenheim, A., Vrousos, C., Subirana, M.: Scintigraphie cisternale. Acta radiol. Diagn. **5**, 804 (1966).
188. Grosjean, M.: À propos de l'emploi du pantopaque dans les myélographies. J. Radiol. Électrol. **38**, 1053 (1957).
189. Grossmann, G.: Tomographie I und II. Fortschr. Röntgenstr. **51**, 191 (1935).
190. Grotjahn, M., French, T.M.: Akinesia after ventriculography; contribution to ego psychology and problem of sleep. Psychoanal. Quart. **7**, 319 (1938).
191. Guerbet, M.: Étude pharmacologique du mono-iodostéarate d'éthyle, produit de contraste pour myélographie. Thérapie **21**, 1219 (1966).
192. Guerbet, A., Gibaud, A., Tilly, G., Joussot, R., Louth, V., Guerbet, M.: Mono-iodostéarate d'éthyle. Préparation et caractères analytiques. Ann. pharm. franç. **23**, 663 (1965).
193. Guillaume, J., Janny, P.: Manométrie intra-crânienne continue. Intérêt de la méthode et premiers résultats. Rev. neurol. **84**, 131 (1951).
194. Guillaume, J., Janny, P., Durand, G.: Effet sur la pression intracrânienne de différentes molécules en solution hypertonique. Neurochirurgie **4**, 264 (1958).
195. Gvozdanovic, V.: Somersault techniques in encephalography and ventriculography. Acta radiol. Diagn. **9**, 160 (1969).
196. Hagalsten, J.: L'anesthésie en neurochirurgie et neuroradiologie pédiatrique. Cah. Anesth. **9**, 189 (1961).
197. Hammer, B., Scherrer, H.: Contribution to the roentgen anatomy of the posterior fossa by pneumotomography. Communication, Annual Meeting of the European Society of Neuroradiology, Bologna 1972.
198. Hanafee, W.N., Lecry, J.W.: Planigraphy during pneumoencephalography. The diagnosis of lesions affecting the optic pathways. Arch. Ophthal. **80**, 161 (1968).
199. Harbert, J.C.: La cisternografia radioisotopica. Aggiornamenti in medicina nucleare. Roma: Il Pensiero Sci. 1971.
200. Harbert, J.C., David, C., McCullough, M.D.: Radionuclide studies in an unusual case of Dandy-Walker cyst. Radiology **101**, 363 (1971).
201. Harbert, J.C., James, A.E., Jr.: Posterior fossa abnormalities demonstrated by cisternography. J. nucl. Med. **13**, 73 (1972).
202. Harbert, J.C., Zeiger, L.S., McCollough, D., Davidson, J.D., Ashburn, W.L.: The dosimetry of ^{131}I-HSA cisternography. J. nucl. Med. **11**, 534 (1970).
203. Hauke, H., Schmitz, H.P., Wenner, J.: Pneumoencephalography: resorption of injected air after oxygen inhalation. Ann. Radiol. **10**, 185 (1967).
204. Heimburger, R.F., Kalsbeck, J.E., Campbell, R.L., Mealy, J.: Positive contrast cerebral ventriculography using water-soluble media. J. Neurol. Neurosurg. Psychiat. **29**, 281 (1966).
205. Heinz, E.R., Davis, D.O., Karp, H.R.: Abnormal isotope cisternography in symptomatic occult hydrocephalus. A correlative isotopic-neuroradiological study in 130 subjects. Radiology **95**, 109 (1970).
206. Heinz, E.R., Karp, H.R., Davis, D.O.: Abnormal isotope cisternography in patients with symptomatic occult hydrocephalus: a correlative isotopic-neuroradiological study of 131 patients. Communication, IX Symposium Neuroradiologicum, Göteborg 1970.
207. Heller, H.: Positive Myelographie mit Äthyl-mono-iodostearat. Fortschr. Röntgenstr. **109**, 69 (1968).
208. Heppner, F.: Air embolism eight hours after ventriculography. A case report. Acta radiol. (Stockh.) **38**, 294 (1952).
209. Hill, M., Wortzman, G., Marshall, B.: Clinical use of droperidol in pneumoencephalography. Canad. med. Ass. J. **98**, 359 (1968).
210. Hill, T., Welch, M.J., Adatepe, M., Potchen, E.J.: A simplified method for the preparation of indium-DTPA brain scanning agent. J. nucl. Med. **11**, 28 (1970).
211. Hodak, J., Chou, S., Loken, M.K.: Scintigraphy of the subarachnoid space. J. nucl. Med. **7**, 344 (1966).
212. Holman, B.L., Davis, D.O.: Progress in Nuclear Medicine. In: Neuro-nuclear medicine. Ed.: Potchen, E.J., St. Louis: McCready, V.R., Sutton Vol. I 1971.
213. Holmes, R.A.: Importanza della proiezione di vertice nella scintigrafia cerebrale. Aggiornamenti in medicina nucleare Roma: Pensiero Sci. 1971.

214. Hosain, E., Reba, R. C., Wagner, H. N.: Ytterbium-169 Diethylenetriaminepentacetic complex: a new radiopharmaceutical for brain scanning. Radiology **91**, 1199 (1968).
215. Howland, W. J., Curry, J. L.: Pantopaque arachnoiditis. Experimental study of blood as a potentiating agent and corticosteroids as an ameliorating agent. Acta radiol. Diagn. **5**, 1032 (1966).
216. Howland, W. J., Curry, J. L., Butler, A. K.: Pantopaque arachnoiditis. Experimental study of blood as a potentiating agent. Radiology **80**, 489 (1963).
217. Hurteau, E. F., Baird, W. C., Sinclair, E.: Arachnoiditis following use of iodized oil. J. Bone Jt Surg. **36**, 393 (1954).
218. Iizuka, J., Wappenschmidt, J.: A combined intracranial diagnosis by means of Conray-Ventriculography and stereo-encephalography. Communication, Annual Meeting of the European Society of Neuroradiology, Bologna 1972.
219. Isherwood, I.: Air meatography. Communication, Annual Meeting of the European Society of Neuroradiology, Bologna 1972.
220. Iwabuchi, T., Suzuki, J.: Pneumoencephalo-roulette tomography with special reference to its application to the diagnosis of auditory nerve tumours. Brain Nerve (Tokyo) **20**, 199 (1968).
221. Kadrnka, S.: Technique de l'encéphalostratigraphie gazeuse. Acta radiol. Diagn. **1**, 587 (1963).
222. Kagen, A., Tsuchiya, G., Patterson, V., Sugar, O.: Test for patency of ventriculo-vascular shunt for hydrocephalus with radioactive iodinated serum albumin. J. Neurosurg. **20**, 1025 (1963).
223. Kaneko, T.: A psychiatric study on disturbances after head injury by means of pneumotomoencephalography. Psychiat. Neurol. jap. **68**, 977 (1966).
224. Kashara, M., Takaishi, S., Tamada, H.: Studien über Liquor cerebrospinalis. VI. Mitteilung: Tierexperimentelle Untersuchungen über die Veränderungen der cerebrospinalen Flüssigkeit nach der Encephalographie. Z. ges. exp. Med. **80**, 347 (1932).
225. Katz, R. A.: Intravenous urea in the therapy of increased intracranial pressure with head encephalopathy. New Engl. J. Med. **262**, 870 (1960).
226. Kieffer, S. A.: Single-sweeps rotation tomography in coronal and lateral planes: its value in pneumoencephalographic diagnosis. Radiology **91**, 372 (1968).
227. Kieffer, S. A., Wolff, J. M., Prentice, W. B., Loken, M. K.: The normal scinticisternogram: a semiquantitative study. Communication, IX Symposium Neuroradiologicum, Göteborg 1970.
228. Kilgore, B. B., Davis, D. O., Potchen, E. J.: Abnormal cerebrospinal fluid dynamics as studied by isotope subarachnoid scintigraphy. Acta radiol. Diagn. **9**, 626 (1969).
229. Kornreich, C. J.: Relief of symptoms following encephalography by combined premedication and use of oxygen. Arch. Neurol. Psychiat. (Chic.) **60**, 512 (1948).
230. Jaeger, R.: Irritating effect of iodized vegetable oils on the brain and spinal cord when divided into small particles. Arch. Neurol. Psychiat. (Chic.) **64**, 715 (1950).
231. James, A. E., De Land, F. H., Hodges, F. J., Wagner, H. N., North, W. A.: Cerebrospinal fluid scanning cisternography. Amer. J. Roentgenol. **110**, 74 (1970).
232. James, A. E., Harbert, J. C., De Land, F. H., McCullough, D. C., Hodges, F. J., Wagner, H. N.: Localized enlargement of the cerebrospinal fluid space demonstrated by cisternography. Neuroradiology **2**, 184 (1971).
233. Janker, R.: Das Röntgenschichtverfahren bei der Darstellung der Hirnräume. Fortschr. Röntgenstr. **53**, 699 (1936).
234. Janny, P., Simon, E.: L'urée en solution hypertonique, nouveau traitement de l'oedème cérébral. Presse méd. **69**, 336 (1961).
235. Javid, M.: Urea in intracranial surgery. J. Neurosurg. **18**, 51 (1961).
236. Javid, M., Settlage, P.: Use of hypertonic urea for the reduction of intracranial pressure. Trans. Amer. neurol. Ass. **80**, 204 (1956).
237. Javid, M., Settlage, P.: Effect of urea on cerebrospinal fluid pressure in human subjects. Preliminary report. J. Amer. med. Ass. **160**, 943 (1956).
238. Jefferson, A., Lewtas, N.: Value of tomography and subdural pneumography in subfrontal fractures. Acta radiol. Diagn. **1**, 118 (1963).
239. Jefferson, A., Occleshaw, J.: The identification of pathological process in the posterior cranial fossa by Myodil ventriculography. Acta neurochir. (Wien) **8**, 468 (1960).
240. Jeppsson, S., Järpe, S.: Intravenous urea as an aid in intracranial surgery. Acta chir. scand. **120**, 137 (1960).
241. Jirout, J.: Changes of size of the subarachnoid spaces after the insufflation of air. Acta radiol. (Stockh.) **46**, 81 (1956).
242. Jüngling, O.: Zur Technik der Sauerstoffüllung der Hirnventrikel zum Zwecke der Röntgendiagnostik. Zbl. Chir. **49**, 833 (1922).
243. Laborit, G., Kind, A.: Une utilisation pratique du 4-hydroxi-butyrate de sodium dans les examens neuroradiologiques. Agressologie **2**, 543 (1961).
244. Lafon, R., Gros, C., Bétoulières, P., Paleirac, R., Bonnet, Y., Bertrand, A.: Pneumostratigraphie encéphalique à «minima». J. Radiol. Électrol. **34**, 388 (1953).
245. Laine, E., Riff, G., Delandtsheer, J. M., Galibert, P.: Intérêt de la ventriculographie fractionée: «tête basse» dans les tumeurs de la fosse postérieure. J. Radiol. Électrol. **38**, 86 (1957).
246. Laine, E., Riff, G., Delandtsheer, J. M., Galibert, P.: Ventriculographie fractionée tête basse. Acta radiol. (Stockh.) **50**, 48 (1958).
247. Langfitt, T. W.: Possible mechanisms of action of hypertonic urea in reducing intracranial pressure. Neurology (Minneap.) **11**, 196 (1961).
248. Lefèvre, J., Fauré, C., Salamon, G.: Étude radiologique des gliomes infiltrants du tronc cérébral. Acta radiol. Diagn. **1**, 343 (1963).
249. Le May, M.: Changes in ventricular size during and after pneumoencephalography. Radiology **88**, 57 (1967).
250. Lenzi, M.: Semeiotica neuroradiologica. Milano: Sormani 1954.
251. Lenzi, M., Canossa, G., Bassani, G.: Pneumostratigrafia normale cerebrale. Torino: Minerva Medica 1959.
252. Liberson, F.: The use of various gases in encephalography: summary of 210 cases, using simultaneous displacement apparatus. Amer. J. med. Sci. **185**, 478 (1933).
253. Lindblom, A.: On the effect of lipiodol on the meninges. Acta radiol. (Stockh.) **5**, 129 (1926).
254. Lindgren, E.: A pneumographic study of the temporal horn. Acta radiol. (Stockh.) Suppl. **69** (1948).
255. Lindgren, E.: Some aspects of the technique of encephalography. Acta radiol. (Stockh.) **31**, 161 (1949).
256. Lindgren, E.: Encephalography in cerebral atrophy. Acta radiol. (Stockh.) **35**, 277 (1951).
257. Lindgren, E.: Röntgenologie. Handbuch der Neurochirurgie, Bd. II. Berlin-Göttingen-Heidelberg: Springer 1954.

258. LINDGREN, E.: Radiologic examination of the brain and spinal cord. Acta radiol. (Stockh.) Suppl. **151** (1957).
259. LINDGREN, E.: Convertible chair-couch for roentgen examinations. Acta radiol. (Stockh.) **55**, 269 (1961).
260. LINDGREN, E., MATTSSON, O.: Tomography with the Mimer. Acta radiol. Diagn. **3**, 453 (1965).
261. LING LEE, H.: Positive contrast myelography in the diagnosis of cerebello-pontine angle tumours. Communication, XII World Congress of Radiology, Tokyo 1969.
262. LITTLETON, J.T.: Some blurring characteristics of small-angle tomography. Medica Mundi **10**, 10 (1964).
263. LOSSIUS, H.M.: Transitory visual disturbances after ventriculography. Acta psychiat. scand. **31**, 81 (1956).
264. LUCE, J.C., LEITH, W., BURRAGE, W.S.: Pantopaque meningitis due to hypersensitivity. Radiology **57**, 878 (1951).
265. LUCKETT, W.H.: Air in the ventricles of the brain following a fracture of the skull; report of a case. Surg. Gynec. Obstet. **17**, 237 (1913).
266. LUNDBERG, N.: Continuous recording and control of ventricular fluid pressure in neurosurgical practice. Acta psychiat. scand. Suppl. **149** (1960).
267. LUTZ, W., TURNER, O.: Planigraphic study of ventricular system; fourth ventricle and adjacent structures. Yale J. Biol. Med. **12**, 399 (1940).
268. LYSHOLM, E.: Das Ventrikulogramm. III. Teil. Dritter und vierter Ventrikel. Acta radiol. (Stockh.) Suppl. **26** (1935).
269. LYSHOLM, E.: Das Ventrikulogramm. I. Teil. Röntgentechnik. Acta radiol. (Stockh.) Suppl. **24** (1937).
270. LYSHOLM, E.: Das Ventrikulogramm. II. Teil. Die Seitenventrikel. Acta radiol. (Stockh.) Suppl. **25** (1937).
271. LYSHOLM, E.: Experience in ventriculography of tumours below the tentorium. Brit. J. Radiol. **19**, 437 (1946).
272. MACLAIRE, A.S.: Lipiodol in neurosurgery with a report of a case with deleterious results. Amer. J. med. Sci. **170**, 874 (1925).
273. MALIS, L.I.: Myelographic examination of foramen magnum. Radiology **70**, 196 (1958).
274. MALMROS, R.: A simple method of producing a special picture of the posterior part of the third ventricle. Acta psychiat. scand. **24**, 587 (1949).
275. MAMO, L., COPHIGNON, J., REY, A., HOUDART, R.: Intérêt de la cisternographie isotopique dans le diagnostic des tumeurs de l'angle ponto-cérébelleux. Presse méd. **79**, 627 (1971).
276. MANFREDI, R., KRUSE, F.: Laminography with central pneumography. J. Neurosurg. **14**, 374 (1957).
277. MANIERI, R., DI CARLANTONIO, G.: L'infusione di soluzioni ipertoniche di urea nel trattamento della ipertensione endocranica. Gazz. int. Med. Chir. **68**, 636 (1963).
278. MANZIN, E., CECOTTO, C.: Considerazioni sull'uso dell'urea nei malati neurochirurgici. Minerva anest. **28**, 52 (1962).
279. MARCOVITCH, A.W., WALKER, A.E., JESSICO, C.M.: Immediate and late effects of intrathecal injection of iodized oil. J. Amer. med. Ass. **116**, 2247 (1941).
280. MARIN, A., ANDRIOLI, G.C., ZACCHI, C.: Stratigraphy as a standard procedure in pneumoencephalographic examinations. Chir. ital. **20**, 1857 (1968).
281. MARKESBERY, W., WILSON, C.B.: Emulsified pantopaque for cerebral ventriculography. Surg. Forum **15**, 419 (1964).
282. MARTIN, P., LECOMTE, P., PASCHETTA, CH., SARRAZIN, R., OLLIER, A.: Myéloencéphalographie par moyens de contraste opaque. J. Radiol. Électrol. **47**, 197 (1966).
283. MARTIN, P., LECOMTE, P., PASCHETTA, CH., SARRAZIN, R., OLLIER, A.: Exploration de l'angle ponto-cérébelleux par moyens de contraste opaque. J. Radiol. Électrol. **47**, 719 (1966).
284. MARTINI, T., OBERSON, R.: Cisternographie radio-isotopique chez les hydrocéphales posttraumatiques; contribution à l'étude de la dynamique pathologique du L.C.R. Acta radiol. Diagn. **9**, 635 (1969).
285. MASCHERPA, F., LOMBARDI, G.: Risultati della stratigrafia applicata alla cisternoencefalografia. Radiol. med. (Torino) **38**, 1160 (1952).
286. MASON, M.S., RAAF, J.: Complications of pantopaque myelography. J. Neurosurg. **19**, 302 (1962).
287. MASSON, C.B.: The disturbances in vision and in visual fields after ventriculography. Bull. neurol. Inst. N.Y. **3**, 190 (1933).
288. MATIN, P., GOODWIN, D.A., DE NARDO, G.L.: Cerebrospinal fluid scanning and ventricular shunts. Radiology **94**, 435 (1970).
289. MATSUBARA, T., NOMURA, T.: Emulsified iodized oil ventriculography. Amer. J. Roentgenol. **84**, 48 (1960).
290. MAUPIN, R.A., BAKER, H.L., JR., KERR, F.W.: Emulsified Pantopaque: its possible application for myelography. Radiology **86**, 509 (1966).
291. MCALISTER, J.: Radiation dose in isotope encephalography. Lancet i, 527 (1968).
292. MCCONNELL, A.A.: Ventriculography as an aid in localization of intracranial tumours. Brit. med. J. **2**, 796 (1923).
293. MCCONNELL, A.A.: Subdural air after pneumoencephalography. Brain **76**, 485 (1953).
294. MCLACHLAN, M.S.: Polytome encephalography in investigation of pituitary tumours. Proc. roy. Soc. Med. **63**, 464 (1970).
295. MCQUEEN, J.D., ABBASSIOUN, K.: Cisternal brain scanning with positron-emitting isotopes. J. Neurosurg. **29**, 597 (1968).
296. MEACHAM, W.F., TOLCHIN, S.: The ependymal response to long-term intraventricular Pantopaque. J. Neurol. Neurosurg. Psychiat. **26**, 559 (1963).
297. MEALEY, J., JR.: Gamma-ray image of subdural effusions. J. Neurosurg. **19**, 934 (1962).
298. MEALEY, J., JR., CAMBELL, J.A.: Scintillography of infantile subdural effusions and its clinical application. Acta radiol. Diagn. **5**, 871 (1966).
299. MERCADER, J.M., CABARROCAS, E.: Effect of Ketamine in cerebral angiography. Communication, Annual Meeting of the European Society of Neuroradiology, London 1971.
300. MERRITT, H. H., FREMONT-SMITH, F.: The cerebrospinal fluid. Philadelphia: Saunders 1937.
301. METZGER, J., ERNEST, C., CABANIS, E., PAUL, D., AUBIN, M.L.: Examen de la tige pituitaire. Communication, Annual Meeting of the European Society of Neuroradiology, Bologna 1972.
302. METZGER, J., ENGEL, PH., BONNEMAZOU, A., FISCHGOLD, H.: La tomographie hypocicloide. Neurochirurgie **13**, 73 (1967).
303. METZGER, J., ENGEL, PH., PRADAT, P., FISCHGOLD, H.: Tomographie hypocicloide du chiasma normal et des adenomas hypophysaire. Communication, VIII Symposium Neuroradiologicum, Paris 1967.
304. MICHELSEN, W.T., SCHLESINGER, E.B., BAILEY, S.: Factors involved in the surgical management of the syndrome of normal pressure hydrocephalus. Communication, IX Symposium Neuroradiologicum, Göteborg 1970.

305. MIGLIORE, A., PAOLETTI, P., VILLANI, R.: L'impiego degli isotopi radioattivi nello studio della dinamica liquorale. Minerva med. **31**, 37 (1961).

306. MIGLIORE, A., PAOLETTI, P., VILLANI, R.: Radioisotopic method for evaluating the patency of the Spitz-Holter valve. J. Neurosurg. **19**, 605 (1962).

307. MONES, R., WERMANN, R.: Pantopaque myelography. Radiology **72**, 803 (1959).

308. MORETTE DE PARDAL, M. L., PARDAL, E.: Mise au point de l'iodoventriculographie. Acta radiol. (Stockh.) **50**, 34 (1958).

309. MANGENEY, F., MUHLMANN WEILL, M., GAUTHIER-LA FAYE, J. P.: Notre expérience du Kétalar en neuro-radiologie. Anesth. Analg. Réanim. **28**, 923 (1971).

310. MURPHY, G., FISHBEIN, R., RUSH, B.: The effect of urea on the postoperative excretion of electrolytes. Surgery **48**, 485 (1960).

311. MURRACK, D., MARKS, V., COUCH, R. S.: Changes in the lumbar C.S.F. during encephalography. Brit. J. Radiol. **34**, 635 (1961).

312. NEUMANN, J.: Demonstration of intradural cranial nerve sections in the pneumoencephalography. Radiol. diagn. (Berl.) **10**, 209 (1969).

313. NEW, P. F., WEBSTER, E. W.: Physical and anatomical considerations in autotomography. Acta radiol. Diagn. **3**, 370 (1965).

314. NEWMAN, H. W.: Encephalography with ethylene. J. Amer. med. Ass. **108**, 461 (1937).

315. NICOL, C. F.: A second case of aseptic meningitis following isotope cisternography using ^{131}I human serum albumin. Neurology (Minneap.) **17**, 199 (1967).

316. NOSIK, W. A.: Contrast myelography with emulsified pantopaque. Amer. J. Roentgenol. **65**, 374 (1951).

317. NOTERMAN, J.: La circulation du liquide cephalo-rachidien et la cisternographie isotopique. Acta chir. belg. **5**, 342 (1969).

318. NOVAK, Z.: "Roto.-veg SG"-apparatus for rotational cerebral pneumography. Neuropsihijatrija **14**, 143 (1966).

319. OBERSON, R., MARTINI, T., FOROGLOU, G.: Scintigraphic patterns of normal pericerebral cerebrospinal fluid circulation. Communication, IX Symposium Neuroradiologicum, Göteborg 1970.

320. OLDHAM, R. K., STAAB, E. V.: Aseptic meningitis following the intrathecal injection of radioiodinated serum albumin. Radiology **97**, 317 (1970).

321. OMMAYA, A. K., DI CHIRO, G., BALDWIN, M., PENNYBACKER, J. B.: Nontraumatic cerebrospinal fluid rhinorrhoea. J. Neurol. Neurosurg. Psychiat. (Chic.) **31**, 214 (1968).

322. ORTIZ BERROCAL, J., ARNAIZ-BUENO, F., GIMENO-ALAVA, A., ESCUDERO-PÉREZ, L.: Estudio del espacio subaracnoideo y de los ventriculos cerebrales con materiales radioactivos. Rev. clin. esp. **101**, 108 (1966).

323. PACIFICO, L.: Il Gamma-idrossi-butirrato di sodio (Gamma-OH) in neurochirurgia. Anest. Rian. Ass. Anest. lomb. **10**, 353 (1969).

324. PACIFICO, L.: Problemi di tecnica anestesiologica in encefalografia. Acta anaesth. (Padova) **20**, 1021 (1969).

325. PACIFICO, L., GIANASI, G.: La Ketamina in neuroradiologia. Personal communication, Annual Meeting of the European Society of Neuroradiology, Bologna 1972.

326. PALEIRAC, R., LABAUGE, R., BASSEDE, J., MINVIELLE, J.: Premiers résultats de la tomo-cisternographie. J. Radiol. Électrol. **34**, 98 (1953).

327. PALUMBO, R., SENIN, V., SIGNORINI, E., CASAMASSIMA, F., GAINOTTI, G.: Recenti progressi in neuroscintigrafia. Ann. Fac. Med. Perugia **59**, 675 (1968).

328. PATTEN, DH., BENSON, DF.: Diagnosis of normal pressure hydrocephalus by RIHSA cisternography. J. nucl. Med. **9**, 457 (1968).

329. PAUL, L. W., ERICKSON, T. C.: Observations on the presence of subdural gas after pneumoencephalography. Radiology **46**, 139 (1946).

330. PEACHER, W. G., ROBERTSON, R. C.: Pantopaque myelography: results, comparison of contrast media, and spinal fluid reaction. J. Neurosurg. **2**, 220 (1945).

331. PEET, M. M.: Injuries of the skull, brain and spinal cord. Neuropsychiatric, surgical and medico-legal aspects. Baltimore: Williams & Wilkins Co. 1940.

332. PEIPER, H., KLOSE, H.: Über die Grundlagen einer Myelographie. Langenbecks Arch. klin. Chir. **134**, 303 (1925).

333. PENDERGRASS, E. P., HODES, P. J.: Encephalography: value of second-day examination. Radiology **26**, 146 (1936).

334. PENDERGRASS, E. P., PERRYMAN, C. R.: Poroencephaly. Amer. J. Roentgenol. **56**, 441 (1946).

335. PENDERGRASS, E. P., SCHAEFFER, J. P., HODES, P. J.: The head and neck in roentgen diagnosis. Springfield: Charles C. Thomas 1956.

336. PENFIELD, W.: Cerebral pneumography, its danger and uses. Arch. Neurol. Psychiat. (Chic.) **13**, 580 (1925).

337. PENNING, L., KERCKHOFFS, H. P.: L'effet des èmulsions d'huiles iodées dans l'espace sous-arachnoidien. Neurochirurgie **12**, 831 (1966).

338. PENNING, L., KERCKHOFFS, H. P.: Comparative experimental evaluation of several types of emulsified oily radiopaque materials with cranial subarachnoid space. Radiology **88**, 730 (1967).

339. PENNING, L., KERCKHOFFS, H. P.: Recherches expérimentales d'un nouveau moyen de contraste opaque (Duroliopaque). Psychiat. Neurol. Neurochir. (Amst.) **71**, 105 (1968).

340. PENNING, L., KERCKHOFFS, H. P., HUIZINGA, T.: Experimental evaluation of emulsified iophendylate in the cranial subarachnoid space. Invest. Radiol. **1**, 264 (1966).

341. PENNING, L., KERCKHOFFS, H. P., TEN NAPEL, WOLDRING, M. G.: Experimental investigation of shake emulsion of radiopaque oils in the cranial subarachnoid space. Radiol. clin. Biol. **57**, 103 (1968).

342. PEN-TZE LIN: Radioiodinated serum albumin (RIHSA) cisternography in the diagnosis of incisural block and occult hydrocephalus. Radiology **90**, 36 (1968).

343. PHILIPPART, C.: Effets du mélange gazeux inhalé sur la composition du moyen de contraste utilisé dans myélographie gazeuse. Communication, Meeting of Deutsche Neuroradiologische Gesellschaft, Cologne 1968.

344. PHILIPPART, C.: Résorption du protoxyde d'azote utilisé comme gas de contraste au cours des examens neuroradiologiques. Acta radiol. Diagn. **9**, 199 (1969).

345. PHILIPPART, C., THIBAUT, A.: Utilisation du N_2O au cours de l'encéphalographie gazeuse. Une nouvelle technique. Acta anaesth. belg. **17**, 16 (1966).

346. PHILIPPART, C., THIBAUT, A.: Utilisation du protoxyde d'azote en tant que moyen de contraste et d'anesthésie au cours de l'encéphalographie gazeuse. Ann. Anesth. franç. **8**, 631 (1967).

347. PHILIPPART, C., THIBAUT, A.: Intérêt des neuroleptiques pour l'anesthésie de la myélographie gazeuse. J. belge Radiol. **50**, 133 (1967).

348. PHILIPPART, C., THIBAUT, A., BONNAL, J.: Effet de l'inhalation de protoxyde d'azote au cours des explorations neuroradiologiques réalisées a avec l'air. Neurochirurgie **14**, 97 (1968).
349. PIGNATARO, E.: Schichtaufnahmen mit dicker und dünner Schicht bei vielfacher Strahlenrichtungsveränderung. Fortschr. Röntgenstr. **94**, 261 (1961).
350. PINEAS, H.: Hirnbefund nach Ventriculographie mit Lipiodol ascendens. Zbl. ges. Neurol. Psychiat. **110**, 337 (1927).
351. PIRKEY, E.L., REED, E.S., SMITH, W.H.: Clinical studies of the use of emulsion of ethyl iodophenylundecylate (Pantopaque). Radiology **55**, 89 (1950).
352. PITTINGER, C.R., VAN EPPS, E.S., UTTERBACH, R.A.: Xenon in the encephalography. Neurology (Minneap.) **6**, 429 (1956).
353. POPPEL, M., JACOBSON, H., DEWING, S.: Value of lateral mid-line tomogram in encephalography and ventriculography. Radiology **60**, 236 (1953).
354. PORTERA, A.: Pan-ventriculografia: nuevo metodo con pantopaque emulsionado. Acta ibér. radiol.-cancer. **19**, 221 (1964).
355. PORTERA, A.: Pan-ventriculography. A new technique utilizing emulsified Pantopaque. Acta radiol. Diagn. **5**, 693 (1966).
356. PORTERA, A., BRAVO, G., PARERA, C.: Emulsified Pantopaque ventriculography. J. Neurosurg. **21**, 422 (1964).
357. POTTHOFF, P.C.: La tomographie seriée du tronc cérébral. Radiologie **8**, 369 (1968).
358. POTTHOFF, P.C., SCHMIDT, K.: La tomographie du tronc cérébral. Neurochirurgia **11**, 150 (1968).
359. POTTS, G.: Quoted by 313.
360. POTTS, D.G.: A new universal head unit. Amer. J. Roentgenol. **95**, 957 (1965).
361. POTTS, D.G., TAVERAS, J.M.: A new somersaulting chair for cerebral pneumography. Amer. J. Roentgenol. **91**, 1144 (1964).
362. RALSTON, B.L., GROSS, S.W., NEWMAN, C.W.: Pantopaque ventriculography in the localization of surgical lesions of the posterior fossa. Amer. J. Roentgenol. **81**, 972 (1959).
363. REARDON, J.V., LOWMAN, R.M., LEVY, L.L.: Carbon dioxide pneumoencephalography: a preliminary report. Radiology **89**, 142 (1967).
364. REDSLOB, E., DIFFENBACH, M.P.: Accidental cortical blindness after ventriculography case. Bull. Soc. Ophtal. Paris **51**, 307 (1939).
365. REESE, D.F., BULL, J.W.D.: Positive contrast demonstration of normal internal acoustic meatus, Meckel's cavum, and jugular foramen. Amer. J. Roentgenol. **100**, 650 (1967).
366. RICHARDS, P., ATKINS, H.L.: High specific activity Technetium-99m albumin. J. nucl. Med. **8**, 396 (1967).
367. RIESELBACH, R., DI CHIRO, G., FREIREICH, E., RALL, D.: Subarachnoid distribution of drugs following lumbar injection determined by autoradiography and external scanning. New Engl. J. Med. **267**, 1273 (1962).
368. RIGGS, H.W.: The dangers and mortality of ventriculography. Bull. neurol. Inst. N.Y. **3**, 210 (1934).
369. RINALDI, I., BOTTON, J.E., TROLAND, C.: Cortical visual disturbances following ventriculography and/or ventricular decompression. J. Neurosurg. **19**, 568 (1962).
370. ROBERTS, G.W.: Upright planigrams in pneumoencephalography. Amer. J. Roentgenol. **98**, 749 (1966).
371. ROBERTSON, E.G.: Pneumoencephalography. Springfield: Charles C. Thomas 1957.
372. ROSTOTSKAYA, V.I.: Ventrikulografiia sistemoi dletel'nogo drenazha. Vop. Neĭrokhir. **1**, 51 (1958).
373. RUDD, T.C., O'NEAL, J.T., NELP, W.B.: Cerebrospinal fluid circulation following subarachnoid hemorrhage. J. nucl. Med. **12**, 61 (1971).
374. RUGGIERO, G.: L'encéphalographie fractionnée. Paris: Masson et Cie. 1957.
375. RUGGIERO, G.: Technique neuroradiologique. In: Traité de technique chirurgicale, t. III. Paris: Masson et Cie. 1959.
376. RUGGIERO, G., SMALTINO, F.: Appearance of the ventricular system 24 hours after encephalography. A preliminary report. Acta radiol. (Stockh.) **53**, 279 (1960).
377. RUGGIERO, G.: Neuro-radiologie. Editorial, extrait de «Roentgen Europ», N° **6–7**, 10 (1963).
378. RUGGIERO, G.: Encefalografia e ventricólografia nei tumori della fossa posteriore. Bull. Soc. med.-chir. Bologna **1**, 1 (1963).
379. RUGGIERO, G.: Encephalography with urea. Lecture at the Neurological Institute, London: March 18, 1965. Not published.
380. RUGGIERO, G.: Progrès de l'encéphalographie fractionnée. Société franç. Électro-Radiol. med., Paris. 1964.
381. RUGGIERO, G.: Evoluzione della Tecnica dell'encefalografia (con presentazione di un film). Bull. Soc. Med. Chir. Bologna **2**, 225 (1965).
382. RUGGIERO, G.: Note sull'organizzazione di un servizio di neuroradiologia. Radiographie et Photographie med. Kodak-Pathé Milano **4**, 12 (1964).
383. RUGGIERO, G.: Encephalography today. Acta radiol. Diagn. **5**, 705 (1966).
384. RUGGIERO, G.: Editorial. Neurology and neuroradiology. Neuroradiology **2**, 125 (1971).
385. RUGGIERO, G.: Round table on the technique of encephalography. Discussion, Annual Meeting of the European Society of Neuroradiology, Bologna 1972.
386. RUGGIERO, G., CRISTI, G., TREVISAN, C.: Clinical aspects of encephalography. Acta radiol. Diagn., Suppl. 292 (1969).
387. RUGGIERO, G., DETTORI, P., LEIGHTON, R., PACIFICO, L.: Encefalografia con urea. Bull. Soc. Med. Chir. Bologna **4**, 1 (1963).
388. RUGGIERO, G., DETTORI, P., LEIGHTON, R., PACIFICO, L.: Encephalography with urea. Acta radiol. Diagn. **3**, 161 (1965).
389. RUGGIERO, G., MAZZACURATI, M.: Subtraction technique in encephalography. Invest. Radiol. **2**, 326 (1967).
390. RUGGIERO, G., MAZZACURATI, M.: Soustraction d'image en encéphalographie. Acta radiol. Diagn. **9**, 205 (1969).
391. RUGGIERO, G., MAZZACURATI, M.: Sottrazione in encefalografia. Bull. Soc. Med. Chir. Bologna **3**, 329 (1967).
392. RUGGIERO, G., PACIFICO, L.: Quelques aspects techniques nouveaux de l'encéphalographie fractionnée. Neurochirurgie Paris **9**, 92 (1963).
393. RUGGIERO, G., SCIALFA, G., CRISTI, G., SABATTINI, L.: Further experiences with late radiographic control in encephalography. Communication, Annual Meeting of the European Society of Neuroradiology, Bologna 1972.
394. RUGGIERO, G., TREVISAN, C.: Refinements of the radiologic technique in encephalography. Communication, Annual Meeting of the European Society of Neuroradiology, Bologna 1972.
395. SALAMON, G., BINNERT, D., CAILLE, J.M., GIUDICELLI, G.: Technique d'examen des cisternes périsellaires. Communication, Annual Meeting of the European Society of Neuroradiology, Bologna 1972.

396. SANS, R., PORCHER, J.: Le Polytome. J. Radiol. Électrol. **31**, 604 (1950).
397. SANSONE, G., DE MAESTRI, A., DURAND, P., MACARINI, N.: Pneumoencefalografia e stratigrafia assiale trasversa nel bambino. Minerva pediat. **3**, 358 (1951).
398. SCANLAN, R.L.: Positive contrast medium (Iophendylate) in diagnosis of acoustic neurinomas. Arch. Otolaryng. **80**, 698 (1964).
399. SCHATZKI, T., BAXTER, D.H., TROLAND, C.: Second-day encephalography with particular reference to size of ventricles. New Engl. J. Med. **236**, 419 (1947).
400. SCHECHTER, M.M., GUTIÉRREZ-MAHONEY, C.G.: Autotomography—showing the normal and abnormal mid-line ventricular structure and basal cisterns. Brit. J. Radiol. **35**, 438 (1962).
401. SCHECHTER, M.M., JING, B.S.: Improved visualization of the ventricular system with the technique of autotomography. Radiology **74**, 593 (1960).
402. SCHECHTER, M.M., STRENGER, L.: Three simple devices to facilitate contrast neuroroentgenography. Amer. J. Roentgenol. **87**, 363 (1962).
403. SCHLESINGER, E.B., DEBOVES, S., STEIN, B.: A means of evaluating the efficiency of shunts. Communication, Annual Meeting of the Harvey Cushing Society, Philadelphia 1963.
404. SCHNITKER, M.T., ULRICH, R.P.: Observations on the twenty-four-hour pneumoencephalogram with special reference to the diagnosis of cortical atrophy. Radiology **70**, 15 (1958).
405. SCHOBER, R.: Morphologische Veränderungen am Gehirn nach intrathekaler Anwendung von Röntgenkontrastmitteln (Iodester). Fortschr. Röntgenstr. **101**, 55 (1964).
406. SCHOBER, R.: Röntgenkontrastmittel und Liquorraum. Berlin-Göttingen-Heidelberg: Springer 1964.
407. SCHOBER, R.: Morphologic changes of the brain following intrathecal application of contrast media. Acta radiol. Diagn. **5**, 509 (1966).
408. SCHOENFELD, H., FREEMAN, W.: Ventriculography and encephalography by means of thorium dioxide solution. Med. Ann. D. C. **2**, 279 (1933).
409. SCHUPFER, F.: Retinal hemorrhage after ventriculography; cases. Gazz. int. Med. cir. **50**, 3 (1940).
410. SCHÜRMANN, K.: Cisternos and ventriculo-tomography. Zbl. Neurochir. **28**, 1 (1967).
411. SCHVARCZ, J.: Autotomography of the fourth ventricle and the floor of the third ventricle. Acta radiol. (Stockh.) **52**, 465 (1959).
412. SCHWAB, R.S., FINE, J., MIXTER, W.J.: Reduction of postencephalographic symptoms by inhalation of 95 per cent oxygen. Arch. Neurol. Psychiat. (Chic.) **37**, 1271 (1937).
413. SCHWARZ, G.A., ROSNER, A.A.: Displacement and herniation of the hippocampal gyrus through the incisura tentorii. A clinicopathologic study. Arch. Neurol. Psychiat. (Chic.) **46**, 297 (1941).
414. SCIALFA, G.: Neuroradiologia dell'idrocefalo non tumorale. Acta neurol. (Napoli) **3**, 332 (1970).
415. SCIALFA, G.: Un contributo recente della neuroradiologia alla diagnosi dell'encefalopatia traumatica: la cisternoencefalografia con radioisotopi. Comunicazione, V Congresso Regionale di Neuropsichiatria, Messina 1970.
416. SENIN, U., PALUMBO, R., CASAMASSIMA, F.: L'impiego di nuovi radiocomposti nella visualizzazione scintigrafica dello spazio subaracnoideo spinale. Progr. med. **22**, 90 (1966).
417. SHAPIRO, R., ROBINSON, E.: Controlled pneumoencephalography. A consideration of head position and gas-fluid replacement. J. Neurosurg. **2**, 122 (1954).
418. SHAPIRO, R., ROBINSON, F.: Controlled fractional pneumoencephalography. Radiology **72**, 651 (1959).
419. SHARRON, M., WIENER, S.N.: Pantopaque examination of the cerebello-pontine angle. Radiology **85**, 921 (1965).
420. SHEALY, C.N., NEW, P.F.: Cerebrospinal fluid pressure changes in fractional pneumoencephalography without removal of cerebrospinal fluid. Radiology **81**, 495 (1963).
421. SHIPSS, F., RAAT, J.: Lateral mid-line laminography in encephalography and ventriculography. Amer. J. Roentgenol. **80**, 98 (1958).
422. SICARD, J.A., FORESTIER, J.: Méthode radiographique d'exploration de la cavité épidurale par le lipiodol. Rev. neurol. **12**, 1264 (1921).
423. SICARD, J.A., FORESTIER, J.: Méthode général d'exploration radiologique par l'huile iodée (Lipiodol). Bull. Soc. med. Hôp. Paris **46**, 463 (1922).
424. SICARD, J.A., PARAF, J., LAPLANE, L.: Radiodiagnostic rachidien lipiodole. Ponction atloidooccipitale et cervicale. Presse méd. **31**, 885 (1923).
425. SIEBNER, M.: Pachymeningitis cervicalis hypertrophica und akute Schädigung durch Myelographie. Chirurg **7**, 177 (1935).
426. SIGNORINI, E., CASAMASSIMA, F., GAINOTTI, G., PALUMBO, R., SENIN, U.: L'esplorazione scintigrafica delle cisterne cerebrali. Considerazioni tecniche e rilievi anatomici. Nunt. radiol. (Roma). **9**, 911 (1968).
427. SIGNORINI, E., SENIN, U., GAINOTTI, G., QUATTRINI, A.: La cisternografia nella diagnostica dei tumori endocranici. Riv. Pat. nerv. ment. **15**, 289 (1969).
428. SIMON, J.: Quoted by 17.
429. SIMON, J., RAMEE, A., SIGNARGOUT, J.: La photographie 70 mm en encéphalographie gazeuse. Intérêt et limites actuelles de la méthode. Communication, Annual Meeting of the European Society of Neuroradiology, Bologna 1972.
430. SIMONE, F., TRONCONE, L., DE ROSSI, G., MONTESANTI, I.: Use of intrathecally administered RIHSA ^{131}I in the study of cerebrospinal fluid dynamics, brain atrophy and "normal pressure" hydrocephalus. Communication, IX Symposium Neuroradiologicum, Göteborg 1970.
431. SMALTINO, F., MAZZARELLA, B.: Personal communication.
432. SPINA, F., ASCANIO, C., CONSOLI, V., RICCIARDI, N.: L'uso dell'Itterbio 169-DTPA nella scintigrafia cerebrale. Nunt. radiol. (Roma) **35**, 543 (1969).
433. STAAB, E.V., JOHNSTON, R. E., ALLEN, J.H., BRILLEN, A.B.: Radiation dosimetry associated with radioisotope cisternography. Communication, IX Symposium Neuroradiologicum, Göteborg 1970.
434. STEARS, J.C., SANDERS, B.B.: Tomographic anatomy of suprasellar cistern. Communication, IX Symposium Neuroradiologicum, Göteborg 1970.
435. STEINHAUSEN, T.B., DUNGAN, C.E., FURST, J.B., PLATI, J.T., SMITH, S.W., DARLING, A.P., WOLCOTT, E.C., JR.: Iodinated organic compounds as contrast media for radiographic diagnosis. Experimental and clinical myelography with ethyl-iodophenyl-undecylate (Pantopaque). Radiology **43**, 230 (1944).
436. STERN, H.S., ZOLLE, I., MCAFEE, J.B.: Preparation of Technetium ($Tc99^m$) labeled (Serum Albumin Human). Int. J. appl. Radiat. **16**, 283 (1965).
437. STEWART, J.A.: Second-day pneumoencephalography. Amer. J. Roentgenol. **68**, 749 (1952).

438. STIEVE, F.E.: La technique radiographique en coupe et les divers modes d'effacements. J. Radiol. Électrol. **38**, 49 (1957).
439. STOJANOVIC, M.: Alteration in the cerebrospinal fluid during pneumoencephalography. An. Bolnice **2/3**, 259 (1963).
440. STRAIN, W.H., FRENCH, J.D., JONES, G.E.: Iodinated organic compounds as contrast media for radiographic diagnosis. Radiology **47**, 47 (1946).
441. STUBBS, J., PENNYBACKER, J.: Reduction of intracranial pressure with hypertonic urea. Lancet ii, 1094 (1960)
442. SUBIRANA, M., VROUSOS, C.: Pneumostratigraphie frontale des hémisphères cérébelleux. J. Radiol. Électrol. **45**, 225 (1964).
443. SUTHERLAND, G.R.: Inclined plane zonography. Brit. J. Radiol. **43**, 492 (1970).
444. SVOBODA, M.: Zonographische Wirbelsäulenuntersuchung. Röntgen-Bl. **18**, 13 (1965).
445. SWANN, G.F.: Editorial: Autotomography. Brit. J. Radiol. **35**, 415 (1962).
446. SWEET, W.H., BROWNELL, G.L., SCHOLL, J.A., BOWSHER, D.R., BENDA, P., STICKLEY, E.E.: The formation, flow, and absorption of cerebrospinal fluid: newer concepts based on studies with isotopes. Proc. Assoc. Res. nerv. Dis. **34**, 101 (1954).
447. SWEET, W.H., LOCKSLEY, H.B.: Formation, flow, and reabsorption of cerebrospinal fluid in man. Proc. Soc. exp. Biol. (N.Y.) **84**, 397 (1953).
448. TAKAHASU, S., ANZAI, S., OBARA, J.: Rotatory crossgraphy (rotatory cross-section radiography) of ventricles and subarachnoid cisterns. Tokohu J. exp. Med. **56**, 161 (1952).
449. TANAKA, T.: Pneumoencephalo-roulette tomography for the diagnosis of suboccipital lesions especially combined with pneumo-ventriculography. Brain Nerve (Tokyo) **21**, 1353 (1969).
450. TARLOV, I.M.: Pantopaque meningitis disclosed at operation. J. Amer. med. Ass. **129**, 1014 (1945).
451. TATOR, C.H., FLEMING, J.F.R., SHEPPARD, R.H., TURNER, V.M.: A radioisotopic test for communicating hydrocephalus. J. Neurosurg. **28**, 327 (1968).
452. TAUYA, E.: New radiopharmaceutical for subarachnoid space scintillography (Colloidal ^{113m}In). J. nucl. Med. **10**, 376 (1969).
453. TAVERAS, J.M., WOOD, E.H.: Diagnostic neuroradiology. Baltimore: Williams & Wilkins Co. 1964.
454. TEPLICK, J.G., HASKIN, M.E., SKELLEY, J., WOHL, G.T., SANEN, F.: Experimental studies with a new radiopaque emulsion. Radiology **82**, 478 (1964).
455. THIÉBAUT, F., WACKENHEIM, A., VROUSOS, C.: Atrophies cérébelleuses. La pneumostratigraphie sagittale médiane du cervelet. Atlas de Radiologie clinic. p. 120. : 1959.
456. THIÉBAUT, F., WACKENHEIM, A., VROUSOS, C., SUBIRANA, M.: Atrophies du vermis cérébelleux. Acta radiol. Diagn. **5**, 716 (1966).
457. THIÉBAUT, F., WACKENHEIM, A., WALTER, J.P., VROUSOS, C.: La pneumostratigraphie sagittale médiane du vermis cérébelleux. Technique de radioanatomie normale et pathologique. J. Radiol. Électrol. **40**, 385 (1959).
458. TOLPEZHNIKOV, Y.F.: Autotomography in pneumoencephalography. Vop. Neĭrokhir. **31**, 39 (1967).
459. TSCHUGUNOFF, S.A.: Zur Frage über die Veränderungen der cerebrospinalen Flüssigkeit nach der Encephalographie. Z. ges. Neurol. Psychiat. **122**, 452 (1929).
460. TSUBOKAWA, T.: Effects of Ketalar upon cerebral circulation and metabolism. Jap. J. Anesth. **19**, 1247 (1970).
461. TWINING, E.W.: Radiology of the third and fourth ventricles. Part I. Brit. J. Radiol. **12**, 385 (1939).
462. TWINING, E.W.: Radiology of the third and fourth ventricles. Part II. Brit. J. Radiol. **12**, 569 (1939).
463. TWINING, E.W., ROWBOTHAM, G.F.: Ventriculography by opaque injection. Lancet ii, 122 (1935).
464. VALENTINO, V.: Some experiences with tomography in neuroradiology. Acta radiol. (Stockh.) **45**, 101 (1956).
465. VALLEBONA, A.: Una modalità di tecnica per la dissociazione radiografica delle ombre applicata allo studio del cranio. Radiol. med. (Torino) **17**, 1090 (1930).
466. VALVASSORI, E.G.: The abnormal internal auditory canal: diagnosis of acoustic neurinoma. Radiology **92**, 449 (1969).
467. VAN WART, A.A., DUPONT, J.R., KRAINTZ, L.: Transfer of RIHSA from C.S.F. to blood plasma. Proc. Soc. Exp. Biol. (N.Y.) **103**, 708 (1960).
468. VERBIEST, H.: Le remplissage isolé d'air de la partie postérieure du troisième ventricule dans les obstructions de l'aqueduc de Sylviüs. Rev. neurol. **79**, 526 (1947).
469. VERBIEST, H.: Le remplissage isolé d'air de la partie postérieure du troisième ventricule dans les obstructions de l'aqueduc de Sylvius. Acta radiol. (Stockh.) **34**, 380 (1950).
470. VILLACA, C.M.: Ventriculography, encephalography and myelography with Thorotrast. Rev. Neurol. Psiquiat. S. Paulo **1**, 323 (1935).
471. WACKENHEIM, A., BRAUN, J.P., BABIN, E., MEGRET, M.: Technique d'examen de la citerne pericarotidienne. Communication, Annual Meeting of the European Society of Neuroradiology, Bologna 1972.
472. WAGNER, H.N., HOSAIN, F., DE LAND, F.H., SOM, P.: A new radiopharmaceutical for cisternography. Chelated Ytterbium 169. Radiology **95**, 121 (1970).
473. WEED, L., MCKIFFEN, P.: Pressure changes in the cerebrospinal fluid following intravenous injections of various concentrations. Amer. J. Physiol. **48**, 512 (1919).
474. WEIGELDT, W.: Die röntgenographische Darstellung des Gehirns durch Luftfüllung der liquorführenden Räume. Münch. med. Wschr. **69**, 1764 (1922).
475. WENDE, S., LÜDECKE, B.: Technique and value of gas and pantopaque cisternography in the diagnosis of cerebellopontine angle tumours. Neuroradiology **2**, 24 (1971).
476. WESTRA, D.: Zonographie, die Tomographie mit sehr geringer Verwischung. Fortschr. Röntgenstr. **97**, 605 (1962).
477. WESTRA, D.: Zonography. The narrow-angle tomography. Excerpta med. (Amst.), Sect. XIV (1966).
478. WESTRA, D., ZIEDSES DES PLANTES, B.G.: Anwendungsmöglichkeiten der Planigraphie mit geringer Verwischung. Communication, IX International Congress of Radiology, München 1959.
479. WEYER, K.H., SAMII, M., SCHÜRMANN, K.: Kombinierte ventrikulolumbale Luftfüllung in der Diagnostik der hinteren Schädelgrube. Fortschr. Röntgenstr. **108**, 162 (1968).
480. WICKBOM, I., SHELDON, P.: Some aspects of the radiologic diagnosis of posterior fossa and suprasellar tumours. Acta radiol. (Stockh.). **40**, 249 (1953).
481. WOLFSON, B., SIKER, E., GRAY, G.: Post-pneumoencephalography headache. A study of incidence and an attempt at therapy. Anaesthesia **25**, 328 (1970).
482. ZELLER, O.: Dreijährige Erfahrungen mit der Azetylenausblasung des Subarachnoidalraums bei eitriger Meningitis. Münch. med. Wschr. **82**, 47 (1935).
483. ZIEDSES DES PLANTES, B.G.: Een bijzondere methode voor het maken van röntgenfoto's van schedel en wervelkolom. Ned. T. Geneesk. **75**, 5219 (1931).

484. Ziedses des Plantes, B. G.: Subtraktion. Eine röntgenographische Methode zur separaten Abbildung bestimmter Teile des Objekts. Fortschr. Röntgenstr. **52**, 69 (1935).
485. Ziedes des Plantes, B. G.: Discussion at Dyes Communication: Das Röntgenbild der Hirnkammern als Ausdruck des Tumorwachstums. Fortschr. Röntgenstr. **56**, 8 (1937).
486. Ziedses des Plantes, B. G.: Ventriculographie van de derde en vierde ventrikel met weinig lucht. Folia psychiat. neerl. **52**, 160 (1949).
487. Ziedses des Plantes, B. G.: Examen du troisième et du quatrième ventricule au moyen de petites quantités d'air. Acta radiol. (Stockh.) **34**, 399 (1950).
488. Ziedses des Plantes, B. G.: Ventriculography with small amounts of air. Acta radiol. (Stockh.) **40**, 261 (1953).
489. Ziedses des Plantes, B. G.: Somersault technique for encephalography, myelography, and cisternography. Communication, Annual Meeting of the European Society of Neuroradiology, Bologna 1972.

Index of Illustrations

Index

Note: If an Author is quoted more than one time in the same page, the number of such page is indicated in the Index only once.

Abbreviations

C.S.F. = Cerebrospinal fluid
exam. = examination
exp.w. = experimental work
f.e. = fractional encephalography
i.o. = iodinated oils
p.c. = positive contrast
rad.c. = radioisotope cisternography
t.e. = total encephalography
tom. = tomography
ventr. = ventriculography

Angiography Scintigraphy

Symposium of the European Association of Radiology, Mainz 1-3 October 1970
Editor: L. Diethelm
262 figures. XX, 445 pages. 1972
Cloth DM 78,–; US $30.10
ISBN 3-540-05804-4

Results presented at an international symposium compare the diagnostic capabilities and limitations of angiography/scintigraphy, and angioscintigraphy in regard to the brain, spinal cord, lungs, liver, spleen, pancreas, kidneys, and adrenal glands.

T. Nomura

Atlas of Cerebral Angiography

24 figures. 1 color plate. 212 special plates, 6 angiograms. XI, 322 pages. 1970
Cloth DM 90,–; US $34.70
ISBN 3-540-05222-4
Published by Igaku Shoin Ltd., Tokyo. Sole distribution rights in all countries except the Far East: Springer-Verlag

The recent advances in neurosurgery are due in large part to the advancement of neuroradiology. Improvements in contrast media, x-ray tubes and photographic apparatus have made neuroradiology into one of the important fields of radiology.
Cerebral angiography is the best method of investigating the internal structure of the brain, yet its potential is not easily understood. This book is intended to help the reader to understand the normal three-dimensional angiogram.

A. Wackenheim/J. P. Braun

Angiography of the Mesencephalon

Normal and Pathological Findings
128 figures. XI, 154 pages. 1970
Cloth DM 98,–; US $37.80
ISBN 3-540-05266-6

Normal arteriography and venography of the midbrain region. Diagnosis for surgical and medical purposes based upon angiographic analysis of the blood vessels.

A. Wackenheim

Roentgen Diagnosis of the Craniovertebral Region

Approx. 500 figures. Approx. 660 pages. 1974
In preparation
ISBN 3-540-06615-2
Distribution rights for Japan:
Igaku Shoin Ltd., Tokyo

The author first presents a very detailed radio-anatomical study of the bones, ligaments, meninges, and nervous system of the cranio or vertebral region in children and adults. The work is well and clearly illustrated and is supported by a very full bibliography of over 1000 references. It will prove an indispensable reference work for radiologists, neurologists, neurosurgeons, and orthopedic surgeons.

Prices are subject to change without notice

Springer-Verlag
Berlin · Heidelberg · New York
München · Johannesburg · London · Madrid · New Delhi · Paris · Rio de Janeiro
Sydney · Tokyo · Utrecht · Wien

Organ of the European
Society of Neuroradiology

Neuroradiology

Editorial Board
P. Amundsen, Oslo
N. Azambuja, Montevideo
J. Bories, Paris
J. W. D. Bull, London
R. Chrzanowski, Krakow
G. Cornelis, Louvain
S. Cronqvist, Lund
D. O. Davis, Salt Lake City, Utah
G. Di Chiro, Bethesda, Md.
R. Djindjian, Paris
R. Ethier, Montreal
K. Hara, Osaka
P. Huber, Berne
J. Jirout, Prague
E. M. Klausberger, Vienna
G. Lombardi, Milan
T. H. Newton,
San Francisco, Calif.
G. Ruggiero, Bologna
M. M. Schechter, New York, N.Y.
M. Takahashi, Akita
J. Solé Llenas, Barcelona
J. Taveras, Boston, Mass.
A. Wackenheim, Strasbourg
S. Wende, Mainz
B. G. Ziedses des Plantes,
Amsterdam
L. H. Zingesser, New York, N.Y.

Editorial Secretaries
M. M. Schechter, New York, N.Y.
A. Wackenheim, Strasbourg
S. Wende, Mainz

Advances in angiography and new insights gained from the increasing use of isotopes for diagnosis are mainly responsible for the rapid development of neuroradiology as a separate discipline. As a result of close cooperation among radiologists, neurologists, and neurosurgeons, new light is constantly being shed on this promising field. New knowledge about the morphological and functional relationships of the organs contained within the skull and the vertebral canal under normal and pathological conditions continues to be reported by research workers throughout the world. NEURORADIOLOGY by making these reports readily available provides vital information for assuring proper diagnosis.

1974, Vols. 7-8 (5 issues each): DM 192,–
approx. US $74.00, plus postage and handling
Vols. 1-6 (1970-1973) available. Price per volume:
DM 96,–; approx. US $37.00
Prices are subject to change without notice

Springer-Verlag
Berlin · Heidelberg · New York
München Johannesburg London Madrid New Delhi
Paris Rio de Janeiro Sydney Tokyo Utrecht Wien

MIX
Papier aus verantwortungsvollen Quellen
Paper from responsible sources
FSC® C105338

If you have any concerns about our products,
you can contact us on
ProductSafety@springernature.com

In case Publisher is established outside the EU,
the EU authorized representative is:
Springer Nature Customer Service Center GmbH
Europaplatz 3, 69115 Heidelberg, Germany

Printed by Libri Plureos GmbH
in Hamburg, Germany